Teen Health Series

Stress-Related Disorders SOURCEBOOK

Third Edition

Health Reference Series

Third Edition

Stress-Related Disorders SOURCEBOOK

Basic Consumer Health Information about Stress and Stress-Related Disorders, Including Signs, Symptoms, Types, and Sources of Acute and Chronic Stress, the Impact of Stress on the Body, and Mental Health Problems Associated with Stress, Such as Depression, Anxiety Disorders, Bipolar Disorder, Obsessive-Compulsive Disorder, Substance Abuse, Posttraumatic Stress Disorder, and Suicide

Along with Advice about Getting Help for Stress-Related Disorders, Managing Stress and Coping with Trauma, a Glossary of Stress-Related Terms, and a Directory of Resources for Additional Help and Information

Edited by
Amy L. Sutton

Omnigraphics

P.O. Box 31-1640, Detroit, MI 48231

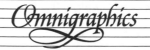

Bibliographic Note
Because this page cannot legibly accommodate all the copyright notices, the Bibliographic Note portion of the Preface constitutes an extension of the copyright notice.

Edited by Amy L. Sutton

Health Reference Series

Karen Bellenir, *Managing Editor*
David A. Cooke, MD, FACP, *Medical Consultant*
Elizabeth Collins, *Research and Permissions Coordinator*
Cherry Edwards, *Permissions Assistant*
EdIndex, Services for Publishers, *Indexers*

* * *

Omnigraphics, Inc.
Matthew P. Barbour, *Senior Vice President*
Kevin M. Hayes, *Operations Manager*

* * *

Peter E. Ruffner, *Publisher*

Copyright © 2011 Omnigraphics, Inc.

ISBN 978-0-7808-1148-5

Library of Congress Cataloging-in-Publication Data

Stress-related disorders sourcebook : basic consumer health information about stress and stress-related disorders, including signs, symptoms, types, and sources of acute and chronic stress, the impact of stress on the body, and mental health problems associated with stress, such as depression, anxiety disorders, bipolar disorder, obsessive-compulsive disorder, substance abuse, posttraumatic stress disorder, and suicide; along with advice about getting help for stress-related disorders, managing stress and coping with trauma, a glossary of stress-related terms, and a directory of resources for additional help and information / edited by Amy L. Sutton. -- 3rd ed.
   p. cm.
 Includes bibliographical references and index.
 Summary: "Provides basic consumer health information about the physical and mental health effects of stress and trauma, related therapies and stress management techniques, and coping tips for adults and children. Includes index, glossary of related terms, and other resources"-- Provided by publisher.
 ISBN 978-0-7808-1148-5 (hardcover : alk. paper) 1. Stress management--Popular works. 2. Stress (Physiology)--Popular works. 3. Stress (Psychology)--Popular works. I. Sutton, Amy L.
 RA785.S78 2011
 616.9'8--dc22

                                                                    2011011839

Table of Contents

Visit www.healthreferenceseries.com to view *A Contents Guide to the Health Reference Series*, a listing of more than 15,000 topics and the volumes in which they are covered.

Part V: Stress Management

Part VI: Additional Help and Information

Preface

About This Book

Nearly half of U.S. adults report their stress has increased in the last year. Work and money lead the list of major stressors, followed closely by concerns about the economy and family responsibilities. Stress takes its toll on the body by eroding sleep quality and mental focus, leaving its victims impatient, irritable, fatigued, and prone to overeating and substance abuse. Prolonged stress adversely affects immune system function, worsening conditions such as chronic pain disorders, diabetes, and heart problems. Mental health disorders, including depression, anxiety, and posttraumatic stress disorder, are also linked to serious problems coping with stress. As stress levels in adults rise, so do those in children and adolescents who struggle to cope with worries about family and school.

Stress-Related Disorders Sourcebook, Third Edition provides updated information about the origins and types of stress and describes physical and mental health disorders that may develop during and after stressful situations. Readers will learn about how stress worsens asthma, digestive disorders, infertility, and chronic pain. The *Sourcebook* also discusses how stress contributes to mental health problems, including depression, anxiety disorders, posttraumatic stress disorder, and addiction to tobacco, alcohol, and drugs. Information about trauma, loss, and grief is presented, along with suggestions for managing stressful situations, such as aggressive driving, caregiver stress, economic hardship, return from active military duty, and occupational stress.

Tips on helping children and teens cope with stress are also offered, along with a glossary of related terms and a directory of resources.

How to Use This Book

This book is divided into parts and chapters. Parts focus on broad areas of interest. Chapters are devoted to single topics within a part.

Part I: Introduction to Stress and Stress-Related Disorders identifies signs and symptoms of acute, chronic, and posttraumatic stress and discusses life events and risk factors that increase vulnerability to developing stress-related disorders. Facts about the impact of financial, emotional, and physical stress on the American population are also included.

Part II: How Stress Affects the Body provides information about health conditions exacerbated by stress. These include asthma, diabetes, gastrointestinal problems, headache, multiple sclerosis, obesity, sleep disorders, and chronic pain disorders.

Part III: How Stress Affects Mental Health discusses how stress erodes emotional well-being and contributes to the development of mental health disorders, such as depression, anxiety disorders, bipolar disorder, disordered eating, obsessive-compulsive disorder, and substance abuse and addiction. Trauma survivors and their families will also find information about common reactions after trauma and types of stress-related disorders that develop after exposure to violence, disaster, assault, or war.

Part IV: Treating Stress-Related Disorders offers information about treatments for stress-related disorders, including psychological therapies, medications, and complementary and alternative medicine. For people coping with a loved one's stress-related responses, this part offers tips on helping someone with posttraumatic stress disorder and recognizing when someone needs help from mental health and other medical professionals.

Part V: Stress Management identifies strategies for combating stress in everyday life. People coping with emotional and physical reactions to stress will find suggestions on healthy habits that alleviate stress and tips for coping with stressful situations at home, at work, and on the road. Information about developing resilience is also included, along with tips on stress management for children, teens, families, and older adults.

Part VI: Additional Help and Information provides a glossary of important terms related to stress and stress-related disorders. A directory of organizations that provide health information about stress-related disorders is also included.

Bibliographic Note

This volume contains documents and excerpts from publications issued by the following U.S. government agencies: Centers for Disease Control and Prevention (CDC); Drug Enforcement Administration (DEA); Federal Bureau of Investigation (FBI); National Cancer Institute (NCI); National Center for Complementary and Alternative Medicine (NCCAM); National Center for Posttraumatic Stress Disorder (NCPTSD); National Health Information Center (NHIC); National Heart, Lung, and Blood Institute (NHLBI); National Highway Traffic Safety Administration (NHTSA); National Institute of Arthritis and Musculoskeletal and Skin Diseases (NIAMS); National Institute of Diabetes and Digestive and Kidney Diseases (NIDDK); National Institute of Mental Health (NIMH); National Institute of Neurological Disorders and Stroke (NINDS); National Institute on Aging (NIA); National Institute on Alcohol Abuse and Alcoholism (NIAAA); National Institute on Drug Abuse (NIDA); National Institutes of Health (NIH); Office of the Surgeon General (OGS); Office on Women's Health (OWH); Substance Abuse and Mental Health Services Administration (SAMHSA); U.S. Army Center for Health Promotion and Preventive Medicine (USACHPPM); and the U.S. Food and Drug Administration (FDA).

In addition, this volume contains copyrighted documents from the following organizations: A.D.A.M., Inc.; American Heart Association; American Institute of Stress; American Psychological Association; Centre for Clinical Interventions; *Cornell Chronicle* / Cornell University News Service; Delta Society; Emory University; Franklin Institute; Iowa State University Extension; March of Dimes Birth Defects Foundation; Meals Matter; Mendosa.com; National Alliance on Mental Illness; National Multiple Sclerosis Society; National Psoriasis Foundation; Nemours Foundation; Pennsylvania State University; ProjectAware; Psych Central; Regents of the University of Michigan; Remedy Health Media; Talk About Sleep; University of California at Irvine; University of California–San Francisco News Office; University of Pennsylvania Health System; and Wake Forest University Baptist Medical Center.

Full citation information is provided on the first page of each chapter or section. Every effort has been made to secure all necessary rights to reprint the copyrighted material. If any omissions have been made, please contact Omnigraphics to make corrections for future editions.

Acknowledgements

Thanks go to the many organizations, agencies, and individuals who have contributed materials for this *Sourcebook* and to medical consultant Dr. David Cooke and prepress service provider WhimsyInk. Special thanks go to managing editor Karen Bellenir and research and permissions coordinator Liz Collins for their help and support.

About the Health Reference Series

The *Health Reference Series* is designed to provide basic medical information for patients, families, caregivers, and the general public. Each volume takes a particular topic and provides comprehensive coverage. This is especially important for people who may be dealing with a newly diagnosed disease or a chronic disorder in themselves or in a family member. People looking for preventive guidance, information about disease warning signs, medical statistics, and risk factors for health problems will also find answers to their questions in the *Health Reference Series*. The *Series*, however, is not intended to serve as a tool for diagnosing illness, in prescribing treatments, or as a substitute for the physician/patient relationship. All people concerned about medical symptoms or the possibility of disease are encouraged to seek professional care from an appropriate health care provider.

A Note about Spelling and Style

Health Reference Series editors use *Stedman's Medical Dictionary* as an authority for questions related to the spelling of medical terms and the *Chicago Manual of Style* for questions related to grammatical structures, punctuation, and other editorial concerns. Consistent adherence is not always possible, however, because the individual volumes within the *Series* include many documents from a wide variety of different producers and copyright holders, and the editor's primary goal is to present material from each source as accurately as is possible following the terms specified by each document's producer. This sometimes means that information in different chapters or sections may follow other guidelines and alternate spelling authorities. For example, occasionally a copyright holder may require that eponymous terms be shown in possessive forms (Crohn's disease *vs.* Crohn disease) or that British spelling norms be retained (leukaemia *vs.* leukemia).

Locating Information within the Health Reference Series

The *Health Reference Series* contains a wealth of information about a wide variety of medical topics. Ensuring easy access to all the fact sheets, research reports, in-depth discussions, and other material contained within the individual books of the *Series* remains one of our highest priorities. As the *Series* continues to grow in size and scope, however, locating the precise information needed by a reader may become more challenging.

A *Contents Guide to the Health Reference Series* was developed to direct readers to the specific volumes that address their concerns. It presents an extensive list of diseases, treatments, and other topics of general interest compiled from the Tables of Contents and major index headings. To access A *Contents Guide to the Health Reference Series*, visit www.healthreferenceseries.com.

Medical Consultant

Medical consultation services are provided to the *Health Reference Series* editors by David A. Cooke, MD, FACP. Dr. Cooke is a graduate of Brandeis University, and he received his M.D. degree from the University of Michigan. He completed residency training at the University of Wisconsin Hospital and Clinics. He is board-certified in Internal Medicine. Dr. Cooke currently works as part of the University of Michigan Health System and practices in Ann Arbor, MI. In his free time, he enjoys writing, science fiction, and spending time with his family.

Our Advisory Board

We would like to thank the following board members for providing guidance to the development of this *Series*:

- Dr. Lynda Baker, Associate Professor of Library and Information Science, Wayne State University, Detroit, MI

- Nancy Bulgarelli, William Beaumont Hospital Library, Royal Oak, MI

- Karen Imarisio, Bloomfield Township Public Library, Bloomfield Township, MI

- Karen Morgan, Mardigian Library, University of Michigan-Dearborn, Dearborn, MI

- Rosemary Orlando, St. Clair Shores Public Library, St. Clair Shores, MI

Health Reference Series *Update Policy*

The inaugural book in the *Health Reference Series* was the first edition of *Cancer Sourcebook* published in 1989. Since then, the *Series* has been enthusiastically received by librarians and in the medical community. In order to maintain the standard of providing high-quality health information for the layperson the editorial staff at Omnigraphics felt it was necessary to implement a policy of updating volumes when warranted.

Medical researchers have been making tremendous strides, and it is the purpose of the *Health Reference Series* to stay current with the most recent advances. Each decision to update a volume is made on an individual basis. Some of the considerations include how much new information is available and the feedback we receive from people who use the books. If there is a topic you would like to see added to the update list, or an area of medical concern you feel has not been adequately addressed, please write to:

Editor
Health Reference Series
Omnigraphics, Inc.
P.O. Box 31-1640
Detroit, MI 48231
E-mail: editorial@omnigraphics.com

Part One

Introduction to Stress and Stress-Related Disorders

Chapter 1

What Is Stress?

Stress is the emotional and physical strain caused by the response to pressure from the outside world. Unfortunately, there is not a universally agreed upon definition of stress, and individuals react differently to stress. What is stressful for one person may be pleasurable or have little effect on others. Stress is not necessarily bad; in small doses, it can help people perform under pressure and motivate them to do their best. But, beyond a certain point, stress stops being helpful and starts causing damage to health, mood, productivity, relationships, and quality of life.

Stress is a normal physical response to events that make a person feel threatened or upset. When danger is sensed—whether it is real or imagined—the body's defenses kick into high gear in a rapid, automatic process known as the fight-or-flight reaction, or the stress response. The brain signals the release of stress hormones. These chemical substances trigger a series of responses that gives the body extra energy: Blood sugar levels rise, the heartbeat speeds up, and blood pressure increases. The muscles tense for action. The blood supply is diverted away from the core to the extremities to help the body deal with the situation at hand. The stress response is the body's way of protecting itself.

From "Stress and Stress Management," by the Substance Abuse and Mental Health Services Administration (SAMHSA, mentalhealth.samhsa.gov), part of the U.S. Department of Health and Human Services, 2009.

3

Are There Different Types of Stress?

Stress management can be complicated and confusing because there are different types of stress: Acute stress, episodic acute stress, chronic stress, and posttraumatic stress, each with its own characteristics, symptoms, duration, and treatment approaches.

Acute stress is the most common form of stress. It comes from demands and pressures of the recent past and anticipated demands and pressures of the near future. Because it is short-term, acute stress does not have enough time to do the extensive damage associated with long-term stress. Acute stress can crop up in anyone's life, and it is highly treatable and manageable.

Those who suffer acute stress frequently are dealing with episodic acute stress. It is common for people with episodic acute stress to be over-aroused, short-tempered, irritable, anxious, and tense. Interpersonal relationships deteriorate rapidly when others respond with real hostility. Work becomes a very stressful place for them. Often, lifestyle and personality issues are so ingrained and habitual with these individuals that they see nothing wrong with the way they conduct their lives. They blame their woes on other people and external events. Frequently, they see their lifestyles, patterns of interacting with others, and ways of perceiving the world as part and parcel of who and what they are. Without proper coping strategies, episodic acute stress develops into chronic stress.

Chronic stress is the grinding stress that wears people away day after day, year after year. It destroys bodies, minds, and lives. It is the stress of unrelenting demands and pressures for seemingly interminable periods of time. The worst aspect of chronic stress is that people get used to it. They forget it is there. People are immediately aware of acute stress because it is new. Chronic stress is ignored because it is familiar and almost comfortable.

Posttraumatic stress disorder (PTSD) stems from traumatic experiences that become internalized and remain forever painful and present. Individuals experiencing PTSD could exhibit signs of hypervigilance (an easily triggered startle response). People with an exaggerated startle response are easily startled by any number of things (e.g., loud noises, doors slamming, shouting). They usually feel tense or on edge. Along with hypervigilance, people experiencing PTSD symptoms also could be dealing with avoidance issues including staying away from places, events, or objects that are reminders of the experience; feeling emotionally numb; feeling strong guilt, depression, or worry; losing interest in activities that were enjoyable in the past; and having trouble remembering the dangerous event. People experiencing PTSD symptoms wear down to breaking points because physical and mental resources are depleted through long-term attrition. The symptoms of posttraumatic stress are difficult to treat and may require the help of a doctor or mental health professional.

What Are Some Common Myths Surrounding Stress?

[Editor's Note: The text under this heading is adapted from the American Psychological Association, 2008.]

Myth: Stress is the same for everyone.

Stress is different for everyone. What is stressful for one person may or may not be stressful for another. Each person may respond to stress in an entirely different way.

Myth: Stress is always bad.

According to this view, zero stress makes us happy and healthy. This is wrong—stress is a normal part of life. Stress can be the kiss of death or the spice of life. The issue is how to manage it. Managed stress makes people productive and happy. Mismanaged stress hurts and even kills.

Myth: Stress is everywhere, so nothing can be done about it.

Not so. Life can be planned so that stress does not become overwhelming.

Myth: The most popular techniques for reducing stress are the best ones.

No universally effective stress reduction techniques exist, because each individual reacts differently.

Myth: No symptoms, No stress.

Absence of symptoms does not mean the absence of stress. In fact, camouflaging symptoms with medication may deprive a person of the signals needed for reducing the strain on physiological and psychological systems.

Myth: Only major symptoms of stress require attention.

This myth assumes that minor symptoms, such as headaches or stomach acid, may be safely ignored. Minor symptoms of stress are the early warnings that life is getting out of hand and stress needs to be better managed.

Common Stressors

[Editor's Note: The text under this heading includes data from the American Psychological Association, 2008.]

- Financial issues: 81 percent of Americans worry about this topic.

- Work and job stability: 67 percent of Americans worry about this topic.

- The nation's economy: 80 percent of Americans worry about this topic.

- Health concerns (family and personal): 64 percent of Americans worry about this topic.

- Relationships: 62 percent of Americans worry about this topic.

- Personal safety: 48 percent of Americans worry about this topic.

- Loss: 72 percent of Americans worry about this topic.

How Does Stress Affect People?

Stress is taking a toll on people—contributing to health problems, poor relationships, and lost productivity at work, according to a national survey released by the American Psychological Association (APA). Twenty-eight percent of Americans say that they are managing their stress extremely well. However, many people report experiencing physical symptoms (77 percent) and psychological symptoms (73 percent) related to stress. While Americans deal with high levels of stress on a daily basis, the health consequences are most serious when that stress is poorly managed. The body does not distinguish between physical and psychological threats. Everyone reacts differently to stress, and each body sends out a different set of red flags.

Is Stress Experienced Differently by Genders or Generations?

The APA reported that nearly half of Americans state that their stress levels have increased since November 2007, with as many as

30 percent rating their average stress levels as extreme (8, 9, or 10 on a 10-point scale where 10 means "a great deal of stress"). At the same time, economic conditions take a physical and emotional toll on people nationwide. Compared with men, more women say they are stressed about the following issues:

- Money (83 percent vs. 78 percent)
- The economy (84 percent vs. 75 percent)
- Housing costs (66 percent vs. 58 percent)
- Health problems affecting their families (70 percent vs. 63 percent)

Across the board, women are reporting higher levels of stress, are more likely than men to cite various stressors, and report more physical and emotional symptoms as a result of stress, suggesting that stress is having a significant impact on women.

In reports released by the APA, older adults report having less stress and managing stress better than younger adults. However, the financial crisis is having a greater impact on older generations, and this impact is leading to more stress at work. Many older adults are waiting to retire or coming out of retirement and joining the workforce to make ends meet.

Does Stress Look Different across Cultures?

Stress is common to all people regardless of ethnicity. However, sources of stress vary among cultural groups. All cultural groups are reporting increased stress about money and work. However, as a result of cultural norms, many ethnic groups are having difficulty asking for help regarding coping skills. When it comes to managing stress, the APA reports that several cultural groups say they are doing enough to manage their stress; however, groups do not report that they are managing their stress well. It is important to maintain a sense of identity and social support when feeling overwhelmed and stressed. This includes embracing cultural background when developing a personal strategy for dealing with stress.

What Are the Warning Signs of Stress?

It is important to learn how to recognize when stress levels are dangerously high. The most dangerous thing about stress is how easily it can get out of control. Many factors can cause it, but common triggers tend to be the pressures of work, relationships, money, or family problems, or merely the fact that life suddenly seems to be a constant tough battle. One of the important aids for combating and dealing with stress is to first recognize it. Stress affects minds, bodies, and behaviors in many ways, and everyone experiences stress differently. A body's stress warning signs alert a person that something is not right, much like the glowing "check engine" light on a car's dashboard.

Warning Signs of Stress

[Editor's Note: The text under this heading is adapted from Mental Health America, 2007.]

Cognitive Signs

- Memory problems
- Inability to concentrate
- Poor judgment
- Negativity
- Anxious or racing thoughts
- Constant worrying

Emotional Signs

- Moodiness
- Irritability or short temper
- Agitation, inability to relax
- Feeling overwhelmed
- Sense of loneliness and isolation
- Depression or general unhappiness

Physical Signs

- Aches and pains
- Headaches
- Diarrhea or constipation
- Nausea, dizziness
- Chest pain, rapid heartbeat

- Loss of sex drive
- Frequent colds

Behavioral Signs

- Eating more or less
- Sleeping too much or too little
- Isolating from others
- Procrastinating or neglecting responsibilities
- Using alcohol, cigarettes, or drugs to relax
- Nervous habits (e.g., nail biting, pacing)

Can Stress Be Prevented?

Stressful situations in life cannot be prevented. However, they can be prepared for in a way that allows a positive response. This is done by building and fostering resilience in different areas of life. Resilience implies that after an event, a person or community may not only be able to cope and recover, but also change to reflect different priorities arising from the experience and prepare for the next stressful situation. Fostering resilience, or the ability to bounce back from a stressful situation, builds a proactive mechanism to manage stress. Developing a greater level of resilience will not prevent stressful conditions from happening, but it can reduce the level of disruption a stressor has and the time it takes to recover.

How Can Stress Be Managed?

Stress can be dealt with proactively or reactively. It can be dealt with proactively by building personal resilience to prepare for stressful circumstances, while learning how to recognize signs and symptoms of stress. It can be dealt with reactively by utilizing coping strategies useful for the individual. The key is not to avoid stress altogether, but to manage the stress in such a way that the negative consequences of stress are avoided. There are many positive ways to manage stress.

The best defense against stress is building resilience. Resilience refers to the ability of an individual, family, organization, or community to cope with adversity and adapt to challenges or change. It is a process of drawing on beliefs, behaviors, skills, and attitudes to move beyond stress, trauma, or tragedy. While building defenses through resilience, it also is important to be ready to deal with stress if the internal resilience reservoir is not enough.

Managing stress can include simple ideas, such as recognizing signs of stress, learning breathing techniques, and engaging in spiritual communities, and more advanced interventions with professionals, such as seeking the help of a mental health professional and learning stress inoculation techniques. The goal of stress inoculation is to develop a procedure that will almost instantaneously put a person in a calm state. This is not necessarily a completely relaxed condition since many demanding situations will not allow that. The idea, however, is to be able to step back and look at problematic circumstances in a realistic light without feeling too hassled.

Uncontrolled stress can lead to many problems. Simple headaches, tight muscles, problems with sleeping, or a bad mood can be a prelude to much more severe symptoms. There are many healthy ways to manage and cope with stress, but they all require change: Either changing the situation or changing reactions to the situation. If stress is affecting a person's ability to work or find pleasure in life, help should be sought from a doctor, mental health provider, or other professional.

References

American Psychological Association. (2008). Stress in America. Retrieved March 23, 2009, from http://apahelpcenter.mediaroom.com/ file.php/138/Stress+in+America+REPORT+FINAL.doc

American Institute of Stress. (n.d.). Effects of stress. Retrieved March 23, 2009, from http://www.stress.org/topic-effects.htm?AIS=2ad4f081 4d4d64867b7bb6500e41ea

Mental Health America. (n.d.). Stress: Know the signs. Retrieved March 23, 2009, from http://www.mentalhealthamerica.net/go/mental-health -month/stress-know-the-signs

Chapter 2

Characteristics of Stress

Chapter Contents

Section 2.1

Signs and Symptoms of Stress

"The Effects of Stress," © American Institute of Stress (www.stress.org). Reprinted with permission. This document is undated. Additional information is available at Current and Past Stress Scoops, Current and Past Newsletters, and elsewhere on www.stress.org. Reviewed by David A. Cooke, MD, FACP, November 8, 2010.

Stress is difficult for scientists to define because it is a highly subjective phenomenon that differs for each of us. Things that are distressful for some individuals can be pleasurable for others. We also respond to stress differently. Some people blush, some eat more while others grow pale or eat less. There are numerous physical as well as emotional responses as illustrated by the following list of some 50 common signs and symptoms of stress.

1. Frequent headaches, jaw clenching, or pain

2. Gritting, grinding teeth

3. Stuttering or stammering

4. Tremors, trembling of lips, hands

5. Neck ache, back pain, muscle spasms

6. Lightheadedness, faintness, dizziness

7. Ringing, buzzing, or popping sounds

8. Frequent blushing, sweating

9. Cold or sweaty hands, feet

10. Dry mouth, problems swallowing

11. Frequent colds, infections, herpes sores

12. Rashes, itching, hives, "goose bumps"

13. Unexplained or frequent "allergy" attacks

14. Heartburn, stomach pain, nausea

15. Excess belching, flatulence

16. Constipation, diarrhea

17. Difficulty breathing, sighing

18. Sudden attacks of panic

19. Chest pain, palpitations

20. Frequent urination

21. Poor sexual desire or performance

22. Excess anxiety, worry, guilt, nervousness

23. Increased anger, frustration, hostility

24. Depression, frequent or wild mood swings

25. Increased or decreased appetite

26. Insomnia, nightmares, disturbing dreams

27. Difficulty concentrating, racing thoughts

28. Trouble learning new information

29. Forgetfulness, disorganization, confusion

30. Difficulty in making decisions

31. Feeling overloaded or overwhelmed

32. Frequent crying spells or suicidal thoughts

33. Feelings of loneliness or worthlessness

34. Little interest in appearance, punctuality

35. Nervous habits, fidgeting, feet tapping

36. Increased frustration, irritability, edginess

37. Overreaction to petty annoyances

38. Increased number of minor accidents

39. Obsessive or compulsive behavior

40. Reduced work efficiency or productivity

41. Lies or excuses to cover up poor work

42. Rapid or mumbled speech

43. Excessive defensiveness or suspiciousness

44. Problems in communication, sharing

45. Social withdrawal and isolation

46. Constant tiredness, weakness, fatigue

47. Frequent use of over-the-counter drugs

48. Weight gain or loss without diet

49. Increased smoking, alcohol, or drug use

50. Excessive gambling or impulse buying

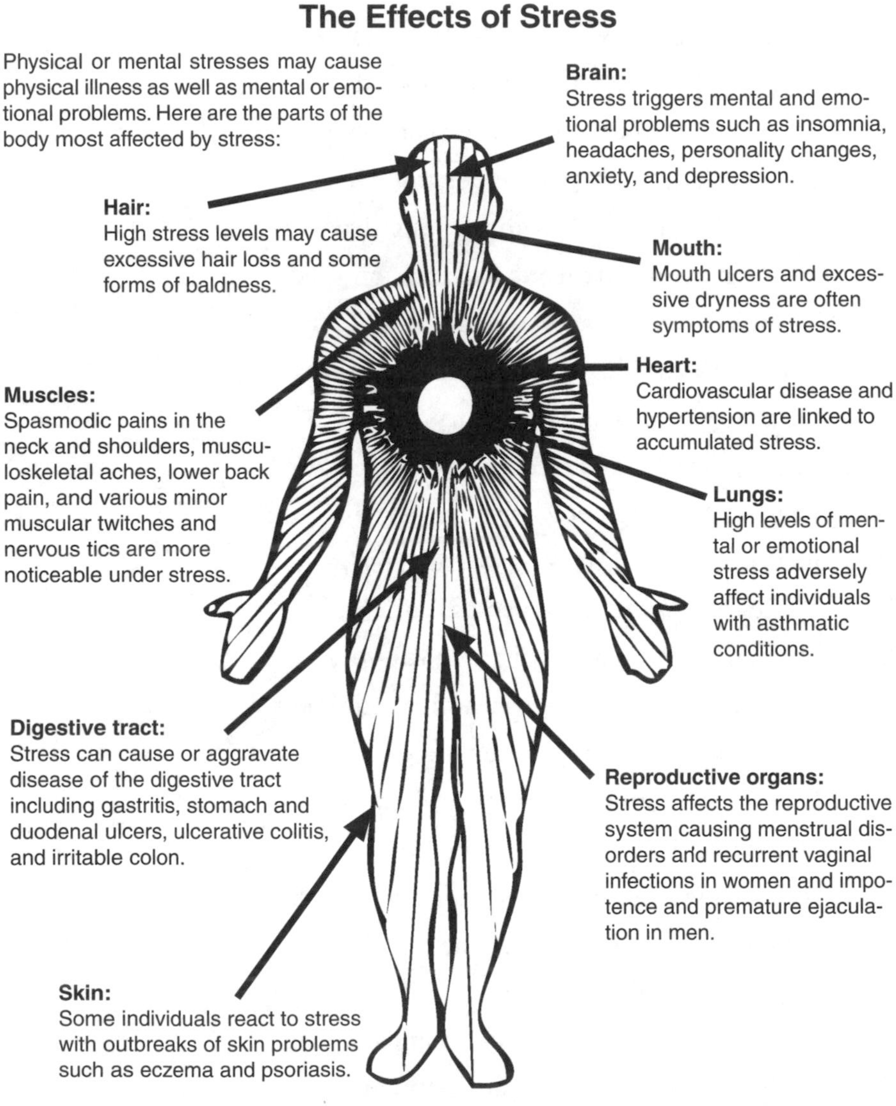

The Effects of Stress

Physical or mental stresses may cause physical illness as well as mental or emotional problems. Here are the parts of the body most affected by stress:

Brain:
Stress triggers mental and emotional problems such as insomnia, headaches, personality changes, anxiety, and depression.

Hair:
High stress levels may cause excessive hair loss and some forms of baldness.

Mouth:
Mouth ulcers and excessive dryness are often symptoms of stress.

Muscles:
Spasmodic pains in the neck and shoulders, musculoskeletal aches, lower back pain, and various minor muscular twitches and nervous tics are more noticeable under stress.

Heart:
Cardiovascular disease and hypertension are linked to accumulated stress.

Lungs:
High levels of mental or emotional stress adversely affect individuals with asthmatic conditions.

Digestive tract:
Stress can cause or aggravate disease of the digestive tract including gastritis, stomach and duodenal ulcers, ulcerative colitis, and irritable colon.

Reproductive organs:
Stress affects the reproductive system causing menstrual disorders and recurrent vaginal infections in women and impotence and premature ejaculation in men.

Skin:
Some individuals react to stress with outbreaks of skin problems such as eczema and psoriasis.

Figure 2.1. Parts of the body most affected by stress.

As demonstrated in the preceding list, stress can have wide ranging effects on emotions, mood, and behavior. Equally important but often less appreciated are effects on various systems, organs, and tissues all over the body, as illustrated by Figure 2.1.

There are numerous emotional and physical disorders that have been linked to stress including depression, anxiety, heart attacks, stroke, hypertension, immune system disturbances that increase susceptibility to infections, a host of viral linked disorders ranging from the common cold and herpes to AIDS [acquired immunodeficiency syndrome] and certain cancers, as well as autoimmune diseases like rheumatoid arthritis and multiple sclerosis. In addition stress can have direct effects on the skin (rashes, hives, atopic dermatitis, the gastrointestinal system (GERD [gastroesophageal reflux disease], peptic ulcer, irritable bowel syndrome, ulcerative colitis) and can contribute to insomnia and degenerative neurological disorders like Parkinson's disease. In fact, it's hard to think of any disease in which stress cannot play an aggravating role or any part of the body that is not affected. This list will undoubtedly grow as the extensive ramifications of stress are increasingly being appreciated.

Section 2.2

Types of Stress

Excerpted from "The Effects of Childhood Stress on
Health across the Lifespan," by the Centers for Disease Control
and Prevention (CDC, www.cdc.gov), 2008.

Stress is an inevitable part of life. Human beings experience stress early, even before they are born. A certain amount of stress is normal and necessary for survival. Stress helps children develop the skills they need to cope with and adapt to new and potentially threatening situations throughout life. Support from parents and/or other concerned caregivers is necessary for children to learn how to respond to stress in a physically and emotionally healthy manner.

The beneficial aspects of stress diminish when it is severe enough to overwhelm a child's ability to cope effectively. Intensive and prolonged stress can lead to a variety of short- and long-term negative health effects. It can disrupt early brain development and compromise functioning of the nervous and immune systems. In addition, childhood stress can lead to health problems later in life including alcoholism, depression, eating disorders, heart disease, cancer, and other chronic diseases.

Positive Stress

Positive stress results from adverse experiences that are short-lived. Children may encounter positive stress when they attend a new daycare, get a shot, meet new people, or have a toy taken away from them. This type of stress causes minor physiological changes including an increase in heart rate and changes in hormone levels. With the support of caring adults, children can learn how to manage and overcome positive stress. This type of stress is considered normal and coping with it is an important part of the development process.

Tolerable Stress

Tolerable stress refers to adverse experiences that are more intense but still relatively short-lived. Examples include the death of a loved one, a natural disaster, a frightening accident, and family disruptions such as separation or divorce. If a child has the support of a caring adult, tolerable stress can usually be overcome. In many cases, tolerable stress can become positive stress and benefit the child developmentally. However, if the child lacks adequate support, tolerable stress can become toxic and lead to long-term negative health effects.

Toxic Stress

Toxic stress results from intense adverse experiences that may be sustained over a long period of time—weeks, months, or even years. An example of toxic stress is child maltreatment, which includes abuse and neglect. Children are unable to effectively manage this type of stress by themselves. As a result, the stress response system gets activated for a prolonged amount of time. This can lead to permanent changes in the development of the brain. The negative effects of toxic stress can be lessened with the support of caring adults. Appropriate support and intervention can help in returning the stress response system back to its normal baseline.

Chapter 3

Stressful Life Events

The most common psychological and social stressors in adult life include the breakup of intimate romantic relationships, death of a family member or friend, economic hardships, racism and discrimination, poor physical health, and accidental and intentional assaults on physical safety. Although some stressors are so powerful that they would evoke significant emotional distress in most otherwise mentally healthy people, the majority of stressful life events do not invariably trigger mental disorders. Rather, they are more likely to spawn mental disorders in people who are vulnerable biologically, socially, and/or psychologically. Understanding variability among individuals to a stressful life event is a major challenge to research. Groups at greater statistical risk include women, young and unmarried people, African Americans, and individuals with lower socioeconomic status.

Divorce is a common example. Approximately one half of all marriages now end in divorce, and about 30 to 40 percent of those undergoing divorce report a significant increase in symptoms of depression and anxiety. Vulnerability to depression and anxiety is greater among those with a personal history of mental disorders earlier in life and is lessened by strong social support. For many, divorce conveys additional economic adversities and the stress of single parenting. Single mothers face twice the risk of depression as do married mothers.

Excerpted from "Mental Health: A Report of the Surgeon General–Chapter 4," by the Office of the Surgeon General (www.surgeongeneral.gov), part of the U.S. Department of Health and Human Services, 2003. Reviewed by David A. Cooke, MD, FACP, November 8, 2010.

The death of a child or spouse during early or mid-adult life is much less common than divorce but generally is of greater potency in provoking emotional distress. Rates of diagnosable mental disorders during periods of grief are attenuated by the convention not to diagnose depression during the first 2 months of bereavement. In fact, people are generally unlikely to seek professional treatment during bereavement unless the severity of the emotional and behavioral disturbance is incapacitating.

A majority of Americans never will confront the stress of surviving a severe, life-threatening accident or physical assault (e.g., mugging, robbery, rape); however, some segments of the population, particularly urban youths and young adults, have exposure rates as high as 25 to 30 percent. Life-threatening trauma frequently provokes emotional and behavioral reactions that jeopardize mental health. In the most fully developed form, this syndrome is called posttraumatic stress disorder. Women are twice as likely as men to develop posttraumatic stress disorder following exposure to life-threatening trauma.

More familiar to many Americans is the chronic strain that poor physical health and relationship problems place on day-to-day well-being. Relationship problems include unsatisfactory intimate relationships; conflicted relationships with parents, siblings, and children; and "falling-out" with coworkers, friends, and neighbors. In mid-adult life, the stress of caretaking for elderly parents also becomes more common.

Relationship problems at least double the risk of developing a mental disorder, although they are less immediately threatening or potentially cataclysmic than divorce or the death of a spouse or child. Finally, cumulative adversity appears to be more potent than stressful events in isolation as a predictor of psychological distress and mental disorders.

Past Trauma and Child Sexual Abuse

Severe trauma in childhood may have enduring effects into adulthood. Past trauma includes sexual and physical abuse, and parental death, divorce, psychopathology, and substance abuse.

Child sexual abuse is one of the most common stressors, with effects that persist into adulthood. It disproportionately affects females. Although definitions are still evolving, child sexual abuse is often defined as forcible touching of breasts or genitals or forcible intercourse (including anal, oral, or vaginal sex) before the age of 16 or 18. Epidemiology studies of adults in varying segments of the community have found that 15 to 33 percent of females and 13 to 16 percent of males were sexually abused in childhood. A large epidemiological study of adults in the general community found a lower prevalence (12.8 percent for females and 4.3 percent for males); however, the definition of sexual abuse was more restricted than in past studies. Sexual abuse in childhood has a mean age of onset estimated at 7 to 9 years of age. In over 25 percent of cases of child sexual abuse, the offense was committed by a parent or parent substitute.

The long-term consequences of past childhood sexual abuse are profound, yet vary in expression. They range from depression and anxiety to problems with social functioning and adult interpersonal relationships. Posttraumatic stress disorder is a common sequela, found in 33 to 86 percent of adult survivors of child sexual abuse. Sexual abuse may be a specific risk factor for adult-onset depression and twice as many women as men report a history of abuse. Other long-term effects include self-destructive behavior, social isolation, poor sexual adjustment, substance abuse, and increased risk of revictimization.

Very few treatments specifically for adult survivors of childhood abuse have been studied in randomized controlled trials. Group therapy and Interpersonal Transaction group therapy were found to be more effective for female survivors than an experimental control condition that offered a less appropriate intervention. In the practice setting, most psychosocial and pharmacological treatments are tailored to the primary diagnosis, which, as noted in the preceding text, varies widely and may not attend to the special needs of those also reporting abuse history.

Domestic Violence

Domestic violence is a serious and startlingly common public health problem with mental health consequences for victims, who are overwhelmingly female, and for children who witness the violence. Domestic violence (also known as intimate partner violence) features a pattern of physical and sexual abuse, psychological abuse with verbal intimidation, and/or social isolation or deprivation. Estimates are that 8 to 17 percent of women are victimized annually in the United States. Pinpointing the prevalence is hindered by variations in the way domestic violence is defined and by problems in detection and underreporting. Women are often fearful that their reporting of domestic violence will precipitate retaliation by the batterer, a fear that is not unwarranted.

Victims of domestic violence are at increased risk for mental health problems and disorders as well as physical injury and death. Domestic violence is considered one of the foremost causes of serious injury to women ages 15 to 44, accounting for about 30 percent of all acute injuries to women seen in emergency departments. According to the U.S. Department of Justice, females were victims in about 75 percent of the almost 2,000 homicides between intimates in 1996. The mental health consequences of domestic violence include depression, anxiety disorders (e.g., posttraumatic stress disorder), suicide, eating disorders, and substance abuse. Children who witness domestic violence may suffer acute and long-term emotional disturbances, including nightmares, depression, learning difficulties, and aggressive behavior. Children also become at risk for subsequent use of violence against their dating partners and wives.

Mental health interventions for victims, children, and batterers are highly important. Individual counseling and peer support groups are the interventions most frequently used by battered women. However, there is a lack of carefully controlled, methodologically robust studies of interventions and their outcomes. There is an urgent need for development and rigorous evaluation of prevention programs to safeguard against intimate partner violence and its impact on children.

Interventions for Stressful Life Events

Stressful life events, even for those at the peak of mental health, erode quality of life and place people at risk for symptoms and signs of mental disorders. There is an ever-expanding list of formal and informal interventions to aid individuals coping with adversity. Sources of informal interventions include family and friends, education, community services, self-help groups, social support networks, religious and spiritual endeavors, complementary healers, and physical activities. As valuable as these activities may be for promoting mental health, they have received less research attention than have interventions for mental disorders. Nevertheless, there are selected interventions to help people cope with stressors, such as bereavement programs and programs for caregivers as well as couples therapy and physical activity.

Couples therapy is the umbrella term applied to interventions that aid couples in distress. The best studied interventions are behavioral couples therapy, cognitive-behavioral couples therapy, and emotion-focused couples therapy. A review article evaluated the body of evidence on the effectiveness of couples therapy and programs to prevent marital discord. The review found that about 65 percent of couples in therapy did improve, whereas 35 percent of control couples also improved. Couples therapy ameliorates relationship distress and appears to alleviate depression. The gains from couples therapy generally last through 6 months, but there are few long-term assessments. Similarly, interventions to prevent marital discord yield short-term improvements in marital adjustment and stability, but there is insufficient study of long-term outcomes.

Physical activities are a means to enhance somatic health as well as to deal with stress. Aerobic physical activities, such as brisk walking and running, have been found to improve mental health for people who report symptoms of anxiety and depression and for those who are diagnosed with some forms of depression. The mental health benefits of physical activity for individuals in relatively good physical and mental health were not as evident, but the studies did not have sufficient rigor from which to draw unequivocal conclusions.

Chapter 4

Factors That Influence Response to Stress

Chapter Contents

Section 4.1

Personality and Stress

Our ability to withstand stress-related, inflammatory diseases may be associated, not just with our race and sex, but with our personality as well.

Researchers discovered low levels of extroversion in aging women may signal that blood levels of a key inflammatory molecule have crossed over a threshold linked to a doubling of risk of death within 5 years.

An emerging area of medical science examines the mind-body connection, and how personality and stress contribute to disease in the aging body. Long-term exposure to hormones released by the brains of people under stress, for instance, takes a toll on organs.

Like any injury, this brings a reaction from the body's immune system, including the release of immune chemicals that trigger inflammation in an attempt to begin the healing process. The same process goes too far as part of diseases from rheumatoid arthritis to Alzheimer's disease to atherosclerosis, where inflammation contributes to clogged arteries, heart attacks, and strokes.

The current study found that that extroverts, and in particular those with high "dispositional activity" or engagement in life, have dramatically lower levels of the inflammatory chemical interleukin 6 (IL-6).

Swiss psychiatrist Carl Jung defined extroverts as focused on the world around them and most happy when active and surrounded by people. Introverts looked inward and were shy.

The definitions of extroversion and other personality traits were refined by American psychologist Gordon Allport beginning in the 1930s. He reviewed all adjectives in the dictionary used to describe personality, and attempted to group them into clusters.

Over the next several decades, researchers statistically analyzed these dictionary terms and discovered that they tended to cluster into five general dimensions: extroversion vs. introversion, emotional stability vs. neuroticism, open- vs. closed-minded, agreeable vs. hostile, and conscientiousness vs. unreliability.

These dimensions, known as the "Five Factor Model" of personality, served to organize hundreds of specific traits like "activity" for psychologists, similar to the way the Periodic Table organizes elements for physicists.

"Our study took the important first step of finding a strong association between one part of extroversion and a specific, stress-related, inflammatory chemical," said Benjamin Chapman, Ph.D., assistant professor within the Rochester Center for Mind-Body Research (RCMBR), part of the Department of Psychiatry at the University of Rochester Medical Center, and lead author of the study.

"The next step is to determine if one causes the other. If we knew the direction and mechanism of causality, and it were low dispositional activity causing inflammation, we could design treatments to help high-risk patients become more engaged in life as a defense against disease."

Some past studies had contended, and the current analysis agreed, that women and minorities have higher levels of IL 6 than white males on average. Women may be more vulnerable to stress because of hormonal differences and minorities because of factors like perceived racism, but those questions have yet to be fully answered.

While these trends exist, variations within these large groups are so great that further risk markers are needed to better determine any given patient's actual risk. The current study looked at whether particular personality traits, including low extroversion, were associated with IL-6 levels in a sample of 103 urban primary care patients aged 40 and older.

You Must Have Been a Calm Baby

According to landmark studies in the early 1990s, extroversion is a personality trait with three parts: A tendency toward happy thoughts, a desire to be around others, and "dispositional energy," a sense of innate vigor or active engagement with life ("I'm bursting with energy; my life is fast-paced"). Other dimensions of extroversion, such as sensation-seeking, have also been proposed.

While the first two extrovert qualities were not found to track with inflammation, the current study found increases in "dispositional activity" came with statistically significant decreases in IL-6 ($p = .001$). P values measure the weight that should be attributed to a finding, with values less than .05 usually deemed significant.

In the current study, a patient's degree of extroversion was determined by standard tests, including the NEO Five-Factor Inventory, an instrument based on the Five Factor Model. The study found that the difference between the 84th percentile of dispositional activity and the 16th translated roughly into a 1.29 picogram (pg) increase in IL-6 per milliliter of blood.

Those findings took on meaning when comparisons revealed that, for both white and minority women, the difference between high and low dispositional energy was enough to shift IL-6 levels above 3.19 pg/ml, the threshold established by a large, epidemiological study (Harris et al., 1999) over which five-year mortality risk was found to double.

"If this aspect of personality drives inflammation, dispositional energy and engagement with life may confer a survival advantage," Chapman said. "But we don't know if low dispositional activity is causing inflammation, or inflammation is taking its toll on people by reducing these personality tendencies, so we must be cautious in our interpretation of this association."

The findings recall an idea described as early as 1911 by French philosopher Henri Bergson that he called élan vitale or "life force," according to the authors. This aspect of adult personality may be linked to childhood temperament as well. Some babies are very relaxed, others active. Activity level may reflect a fundamental, biologically based energy reserve, although no one has explained the biochemistry behind it.

The team gauged the magnitude of IL-6 associations for gender, race/ethnicity, and personality by examining the degree to which each factor was associated with differences between people in IL-6. Of the differences in inflammation found in the patient sample in levels of IL-6, about 9 percent of the difference was due to gender, 6 percent was due to dispositional activity levels, and another 4 percent to race/ethnicity. That a personality trait may contribute more to IL-6 levels than race/ethnicity was "a great surprise."

While it may be difficult for patients to change their nature, part of the solution may be physical exercise as a therapy. The activity component of extroversion has been linked with exercise by past studies, as has daily physical activity with lower IL-6 levels in the aging. Still, the team is not convinced that exercise represents the whole answer.

"Beyond physical activity, some people seem to have this innate energy separate from exercise that makes them intrinsically involved in life," Chapman said.

"It will be fascinating to investigate how we can increase this disposition toward engagement. Potentially, you might apply techniques developed to treat depression like 'pleasurable event scheduling' to patients with low dispositional energy, where you get people more involved in life by filling their time with things they enjoy as a therapy."

The study is published in the July issue of the journal *Brain, Behavior and Immunity*. Source: University of Rochester Medical Center.

Section 4.2

Men and Women Cope with Stress Differently

According to a study that appeared in a 2007 issue of *SCAN (Social Cognitive and Affective Neuroscience)*, researchers at the University of Pennsylvania School of Medicine discussed how men and women differ in their neural responses to psychological stress.

"We found that different parts of the brain activate with different spatial and temporal profiles for men and women when they are faced with performance-related stress," says J.J. Wang, PhD, Assistant Professor of Radiology and Neurology, and lead author of the study.

These findings suggest that stress responses may be fundamentally different in each gender, sometimes characterized as "fight-or-flight" in men and "tend-and-befriend" in women. Evolutionarily, males may have had to confront a stressor either by overcoming or fleeing it, while women may have instead responded by nurturing offspring and affiliating with social groups that maximize the survival of the species in times of adversity. The "fight-or-flight" response is associated with the main stress hormone system that produces cortisol in the human body—the hypothalamic-pituitary-adrenal (HPA) axis.

Thirty-two healthy subjects—16 females and 16 males—received fMRI (functional Magnetic Resonance Imaging) scans before, during, and after they underwent a challenging arithmetic task (serial subtraction of 13 from a 4 digit number), under pressure. To increase the level of stress, the researchers frequently prompted participants for a faster performance and asked them to restart the task if they responded incorrectly. As a low stress control condition, participants were asked to count backward without pressure.

The researchers measured heart rate, cortisol levels (a stress hormone), subjects' perceived stress levels throughout the experiments, and regional cerebral blood flow (CBF), which provides a marker of regional brain function. In men, it was found that stress was associated with increased CBF in the right prefrontal cortex and CBF reduction in the left orbitofrontal cortex. In women, the limbic system—a part of the brain primarily involved in emotion—was activated when they were under stress. Both men and women's brain activation lasted beyond the stress task, but the lasting response in the female brain was stronger. The neural response among the men was associated with higher levels of cortisol, whereas women did not have as much association between brain activation to stress and cortisol changes.

"Women have twice the rate of depression and anxiety disorders compared to men," notes Dr. Wang. "Knowing that women respond to stress by increasing activity in brain regions involved with emotion, and that these changes last longer than in men, may help us begin to explain the gender differences in the incidence of mood disorders."

Additional researchers involved with this study are Marc Korczykowski, Penn; Hengyi Rao, Penn; Yong Fan, Penn; John Pluta, Penn; Ruben Gur, Penn; Bruce McEwen, The Rockefeller University; and John Detre, Penn. This study was conducted at the Center for Functional Neuroimaging at the University of Pennsylvania.

Section 4.3

Resistance Mechanisms in Brain May Prevent Stress-Related Illness

From "Stress: Brain Yields Clues About Why Some Succumb
While Others Prevail," by the National Institutes of Health
(NIH, www.nih.gov), October 18, 2007.

Results of a study may one day help scientists learn how to enhance a naturally occurring mechanism in the brain that promotes resilience to psychological stress. Researchers funded by the National Institutes of Health's National Institute of Mental Health (NIMH) found that, in a mouse model, the ability to adapt to stress is driven by a distinctly different molecular mechanism than is the tendency to be overwhelmed by stress. The researchers mapped out the mechanisms—components of which also are present in the human brain—that govern both kinds of responses.

In humans, stress can play a major role in the development of several mental illnesses, including post-traumatic stress disorder and depression. A key question in mental health research is: Why are some people resilient to stress, while others are not? This research indicates that resistance is not simply a passive absence of vulnerability mechanisms, as was previously thought; it is a biologically active process that results in specific adaptations in the brain's response to stress.

Results of the study were published online in *Cell*, on October 18, [2007] by Vaishnav Krishnan, Ming-Hu Han, PhD, Eric J. Nestler, MD, PhD, and colleagues from the University of Texas Southwestern Medical Center, Harvard University, and Cornell University.

Vulnerability was measured through behaviors such as social withdrawal after stress was induced in mice by putting them in cages with bigger, more aggressive mice. Even a month after the encounter, some mice were still avoiding social interactions with other mice—an indication that stress had overwhelmed them—but most adapted and continued to interact, giving researchers the opportunity to examine the biological underpinnings of the protective adaptations.

"We now know that the mammalian brain can launch molecular machinery that promotes resilience to stress, and we know what several major components are. This is an excellent indicator that there are similar mechanisms in the human brain," said NIMH Director Thomas R. Insel, MD.

Looking at a specific part of the brain, the researchers found differences in the rate of impulse-firing by cells that make the chemical messenger dopamine. Vulnerable mice had excessive rates of impulse-firing during stressful situations. But adaptive mice maintained normal rates of firing because of a protective mechanism—a boost in activity of channels that allow the mineral potassium to flow into the cells, dampening their firing rates.

Higher rates of impulse-firing in the vulnerable mice led to more activity of a protein called BDNF [brain-derived neurotrophic factor], which had been linked to vulnerability in previous studies by the same researchers. With their comparatively lower rates of impulse-firing, the resistant mice did not have this increase in BDNF activity, another factor that contributed to resistance.

The scientists found that these mechanisms occurred in the reward area of the brain, which promotes repetition of acts that ensure survival. The areas involved were the VTA (ventral tegmental area) and the NAc (nucleus accumbens).

In a series of experiments, the scientists extended their findings to provide a progressively larger picture of the vulnerability and resistance mechanisms. They used a variety of approaches to test the findings, strengthening their validity.

"The extensiveness and thoroughness of their research enabled these investigators to make a very strong case for their hypothesis," Insel said.

For example, the researchers showed that the excess BDNF protein in vulnerable mice originated in the VTA, rather than in the NAc.

Chemical signals the protein sent from the VTA to the NAc played an essential role in making the mice vulnerable. Blocking the signals with experimental compounds turned vulnerable mice into resistant mice.

The scientists also conducted a genetic experiment which showed that, in resistant mice, many more genes in the VTA than in the NAc went into action in stressful situations, compared with vulnerable mice. Gene activity governs a host of biochemical events in the brain, and the results of this experiment suggest that genes in the VTA of resilient mice are working hard to offset mechanisms that promote vulnerability.

Another component of the study revealed that mice with a naturally occurring variation in part of the gene that produces the BDNF protein are resistant to stress. The variation results in lower production of BDNF, consistent with the finding that low BDNF activity promotes resilience.

The scientists also examined brain tissue of deceased people with a history of depression, and compared it with brain tissue of mice that showed vulnerability to stress. In both cases, the researchers found higher-than-average BDNF protein in the brain's reward areas, offering a potential biological explanation of the link between stress and depression.

"The fact that we could increase these animals' ability to adapt to stress by blocking BDNF and its signals means that it may be possible to develop compounds that improve resilience. This is a great opportunity to explore potential ways of increasing stress-resistance in people faced with situations that might otherwise result in post-traumatic stress disorder, for example," said Nestler.

"But it doesn't happen in a vacuum. Blocking BDNF at certain stages in the process could perturb other systems in negative ways. The key is to identify safe ways of enhancing this protective resilience machinery," Nestler added.

Section 4.4

Chronic Stress and Loneliness Affect Health

Loneliness kills, according to research dating back to the 1970s. In one classic study, published in the *American Journal of Epidemiology* (Vol. 109, No. 2, pages 186–204 [1979]), socially isolated people in Alameda County, California, were between two and three times more likely to die during the 9-year study than those who had many friends.

"The increase in morbidity with social isolation is equal to that of cigarette smoking," notes Martha McClintock, PhD, a University of Chicago psychology professor who researches social isolation and stress.

But while the pathway from smoking to cancer is largely established, the path from loneliness and other forms of chronic stress to many health consequences—including increased risk for cancer, cardiovascular illness, and Alzheimer's disease—is not, she says. In humans, some of the effect may be due to the practical benefits of having a social network, says Gretchen Hermes, a fourth-year MD-PhD student at the University of Chicago. For instance, people with many friends might be more likely to brush their teeth and exercise. And gregarious people may have more friends who bring them food or medicine when they get sick.

But new animal studies suggest that there are direct, physiological pathways from loneliness and other chronic stressors to illness. And those pathways may differ depending on gender and temperament, with male and behaviorally inhibited animals being particularly susceptible, researchers are finding.

Acute Stress: An Immune Booster?

Hermes and her colleagues found that, overall, social isolation suppressed wound healing in male and female rats, according to a study published last year in the *American Journal of Physiology-Regulatory, Comparative, and Integrative Physiology* (Vol. 290, No. 1, pages 273–282 [2005]). However, when they also acutely stressed the rats by trapping them in a small tube, the socially isolated female rats surprised researchers with an enhanced immune response, while the socially isolated male rats showed a further suppression of the immune response.

The researchers housed 60 female and 60 male rats either in groups of five or in isolated cages for more than 3 months. Then they injected half of the animals with a few milligrams of seaweed, right under their skin. The substance is harmless, but the immune system identifies it as foreign and surrounds it with scar tissue before absorbing it back into the body.

Both male and female isolated rats took longer to heal the wound than their group-housed brothers and sisters, the researchers found. While rats don't often face seaweed injections in the wild, the procedure taps into an underlying defense against many common illnesses, McClintock says.

"The basic inflammatory response is involved in a whole variety of different diseases, ranging from heart disease to infectious diseases and some forms of cancer," she notes.

Though socially isolated male and female rats responded similarly to the seaweed test, differences emerged when they were also exposed to an acute stressor. Two weeks before the seaweed injection, the researchers placed half of the socially isolated animals in a restraint tube for 30 minutes, a procedure that mimics the experience of being trapped in a collapsing burrow, says Hermes.

For the female rats, the trial revved up their immune systems—and they healed faster than those who didn't spend time in the restraint tube. The acutely stressed males, conversely, showed a slowed immune response.

"The females were much more resilient," Hermes notes. The results fit with research on humans, says McClintock.

"Men who are lonely, or bereaved, or who lose their partners are known to be more vulnerable to disease and death, whereas women are more resilient," she notes.

The differences in both rats and humans may stem from the evolutionary pressure, McClintock theorizes. To pass on their genes, male animals only need to live long enough to mate. Female animals have to make it for the long haul.

"They need to survive to deliver and to take care of their young," she notes. "You can imagine it would be beneficial for evolution to select for females who could respond to a brief stressor with augmenting their immune function."

The Cost of Inhibition

One strength of the study is that they were able to randomly assign animals to social or isolated groups, notes McClintock. "That doesn't happen in nature," she says. For instance, some rats and humans tend to seek out others, while behaviorally inhibited animals will more likely live in isolation.

Even discounting of the effect of isolation, behavioral inhibition does seem to carry a health cost, according to a study published in the July [2006] issue of *Hormones and Behavior* (Vol. 50, No. 1, pages 454–462). In fact, behaviorally inhibited rats—those that tend to explore less because they find novel environments more threatening—died of natural causes a full 6 months earlier than their easygoing sisters, researchers found.

Penn State biobehavioral health professor Sonia Cavigelli, PhD, and her colleagues tested the temperament of 81 female rats when they were 20 days old, by placing them in an unfamiliar room, which included opaque walls and novel objects. Some of the animals moved freely around the room and sniffed the objects, while others huddled in the corner.

The animals then were housed in groups of three and lived out their natural lifespan. The particular strain of rat used in the study tends to live about 2 years, and they usually die of cancerous tumors that begin in their mammary glands, says Cavigelli.

While all the animals tended to die of tumors over time, the gregarious animals developed them about 6 months later than the inhibited ones. This may be because the inhibited animals don't socialize as much as other animals, or they may just get startled more often.

"Individuals that go through the stress response more frequently go through faster wear and tear on the system," Cavigelli notes.

Both studies shed light on the intricate mechanisms through which chronic stress, due to either social isolation or hypervigilance, can kill, says McClintock.

"They really begin to get to the richness of the dynamic," she notes. "In the area of stress, immunity, social context, and sex, one shouldn't expect simple main effects."

Section 4.5

Media Coverage Linked to Stress

From "Media Coverage of Traumatic Events,"
from the National Center for PTSD (www.ptsd.va.gov),
part of the Veterans Administration, June 15, 2010.

Many people find it hard to resist news of traumatic events, such as disasters and terrorist attacks. As awful as it is to watch and read about, many still cannot turn away. Why is this kind of news so hard to resist? Some say it is because people are trying to inform themselves, to be prepared in case of future disaster or attacks. Others say that people are watching and reading news in an effort to understand and process the event. Still others say the media is trying to draw you in with exciting images almost like those from an action movie. Whatever the reason, we need to understand the effects that this type of news exposure may have.

Watching Traumatic News Is Related to Stress

Research tells us there is a link between watching news of traumatic events, such as terrorist attacks, and stress symptoms. It could be that watching television of the event makes people worse. It could also be that people who have more severe stress reactions are the ones who choose to watch more television about the event. Here are some examples that show the link:

- Research after the September 11th, 2001, terrorist attacks found that in the first few days, adults watched an average of 8 hours of television related to the attacks. Children watched an average of 3 hours of television related to the attacks. Older teens watched more than younger children. In both children and adults, those who watched the most coverage had more stress symptoms than those who watched less.

- The Oklahoma City bombing was also widely covered in the news. In adults, watching bomb-related news did not relate to increased PTSD symptoms. On the other hand, children who watched more bomb-related news did have more PTSD symptoms. Of note, for most Oklahoma school children in the weeks after the bombing, the bulk of their television viewing was bomb-related. Links were seen between PTSD symptoms and bomb-related television for children who did and did not lose a close family member in the bombing.

- In Israel, those who watched television clips of terrorism reported feeling more anxiety than those who watched clips that were not related to terrorism.

- Adults who lost close friends or family in the Mount St. Helens tragedy said that the news coverage made it harder for them to recover. Adults who only lost property said that the news neither hurt nor helped them.

- Children from Kuwait had increased PTSD symptoms after viewing gruesome televised images of violence and death related to the Gulf War.

It is still unclear why this relationship exists. Media might both hurt and help those who experience trauma. Having news media present is sometimes a burden on family members. For example, the media may show their personal grief on television. Also, watching news about a trauma may make the victims feel even more helpless. It may fix even more firmly in their minds the images of death and damage.

Positive Role of the Media

Although there may be negative effects, clearly the media plays a vital role after a disaster. The media provides needed information and alerts. Media outlets can direct the public to services for victims and their families. They are a resource for the community. They can also be a source of hope. In some ways, being involved with the media might give survivors a sense of power. This could help offset their feeling helpless after the trauma.

Recommendations about Viewing

You may want to limit the amount and type of news you are viewing if you:

- feel anxious or stressed after watching a news program;
- cannot turn off the television;

- cannot take part in relaxing or fun activities;
- have trouble sleeping.

Some useful tips include:

- do not watch the news just before bed;
- read newspapers or magazines rather than watching television;
- inform yourself by talking to other people about the attack.

Children

The research with children shows even more clearly that watching too much trauma-related television can be harmful. Here are some tips for dealing with children and media exposure:

- **Be aware that children in the household may be exposed to traumatic images.** It is common for a television to be on for several hours a day in an American household. Adults should be aware of how much news a child is viewing. This may occur even if no adult has decided that the child can watch trauma-related news.

- **Parents should talk with the child about what they are seeing on the news.** For example, children who watched news about the September 11th attacks may have seen the first plane crash into the building over and over again. These children may have needed it explained to them that they were seeing one single crash that happened on one day, not multiple crashes.

- **Put the news into context.** Explain the following:
  - There are many good people who will do their best to keep them safe if something bad happens. Focus on the firemen and rescue teams and not just on the attack.
  - The news often tells us bad things that happen in the world. Most of the time, though, the country is safe. Most people who fly in airplanes land safely on the ground and have no problems at all.

- **Invite children to talk.** Above all, parents need to allow and even invite children to ask questions. Children may have misplaced fears after watching a news report. This may be because they did not understand something. If the child shares those fears or asks questions, parents can help explain and comfort. Parents can tell the child that a lot of people are working hard to make things safer for the future.

- **Limit the child's news viewing.** Some parents do not allow young children to watch the news at all. If news viewing is allowed, experts suggest that parents watch the news with their children. Also, if a child seems to be watching too much trauma-related news, the parent can direct the child to other more positive activities.

Sadly, it is true that most reported news is bad news. We don't hear about the planes that land safely every day. Children need to be reminded that what they see on the news does not reflect the way things are most often in our country.

Chapter 5

Childhood Stress

As providers and caretakers, adults tend to view the world of children as happy and carefree. After all, kids don't have jobs to keep or bills to pay, so what could they possibly have to worry about?

Plenty! Even very young children have worries and feel stress to some degree. Stress is a function of the demands placed on us and our ability to meet them.

Sources of Stress

Pressures often come from outside sources (such as family, friends, or school), but they can also come from within. The pressure we place on ourselves can be most significant because there is often a discrepancy between what we think we ought to be doing and what we are actually doing in our lives.

Stress can affect anyone who feels overwhelmed—even kids. In preschoolers, separation from parents can cause anxiety. As kids get older, academic and social pressures (especially the quest to fit in) create stress.

Many kids are too busy to have time to play creatively or relax after school. Kids who complain about the number of activities they're involved in or refuse to go to them may be signaling that they're overscheduled.

Talk with your kids about how they feel about extracurricular activities. If they complain, discuss the pros and cons of quitting one activity. If quitting isn't an option, explore ways to help manage your child's time and responsibilities so that they don't create so much anxiety.

Kids' stress may be intensified by more than just what's happening in their own lives. Do your kids hear you talking about troubles at work, worrying about a relative's illness, or fighting with your spouse about financial matters? Parents should watch how they discuss such issues when their kids are near because children will pick up on their parents' anxieties and start to worry themselves.

World news can cause stress. Kids who see disturbing images on TV or hear talk of natural disasters, war, and terrorism may worry about their own safety and that of the people they love. Talk to your kids about what they see and hear, and monitor what they watch on TV so that you can help them understand what's going on.

Also, be aware of complicating factors, such as an illness, death of a loved one, or a divorce. When these are added to the everyday pressures kids face, the stress is magnified. Even the most amicable divorce can be a difficult experience for kids because their basic security system—their family—is undergoing a tough change. Separated or divorced parents should never put kids in a position of having to choose sides or expose them to negative comments about the other spouse.

Signs and Symptoms

While it's not always easy to recognize when kids are stressed out, short-term behavioral changes—such as mood swings, acting out, changes in sleep patterns, or bedwetting—can be indications. Some kids experience physical effects, including stomachaches and headaches. Others have trouble concentrating or completing schoolwork. Still others become withdrawn or spend a lot of time alone.

Younger children may show signs of reacting to stress by picking up new habits like thumb sucking, hair twirling, or nose picking; older kids may begin to lie, bully, or defy authority. A child who is stressed may also have nightmares, difficulty leaving you, overreactions to minor problems, and drastic changes in academic performance.

Reducing Stress

How can you help kids cope with stress? Proper rest and good nutrition can boost coping skills, as can good parenting. Make time for your kids each day. Whether they need to talk or just be in the same room with you, make yourself available.

Even as kids get older, quality time is important. It's really hard for some people to come home after work, get down on the floor, and play with their kids or just talk to them about their day—especially if they've had a stressful day themselves. But expressing interest in your kids' days shows that they're important to you.

Help your child cope with stress by talking about what may be causing it. Together, you can come up with a few solutions like cutting back on after-school activities, spending more time talking with parents or teachers, developing an exercise regimen, or keeping a journal.

You can also help by anticipating potentially stressful situations and preparing kids for them. For example, let a child know ahead of time (but not too far ahead of time) that a doctor's appointment is coming up and talk about what will happen there. Keep in mind, though, that younger kids probably won't need too much advance preparation. Too much information can cause more stress—reassurance is the key.

Remember that some level of stress is normal; let kids know that it's OK to feel angry, scared, lonely, or anxious and that other people share those feelings.

Helping Your Child Cope

When kids can't or won't discuss these issues, try talking about your own concerns. This shows that you're willing to tackle tough topics and are available to talk with when they're ready. If a child shows symptoms that concern you and is unwilling to talk, consult a counselor or other mental health specialist.

Books can help young kids identify with characters in stressful situations and learn how they cope. Check out *Alexander and the Terrible, Horrible, No Good, Very Bad Day* by Judith Viorst; *Tear Soup* by Pat Schweibert, Chuck DeKlyen, and Taylor Bills; and *Dinosaurs Divorce* by Marc Brown and Laurene Krasny Brown.

Most parents have the skills to deal with their child's stress. The time to seek professional attention is when any change in behavior persists, when stress is causing serious anxiety, or when the behavior is causing significant problems in functioning at school or at home.

If you need help finding resources for your child, consult your doctor or the counselors and teachers at school.

Chapter 6

Stress and Aging

Increasing scientific evidence suggests that prolonged psychological stress takes its toll on the body, but the exact mechanisms by which stress influences disease processes have remained elusive. Now, scientists report that psychological stress may exact its toll, at least in part, by affecting molecules believed to play a key role in cellular aging and, possibly, disease development.

In the study, published in the December 7, 2004 issue of *Proceedings of the National Academy of Sciences*, the UCSF [University of California–San Francisco]-led team determined that chronic stress, and the perception of life stress, each had a significant impact on three biological factors—the length of telomeres, the activity of telomerase, and levels of oxidative stress—in immune system cells known as peripheral blood mononucleocytes, in healthy premenopausal women.

Telomeres are DNA-protein complexes that cap the ends of chromosomes and promote genetic stability. Each time a cell divides, a

"UCSF-led study suggests link between psychological stress and cell aging," University of California–San Francisco News Office, November 29, 2004. Reprinted with permission. This University of California at San Francisco News Release is based upon the following published manuscript: "Accelerated telomere shortening in response to life stress," by Elissa S. Epel, et al., *Proceedings of the National Academy of Sciences*, December 7, 2004; 101(49), 17312–17315, http://www.pnas .org/content/101/49/17312. The text that follows this document under the heading "Health Reference Series Medical Advisor's Notes and Updates" was provided to Omnigraphics, Inc. by David A. Cooke, MD, FACP, November 8, 2010. Dr. Cooke is not affiliated with the University of California–San Francisco News Office.

portion of telomeric DNA dwindles away, and after many rounds of cell division, so much telomeric DNA has diminished that the aged cell stops dividing. Thus, telomeres play a critical role in determining the number of times a cell divides, its health, and its life span. These factors, in turn, affect the health of the tissues that cells form. Telomerase is an enzyme that replenishes a portion of telomeres with each round of cell division, and protects telomeres. Oxidative stress, which causes DNA damage, has been shown to hasten the shortening of telomeres in cell culture.

The results of the study—which involved 58 women, ages 20–50, all of whom were biological mothers either of a chronically ill child (39 women, so-called "caregivers") or a healthy child (19 women, or "controls")—were dramatic.

As expected, most women who cared for a chronically ill child reported that they were more stressed than women in the control group, though, as a group, their biological markers were not different from those of the controls. However, in one of the study's key findings, the duration of caregiving—after controlling for the age of the women—proved critical: The more years of care giving, the shorter the length of the telomeres, the lower the telomerase activity, and the greater the oxidative stress.

Moreover, the perception of being stressed correlated in both the caregiver and control groups with the biological markers. In fact, in the most stunning result, the telomeres of women with the highest perceived psychological stress—across both groups—had undergone the equivalent of approximately 10 years of additional aging, compared with the women across both groups who had the lowest perception of being stressed. The highest-stress group also had significantly decreased telomerase activity and higher oxidative stress than the lowest-stress group.

"The results were striking," says co-author Elizabeth Blackburn, PhD, Morris Herzstein Professor of Biology and Physiology in the Department of Biochemistry and Biophysics at UCSF. "This is the first evidence that chronic psychological stress—and how a person perceives stress—may damp down telomerase and have a significant impact on the length of telomeres, suggesting that stress may modulate the rate of cellular aging."

The Link from Mind to Body

"Numerous studies have solidly demonstrated a link between chronic psychological stress and indices of impaired health, including cardiovascular disease and weakened immune function," says lead author Elissa Epel, PhD, UCSF assistant professor of psychiatry. "The new findings suggest a cellular mechanism for how chronic stress may cause premature onset of disease. Anecdotal evidence and scientific evidence have suggested that chronic stress can take years off your life; the implications of this study are that this is true at the cellular level. Chronic stress appears to have the potential to shorten the life of cells, at least immune cells."

While it is not yet clear how psychological stress impacts telomeres, the team suspects stress hormones may play a role.

The Next Investigative Steps

A next step in the research will be determining if prolonged psychological stress has an impact on telomeres in other types of cells, such as cells of the lining of the cardiovascular system.

The scientists also plan to further examine the impact of prolonged psychological stress on immune system cells, which mount the body's healing response to wounds, and defenses against illness. When the immune system needs to rev up, it produces more defense cells, which requires high levels of the telomerase enzyme, in order to maintain telomere length, thus allowing for additional rounds of cell division. The current study suggests that, for people under chronic stress, the telomerase activity of their immune cells might be impaired.

The current study represented a one-time snapshot of the biological markers in the women. Both the caregivers and controls were given a standardized 10-item questionnaire assessing their level of perceived stress during the previous month, and measurements of their objective stress (caregiver status, and duration of caregiving stress) were collected. The data was then correlated with the indices of cell aging (telomerase and telomere length).

The team is now conducting a long-term study in which the length of telomeres will be measured repeatedly in participants to test whether the rate of telomere shortening in individuals with higher reported levels of stress is actually faster than in those with lower reported levels of stress.

If the findings bear out, there would be numerous implications for clinical intervention, says Epel. The effect of prolonged psychological stress on telomeres presumably takes many years, which could make it possible to intervene. The team wants to carry out clinical trials to see if stress reduction interventions, such as meditation, yoga, or cognitive-behavioral therapy, would increase telomerase activity and telomere length—or slow the rate of telomere shortening—in individuals.

At this point, there is not a routine test for assessing telomerase activity or telomere length in cells, and scientists are years away from knowing enough about the correlation between chronic psychological stress and these biological markers to proceed in this direction.

However, if the evidence that telomere length is a risk factor for disease becomes more established, it's possible, the scientists say, that prematurely shortened telomeres might someday be a traditional health-risk factor, such as high LDL [low-density lipoprotein] cholesterol. And if this were the case, drugs that activated the telomerase enzyme just enough to forestall over-shortening of telomeres might be administered.

Co-authors of the study were Richard M. Cawthon, MD, PhD, Department of Human Genetics, University of Utah, who also served as a co-senior author; Jue Lin, PhD, UCSF Department of Biochemistry and Biophysics; Firdaus S. Dhabhar, PhD, Department of Oral Biology, College of Dentistry, Molecular Virology, Immunology, and Medical Genetics, College of Medicine, Ohio State University; Nancy E. Adler, PhD, UCSF professor and vice chair of psychiatry, and Jason D. Morrow, PhD, Department of Medicine and Pharmacology, Vanderbilt University School of Medicine.

The study was funded by the John D. & Catherine T. MacArthur Foundation, the Hellman Family Fund, the Steven and Michele Kirsch Foundation, the Burroughs Wellcome Fund Clinical Scientists Award in Translational Research, the Dana Foundation, and the National Institutes of Health.

Health Reference Series Medical Advisor's Notes and Updates

Since the publication of the above text, several other laboratories have reproduced their results. Additional research has supported the authors' theory that psychological stress affects immunologic function. Scientific interest in this topic continues to grow.

Chapter 7

Stress in the United States

About the Stress in America Survey

In July 2009, the American Psychological Association (APA) commissioned its annual nationwide survey to examine the state of stress across the country and understand its impact. The survey included specific questions for people living with chronic health conditions to help establish not only a better understanding of patients' experiences but also the ways lifestyle and behavior factor into disease prevention and management. In addition, an omnibus survey was conducted among youth ages 8–17 to learn more about how stress affects tweens and teens.

Overall, the Stress in America survey measured attitudes and perceptions of stress among the general public, identifying leading sources of stress, common behaviors used to manage stress, and the impact of stress on our lives. The results of the survey draw attention to the serious physical and emotional implications of stress and the inextricable link between the mind and body.

The survey explored:

- perceptions of respondents' personal levels of stress;

- circumstances, situations, and life events that cause stress;

- perceptions of how well people manage stress;

- the impact of stress on families;

- activities, resources, and behaviors people use to deal with stress; and

- the role of lifestyle and behavior in managing chronic illness.

[Editor's Note: Parenthetical references in the text of this chapter prefaced by "Q" refer to specific numbered questions in the survey.]

Methodology

The Stress in America survey was conducted online within the United States by Harris Interactive on behalf of APA between July 21 and August 4, 2009, among 1,568 adults aged 18 and older who reside in the United States, including [the following]:

- 729 men and 839 women

- 1,020 adults who identified as having one or more chronic conditions including high blood pressure, high cholesterol, overweight or obese, arthritis, depression, asthma or other respiratory disease, type 2 diabetes, chronic pain, an anxiety disorder, heart disease or heart attack, cancer, stroke, type 1 (juvenile) diabetes, and 512 adults who do not have a chronic condition

- 504 Millennials (18- to 30-year-olds), 369 Gen Xers (31- to 44-year-olds), 464 Boomers (45- to 63-year-olds), and 231 Matures (64 years and older)

- 235 adults who are parents of children aged 8–17

- 984 people who are employed and 584 people who are not employed.[1] Among those who are not employed, 192 adults are looking for work. Overall, 256 adults are retired and 163 are stay-at-home spouses or partners ("homemakers").

- 820 White, non-Hispanic adults; 333 Black, non-Hispanic adults; and 311 Hispanic adults

- 362 adults who reside in the East, 516 in the South, 340 in the Midwest, and 349 in the West. Respondents were also analyzed by the kind of area they lived in and include 545 adults who live in an urban or city area, 620 who live in a suburban area near a city, and 403 who live in a small town or rural area.

All sample surveys, whether or not they use probability sampling, are subject to multiple sources of error, which are most often not possible to quantify or estimate, including sampling error, coverage error, error associated with nonresponse, error associated with question wording and response options, and post-survey weighting and adjustments.

Therefore, Harris Interactive avoids the words "margin of error" as they are misleading. All that can be calculated are different possible sampling errors with different probabilities for pure, unweighted, random samples with 100 percent response rates. These are only theoretical because no published surveys come close to this ideal.

Respondents for this survey were selected from among those who have agreed to participate in Harris Interactive surveys. The data have been weighted to reflect the composition of the U.S. population aged 18 and older. Because the sample is based on those who agreed to be invited to participate in the Harris Interactive online research panel, no estimates of theoretical sampling error can be calculated.

Key Findings

Stress in the Family

As families across America navigate particularly challenging economic times, findings from the 2009 Stress in America survey suggest that stress and worry[2] are having more of an impact on young people than parents believe. (See Figure 7.1 and Table 7.1.) Parents and young people differ on several key measures related to how much stress or worry young people experience, what is causing the stress or worry, and how their level of stress or worry has changed over the last year. For example, fewer parents than children believe that children's stress has increased in the past year, there is a disconnect between what parents believe causes stress in children and what children consider worrisome, and parents appear to be unaware of the degree to which children report physical symptoms like headaches and difficulties sleeping that are often associated with stress. This possible disconnect within the family could have long-term implications for young people, many of whom don't appear to be getting the support they need to identify and understand stress or to learn healthy strategies for managing stress.

Nearly a quarter of Americans reported experiencing high stress levels in the past month (8, 9, or 10 on a 10-point scale), yet, many parents seem unaware of the impact that their stress has on their children. Nearly two-thirds (63 percent) of parents reported that their stress levels have a slight or no impact on their child's stress levels, which is concerning when considering the number of young people who view their parents as their primary teachers as it relates to learning about healthy habits. Nearly 80 percent of young people say they learn about healthy living from their parents or guardians, suggesting that parents are important role models for children. Yet parents are not modeling healthy behavior when it comes to stress management. Half of parents (50 percent) say their stress has increased in the past year, but less than half of moms (45 percent) and just over half of dads (56 percent) say they're doing enough to manage their stress. And while three-quarters of young people say they're comfortable talking to their parents or guardians about the things they worry about, responses to the youth omnibus indicate that stress may be a real problem for many young people and they may not be getting the family support needed to manage that stress.

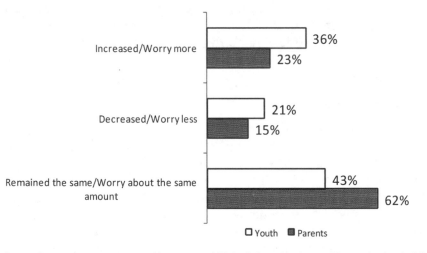

Parents: Compared to one year ago, would you say your child's level of stress has decreased, increased or remained the same?
Youth: *Compared to last summer, do you think you worry more or less now?*

Figure 7.1. *Change in stress level since last year.*

Overall, parents' responses to survey questions about the causes and impacts of stress and worry on their children are out of sync with feedback received by youth.

- Nearly half (45 percent) of teens ages 13–17 said that they worried more this year, but only 28 percent of parents think their teen's stress increased, and while a quarter (26 percent) of tweens ages 8–12 said they worried more this year, only 17 percent of parents believed their tween's stress had increased. (Q220, Q710)

- Only 2–5 percent of parents rate their child's stress as extreme (an 8, 9, or 10 on a 10-point scale) when 14 percent of tweens (ages 8–12) and 28 percent of teens (ages 13–17) say they worry a lot or a great deal. (Q2208, Q705)

- Children were nearly two times more likely to say they worried about their family's financial difficulties than their parents perceived (30 percent of youth say they worried about their family having enough money when only 18 percent of parents reported that this was a source of stress for their child). (Q2215, Q715)

- Parents were much more likely than kids to say that children's relationships with their parents or siblings were top sources of stress or worry (16 percent vs. 8 percent for parents, 17 percent vs. 8 percent for siblings). (Q2215, Q715)

- Children were more likely to report that they worry about things related to school than parents perceived. Forty-four percent of all children ages 8–17 reported that doing well in school was a source of worry compared to only 34 percent of parents reporting this as a source of stress for their child. Over a quarter (29 percent) of children ages 13–17 reported that they worry about getting into a good college and deciding what to do after high school, when only 5 percent of parents of 13- to 17-year-olds agreed that this was a source of stress for their child.

- While 13 percent of parents believe that children experience headaches, 36 percent of children reported headaches in the past month. (Q2218, Q730)

- Children are three times more likely to report having experienced difficulty sleeping in the past month than parents were to report this symptom on behalf of their children (45 percent of children compared with 13 percent of parents). (Q2218, Q730)

- Children (34 percent) were four times more likely to report having eaten too much or too little in the past month than parents were to report these behaviors in their children (8 percent). (Q2218, Q730)

Perceptions of Stress

The perceived impact of stress appears to have peaked in the last year, which started out with daily stories about layoffs, home foreclosures, and the continued effects of last year's financial meltdown. Despite

Table 7.1. Sources of Stress by Age

Sources of Stress by Age	Parents			Youth		
	Total	8–12	13–17	Total	8–12	13–17
n =	235	101	134	1206	536	670
Managing school pressures/respon-sibilities/homework/grades/Doing well in school	34%	31%	36%	44%	44%	43%
Relationships with siblings/Getting along with my brother(s) or sister(s)	17%	17%	16%	8%	14%	2%
Relationships with peers/Getting along with my friends	20%	20%	20%	16%	22%	11%
Relationships with parent(s)/Getting along with my parent(s)/guardian	16%	21%	13%	8%	9%	8%
Your family's financial difficulties/My family having enough money	18%	20%	17%	30%	28%	31%
His/her physical appearance/weight/ The way I look/my weight	17%	17%	17%	22%	17%	26%
Your relationship with your spouse/part-ner/My parent(s)/guardian or other family members arguing or fighting more	12%	16%	9%	10%	14%	7%
Pressure managing extracurricular commitments (e.g., sports, hobbies)/ Managing activities such as sports, music, clubs, etc.	12%	12%	12%	10%	7%	12%
Peer pressure to engage in risky behaviors (e.g., smoking, drink-ing, drugs, sex, etc.)/Pressure from friends who want me to try smoking, drinking, drugs, sex, etc.[3]	6%	1%	10%	2%	—	3%
Getting into a good college/determin-ing future/Getting into a good college/ Deciding what to do after high school	3%	1%	5%	17%	5%	29%
Non-financial pressures on family members (e.g., health, job frustra-tions, getting along with extended family, etc.)	3%	3%	4%	NA	NA	NA
Getting along with my boyfriend or girlfriend	NA	NA	NA	3%	1%	4%
My parent(s)/guardian losing their jobs	NA	NA	NA	6%	7%	6%
Other	8%	10%	6%	10%	12%	8%

the bad news that surrounds them, fewer Americans report that their stress is on the rise—in 2009, 42 percent reported their stress has increased over the past year compared to 47 percent in 2008. Regardless, nearly half (42 percent) of Americans are still reporting that their stress has increased. For the quarter of people who report they are experiencing high levels of stress (24 percent of adults reported stress levels of 8, 9, or 10 on a 10-point scale, where 1 means you have little or no stress and 10 means you have a great deal of stress), this could be a precursor to serious health consequences related to chronic stress.

While some report they do exercise or walk to manage their stress (44 percent), findings from the Stress in America survey show that many Americans are turning to less desirable strategies to manage their stress. Many people rely on sedentary activities to manage their stress (49 percent listen to music, 41 percent read, 36 percent watch television or movies, 33 percent play video games, and 32 percent nap to manage stress). Forty-three percent say they eat too much or eat unhealthy foods because of stress. And, many Americans are feeling the physical effects of stress—nearly half of all adults report that they lie awake at night because of stress (47 percent).

Overall, Americans' levels of stress remain high. People do appear to be recognizing that consistently high levels of stress are unhealthy and, for the first time, people are reporting that having lower levels of stress is good for you—half of Americans report that stress levels in the lower range (1, 2, or 3 on a 10-point scale) are healthy compared to 39 percent of people who believed this in 2008 and 28 percent in 2007. Regardless, it's clear given the consistently high levels of stress that people in the United States are reporting that this is still a health concern for many adults and some children.

- A quarter (24 percent) of Americans reported experiencing high levels of stress (a rating of 8, 9, or 10 on a 10-point scale) and half (51 percent) reported moderate stress levels in 2009 (a rating of 4, 5, 6, or 7 on a 10-point scale). (Q605)

- On a scale of 1 to 10, where 1 means little or no stress and 10 means a great deal of stress, 50 percent of Americans in 2009 consider the bottom range—from 1 to 3—to be a healthy level of stress. In 2008, less than 40 percent considered these lower levels of stress healthy, and less than 30 percent felt this way in 2007. (Q605)

- The percentage of Americans reporting that their level of stress increased in the previous five years is down nearly 10 points compared with the summer of 2008 (45 percent compared with 53 percent). Similarly, the percentage of Americans reporting that their level of stress increased in the past year is down as well (42 percent compared with 47 percent in 2008). (Q623_08, Q620_54)

The Role of Lifestyle and Behavior in Promoting Good Health

Two-thirds (66 percent) of adults living in the United States have been told by a health care provider that they have one or more chronic conditions, most commonly high blood pressure or high cholesterol, and the vast majority of adults indicated that a health care provider recommended lifestyle and behavior changes (70 percent). In particular, health care providers recommended that people exercise more (48 percent), lose weight (38 percent), and eat healthier (36 percent). Unfortunately, few adults say they were offered support to make lasting changes. Less than half of adults who were instructed to make lifestyle changes were given an explanation for the recommendation (46 percent), offered advice or shown techniques to help make changes (35 percent), or referred to another health care provider to support the adoption of lifestyle changes (range: 5–10 percent). And, only half (48 percent) of adults reported that their health care providers followed up with them to check on their progress in making lifestyle and behavior changes.

In general, people reported facing a number of barriers in their efforts to make lasting lifestyle and behavior changes that are recommended by a health care provider. A third (33 percent) cited their own lack of willpower as the reason they were unsuccessful. In addition, not having enough time (20 percent) and lack of confidence (14 percent) were other specific personal barriers people said were preventing them from making lifestyle and behavior changes. More than one in 10 people cited stress as a barrier preventing them from making lifestyle and behavior changes (14 percent of adults report they are too stressed to make these changes).

Patients advised by their health care provider to make lifestyle changes specifically associated with behaviors or symptoms of stress—such as quitting smoking, getting more sleep, or reducing stress overall—were the least likely to report success in making lifestyle changes. Among those who received each recommendation, only 27 percent were successful quitting smoking, 47 percent were successful getting more sleep, and 51 percent were successful reducing stress. In comparison, between 63 percent and 73 percent of adults reported being successful at exercising more, losing weight, and eating a healthier diet. And adults reporting the highest stress levels (8, 9, or 10 on a 10-point scale) were less likely to be successful at making positive lifestyle changes when it came to eating a healthier diet, exercising more, losing weight, reducing stress, and getting more sleep.

2009 Snapshot of Stress in America

Parents and stress: Mothers report higher levels of stress than fathers, are more likely to report a variety of symptoms as a result of stress, and are less likely to believe they're doing enough to manage their stress.

Mothers report higher average stress levels than fathers do, and are five times more likely to report a stress level of 10, indicating that moms are living with a great deal of stress.

- Mothers of children aged 8–17 report higher levels of stress than fathers, with 15 percent of moms rating their stress at a level of 10 in the last month (compared to 3 percent of dads).

- Mothers show concern about finances and are more likely than fathers to cite money (88 percent of mothers vs. 68 percent of fathers), the economy (70 percent vs. 60 percent), and housing costs (67 percent vs. 52 percent) as very or somewhat significant causes of stress.

Mothers also generally report more physical symptoms of stress than fathers.

- During the last month, more mothers than fathers report lying awake (66 percent vs. 55 percent), eating too much or eating unhealthy foods (52 percent vs. 48 percent), or skipping a meal (54 percent vs. 47 percent) because of stress.

- Mothers report experiencing various symptoms more frequently than fathers during that last month including feeling as though they could cry (54 percent vs. 15 percent), headache (54 percent vs. 32 percent), feeling nervous or anxious (44 percent of mothers vs. 27 percent of fathers), and feeling depressed or sad (41 percent vs. 27 percent).

Overall, moms (45 percent) and single parents (36 percent) are less likely to believe they are doing enough to manage their stress (compared with 56 percent of dads and 59 percent of married parents).

Gender and stress: Results indicate that women continue to bear the brunt of stress, particularly in relation to financial concerns and worries over their family's health and family responsibilities, and they consistently report higher levels of stress than men. Of greatest concern is the fact that women report more physical and emotional symptoms of stress, and are more likely to report lacking willpower to make changes recommended by health care providers.

- More women (27 percent) report high levels of stress (an 8, 9, or 10 on a 10-point scale) than men (19 percent). (Q605)

- More women say that financial issues such as money (75 percent women vs. 67 percent men), the economy (66 percent women vs. 59 percent men), and housing costs (51 percent women vs. 43 percent men) are a significant source of stress in their lives. (Q625_61)

- Regardless of their levels of stress or concern about stress, women are much less likely (49 percent) than men (60 percent) to report that work-related demands have interfered with responsibilities at home in the past 3 months. (Q920)

- Women are also more likely than men to say issues related to their family are a significant source of stress, including family responsibilities (60 percent women vs. 50 percent men) and health problems affecting their families (51 percent women vs. 43 percent men). (Q625_61)

- More women than men say that stress has kept them up at night in the past month (52 percent women vs. 42 percent men), or that they have eaten too much or unhealthy foods (52 percent women vs. 33 percent men), or skipped a meal (women 42 percent vs. men 31 percent) as a result of stress. (Q770, Q785, Q800)

- Across the board, women are much more likely to report having experienced symptoms of stress in the past month than men, including irritability or anger (51 percent women vs. 39 percent men); fatigue (49 percent women vs. 37 percent men); lack of interest, motivation, or energy (45 percent women vs. 35 percent men); feeling nervous or anxious (42 percent women vs. 28 percent men); feeling depressed or sad (42 percent women vs. 26 percent men); headache (43 percent women vs. 24 percent men); feeling like crying (46 percent women vs. 16 percent men); upset stomach or indigestion (31 percent women vs. 24 percent men); muscular tension (28 percent women vs. 20 percent men); and change in appetite (24 percent women vs. 15 percent men). (Q810)

- More women than men (37 percent vs. 28 percent) say not having enough willpower keeps them from making the lifestyle changes recommended by their health care provider. (Q2255)

Generations and stress[4]: Regardless of age, general economic and financial concerns continue to be significant sources of stress for most adults, but specific stressors and physical symptoms related to stress vary significantly among generations.

In general, economic and financial concerns continue to be significant sources of stress for the majority of adults across age ranges (range: 54 to 81 percent), but when comparing sources of stress across generations, there are some notable differences. Millennial are most likely to see money as a significant stressor (81 percent compared to 74 percent of Gen Xers, 71 percent of Boomers and 54 percent of Matures), Gen Xers are more likely to view work as a significant source of stress (75 percent compared to 71 percent of Millennials, 73 percent of Boomers and 31 percent of Matures), and Boomers are more likely to cite the economy as a significant source of stress (72 percent compared to 50 percent of Millennials, 66 percent of Gen Xers, and 57 percent of Matures).

Adults report a variety of physical symptoms of stress depending on their age.

- Gen Xers are more likely to report feeling irritable or angry as a result of stress in the past month (53 percent) than Boomers (47 percent) and Millennials (46 percent). Significantly fewer Matures (29 percent) report similar feelings caused by stress. (Q810)

- Similar percentages of Millennials (43 percent) and Gen Xers (41 percent) report that they experience headaches resulting from stress, while Boomers (31 percent) and Matures (16 percent) are less likely to say they have experienced headaches resulting from stress in the past month. (Q810)

Stress by region[5]: Money and work top the list of significant sources of stress across the board in the United States, but there are regional differences in sources of stress and behaviors used to manage stress. (See Table 7.2.) For example, adults living in the South are most likely to cite the economy and family responsibilities as significant sources of stress. Adults living in the East are more likely to report engaging in unhealthy behaviors such as smoking and drinking alcohol to manage stress.

- The economy is more likely to be seen as a significant source of stress in the South (69 percent) than in other regions (62 percent in the East, 57 percent in the Midwest and 60 percent in the West). (Q625_61)

- Family responsibilities are more often considered a significant stressor in the South (64 percent) than in other regions of the country (56 percent in the East, 49 percent in the Midwest, and 48 percent in the West). (Q625_61)

- There was a significant drop since last year in the percentage of people living in the West who report that family health problems are a significant source of stress (41 percent in 2009 vs. 59 percent in 2008). (Q625_61)

While adults across America report similar levels of stress, there are some regional differences in the activities that adults do to help manage stress and their ability to make lifestyle and behavior changes.

- Adults in the East (5.5 on a 10-point scale), Midwest (5.6 on a 10-point scale), South (5.4 on a 10-point scale), and West (5.3 on a 10-point scale) reported similar average stress levels. They also agree that lower levels of stress are healthy. (Q605, Q610)

- Southerners are more likely than adults in other regions to pray (42 percent vs. 23 percent in the East, 31 percent in the Midwest, and 29 percent in the West) as a way to cope with stress and more Westerners say they exercise or walk (50 percent vs. 45 percent in the East, 46 percent in the Midwest, and 37 percent in the South) and spend time with family and friends (42 percent vs. 29 percent in the East, 38 percent in the Midwest, and 36 percent in the South) to manage stress than residents of other regions. (Q965)

- Easterners are more likely to smoke (21 percent) or drink alcohol (19 percent) than adults in the Midwest (15 percent and 14 percent), West (8 percent and 14 percent), and South (12 percent and 11 percent). (Q965)

- Adults living in rural areas are more likely than those in urban areas to cite certain personal barriers to implementing lifestyle and behavior changes, including lack of willpower (39 percent rural vs. 25 percent urban), cost (24 percent vs. 15 percent), and lack of confidence in their ability to make a change (18 percent vs. 10 percent). (Q965)

Table 7.2. Stress Management Techniques, by Region

	East	Midwest	South	West
Exercise or walk	45%	46%	37%	50%
Listen to music	43%	51%	53%	49%
Read	35%	50%	41%	40%
Watch television or movies for more than 2 hours per day	31%	44%	38%	30%
Nap	31%	28%	30%	34%
Spend time with friends or family	29%	38%	36%	42%
Eat	26%	29%	30%	27%
Play video games or surf the internet	25%	38%	36%	32%
Pray	23%	31%	42%	29%
Spend time doing a hobby	23%	29%	29%	26%
Smoke	21%	15%	12%	8%
Drink alcohol	19%	14%	11%	14%
Shop	12%	15%	17%	10%
Go to church or religious services	11%	20%	23%	21%
Meditation or yoga	11%	4%	7%	8%
See a mental health professional	8%	4%	4%	2%
Get a massage/Go to a spa	7%	8%	12%	12%
Play sports	5%	12%	9%	13%
Gamble	2%	5%	4%	3%

Stress in the workplace: Employed Americans continue to say their work is a significant source of stress, even though they report greater satisfaction with their jobs than in 2008. However, about half of workers report having lost productivity due to stress while at work during the past month and the percentages of people overall who report they are pleased with their place of employment are still low.

- Compared to 2008, slightly more employees report feeling satisfied with their jobs (65 percent in 2009 vs. 61 percent in 2008), the health and safety initiatives implemented by their employer (49 percent vs. 46 percent), and ways employers help workers balance work and non-work demands (42 percent vs. 39 percent). While these findings represent an increase in job satisfaction in the last year, the percentage of people who appear to be happy at their job and with their employer is still low. (Q1905_08)

- Just over half of employees (54 percent) would recommend their workplace to others as a good place to work. In 2008, fewer employees (44 percent) said they would have recommended their workplace to others. (Q1905_08)

- However, 51 percent of employees report some amount of lost productivity due to stress while at work (compared to 40 percent in 2008). Interestingly, younger workers are more likely to report some degree of lost productivity due to stress—roughly six in 10 Millennials and Gen Xers report some amount of lost productivity (61 percent and 58 percent, respectively). In contrast, fewer than half (47 percent) of Boomers report some lost productivity and just 22 percent of working adults 64 and older report any degree of lost productivity. (Q945)

- For the first time, more working adults agree (41 percent) than disagree (36 percent) that they typically feel tense or stressed out during their workday (compared to 39 percent who agreed and 39 percent who disagreed in 2008, and 34 percent who agreed and 41 percent who disagreed in 2007). (Q905)

Ethnicity and stress: Hispanics are more likely than Whites or Blacks to report an increase in stress levels over the past year, and Hispanics are also the group most likely to report physical symptoms as a result of stress, indicating that stress may be a serious health concern for the Hispanic population in the United States.

- A greater percentage of Hispanics report that their stress has increased in the past year than said this in 2008 (50 percent compared to 44 percent in 2008).

- A lower percentage of both Whites (40 percent in 2009 compared to 49 percent in 2008) and Blacks (39 percent in 2009 compared to 43 percent in 2008) reported that their stress levels had increased in the past year than said this in 2008. (Q605)

- Money is more likely to be seen as a significant source of stress among Hispanics (77 percent) than for Whites (68 percent) and Blacks (74 percent). (Q625_61)

- More Blacks report personal health concerns (57 percent vs. 46 percent for Whites and 42 percent for Hispanics) and family issues (64 percent of Blacks identified family responsibilities as a source of stress and 58 percent reported family health problems as a source of stress, compared with 53 percent and 45 percent for

Whites and 60 percent and 51 percent for Hispanics, respectively) as significant sources of stress than other groups. (Q625_61)

Hispanics also more commonly report experiencing symptoms of stress than Whites and Blacks.

- More Hispanics report having experienced headaches in the past month as a result of stress (44 percent) than Blacks (34 percent) and Whites (32 percent), and more Hispanics say they have experienced a change in appetite (26 percent) in the last month as a result of stress than Blacks (17 percent) and Whites (18 percent). (Q810)

- Hispanics more commonly say they experienced upset stomach or indigestion (34 percent) than Blacks (22 percent) and Whites (27 percent). (Q810)

- Almost half of Hispanics say they have experienced fatigue in the past month (49 percent) compared to Blacks (32 percent) and Whites (43 percent), and more Hispanics (53 percent) than Whites (45 percent) and Blacks (46 percent) report having lain awake at night in the past month due to stress. (Q810)

- Hispanics are more likely to say they have felt nervous or anxious due to stress in the past month (41 percent) than Blacks (25 percent) and Whites (36 percent). (Q810)

Endnotes

1. By definition, anyone who indicated that they are employed full-time, part-time, or are self-employed are included in the "employed" category, while everyone who did not indicate that they were employed are included in the "not employed" or "not working" category. This report also includes the results of a YouthQuery survey conducted between August 19 and 27, 2009, among 1,206 young people aged 8–17 years old. Results were weighted as needed for age, sex, race/ethnicity, education, region, and household income. Propensity score weighting was also used to adjust for respondents' propensity to be online.

2. Parents were asked to respond to questions about their children's stress throughout the survey; however, youth ages 8 to 17 who responded to the YouthQuery survey were asked about how much they worry, rather than stress, to ensure that youth were able to properly understand and interpret questions.

3. Asked of all parents and youth aged 13–17.

4. Millennials (18- to 30-year-olds), Gen Xers (31- to 44-year-olds), Boomers (45- to 63-year-olds), and Matures (64 years and older)

5. The states included in each region are: East: Connecticut; Delaware; Maine; Maryland; Massachusetts; New Hampshire; Rhode Island; Vermont; New Jersey; New York; Pennsylvania; Washington, DC; West Virginia. South: Alabama, Arkansas, Florida, Georgia, Kentucky, Louisiana, Mississippi, North Carolina, Oklahoma, South Carolina, Tennessee, Texas, Virginia. Midwest: Illinois, Indiana, Iowa, Kansas, Michigan, Minnesota, Missouri, Nebraska, North Dakota, Ohio, South Dakota, Wisconsin. West: Alaska, Arizona, California, Colorado, Hawaii, Idaho, Montana, Nevada, New Mexico, Oregon, Utah, Washington, Wyoming. The urban, suburban, and rural breakdown is based on respondents' self-reported answer asking them to describe the area where they currently reside.

Part Two

How Stress Affects the Body

Chapter 8

Alzheimer Disease

Chapter Contents

Section 8.1

What Is Alzheimer Disease?

Excerpted from "Alzheimer's Disease Fact Sheet," National
Institute on Aging (NIA, www.nia.nih.gov), part of the National
Institutes of Health, February 2010.

Alzheimer disease is an irreversible, progressive brain disease that slowly destroys memory and thinking skills, and eventually even the ability to carry out the simplest tasks. In most people with Alzheimer disease, symptoms first appear after age 60.

Alzheimer disease is the most common cause of dementia among older people. Dementia is the loss of cognitive functioning—thinking, remembering, and reasoning—to such an extent that it interferes with a person's daily life and activities. Estimates vary, but experts suggest that as many as 5.1 million Americans may have Alzheimer disease.

Alzheimer disease is named after Dr. Alois Alzheimer. In 1906, Dr. Alzheimer noticed changes in the brain tissue of a woman who had died of an unusual mental illness. Her symptoms included memory loss, language problems, and unpredictable behavior. After she died, he examined her brain and found many abnormal clumps (now called amyloid plaques) and tangled bundles of fibers (now called neurofibrillary tangles). Plaques and tangles in the brain are two of the main features of Alzheimer disease. The third is the loss of connections between nerve cells (neurons) in the brain.

Changes in the Brain in Alzheimer Disease

Although we still don't know what starts the Alzheimer disease process, we do know that damage to the brain begins as many as 10 to 20 years before any problems are evident. Tangles begin to develop deep in the brain, in an area called the entorhinal cortex, and plaques form in other areas. As more and more plaques and tangles form in particular brain areas, healthy neurons begin to work less efficiently. Then, they lose their ability to function and communicate with each other, and eventually they die. This damaging process spreads to a nearby structure, called the hippocampus, which is essential in forming memories. As the death of neurons increases, affected brain regions begin to shrink. By the final stage of Alzheimer disease, damage is widespread and brain tissue has shrunk significantly.

Very Early Signs and Symptoms

Memory problems are one of the first signs of Alzheimer disease. Some people with memory problems have a condition called amnestic mild cognitive impairment (MCI). People with this condition have more memory problems than normal for people their age, but their symptoms are not as severe as those with Alzheimer disease. More people with MCI, compared with those without MCI, go on to develop Alzheimer disease.

Other changes may also signal the very early stages of Alzheimer disease. For example, brain imaging and biomarker studies of people with MCI and those with a family history of Alzheimer disease are beginning to detect early changes in the brain like those seen in Alzheimer disease. These findings will need to be confirmed by other studies but appear promising. Other recent research has found links between some movement difficulties and MCI. Researchers also have seen links between some problems with the sense of smell and cognitive problems. Such findings offer hope that some day we may have tools that could help detect Alzheimer disease early, track the course of the disease, and monitor response to treatments.

Mild Alzheimer Disease

As Alzheimer disease progresses, memory loss continues and changes in other cognitive abilities appear. Problems can include getting lost, trouble handling money and paying bills, repeating questions, taking longer to complete normal daily tasks, poor judgment, and small mood and personality changes. People often are diagnosed in this stage.

Moderate Alzheimer Disease

In this stage, damage occurs in areas of the brain that control language, reasoning, sensory processing, and conscious thought. Memory loss and confusion increase, and people begin to have problems recognizing family and friends. They may be unable to learn new things, carry out tasks that involve multiple steps (such as getting dressed), or cope with new situations. They may have hallucinations, delusions, and paranoia, and may behave impulsively.

Severe Alzheimer Disease

By the final stage, plaques and tangles have spread throughout the brain and brain tissue has shrunk significantly. People with severe Alzheimer disease cannot communicate and are completely dependent on others for their care. Near the end, the person may be in bed most or all of the time as the body shuts down.

What Causes Alzheimer Disease

Scientists don't yet fully understand what causes Alzheimer disease, but it is clear that it develops because of a complex series of events that take place in the brain over a long period of time. It is likely that the causes include genetic, environmental, and lifestyle factors. Because people differ in their genetic make-up and lifestyle, the importance of these factors for preventing or delaying Alzheimer disease differs from person to person.

The Basics of Alzheimer Disease

Scientists are conducting studies to learn more about plaques, tangles, and other features of Alzheimer disease. They can now visualize plaques by imaging the brains of living individuals. They are also exploring the very earliest steps in the disease process. Findings from these studies will help them understand the causes of Alzheimer disease.

One of the great mysteries of Alzheimer disease is why it largely strikes older adults. Research on how the brain changes normally with age is shedding light on this question. For example, scientists are learning how age-related changes in the brain may harm neurons and contribute to Alzheimer damage. These age-related changes include atrophy (shrinking) of certain parts of the brain, inflammation, and the production of unstable molecules called free radicals.

Genetics

In a very few families, people develop Alzheimer disease in their 30s, 40s, and 50s. Many of these people have a mutation, or permanent change, in one of three genes that they inherited from a parent. We know that these gene mutations cause Alzheimer disease in these "early-onset" familial cases. Not all early-onset cases are caused by such mutations.

Most people with Alzheimer disease have "late-onset" Alzheimer disease, which usually develops after age 60. Many studies have linked a gene called APOE to late-onset Alzheimer disease. This gene has several forms. One of them, APOE [apolipoprotein E] epsilon 4, increases a person's risk of getting the disease. About 40 percent of all people who develop late-onset Alzheimer disease carry this gene. However, carrying the APOE epsilon 4 form of the gene does not necessarily mean that a person will develop Alzheimer disease, and people carrying no APOE epsilon 4 forms can also develop the disease.

Most experts believe that additional genes may influence the development of late-onset Alzheimer disease in some way. Scientists around the world are searching for these genes. Researchers have identified variants of genes that may play a role in risk of late-onset Alzheimer disease.

Lifestyle Factors

A nutritious diet, physical activity, social engagement, and mentally stimulating pursuits can all help people stay healthy. New research suggests the possibility that these factors also might help to reduce the risk of cognitive decline and Alzheimer disease. Scientists are investigating associations between cognitive decline and vascular and metabolic conditions such as heart disease, stroke, high blood pressure, diabetes, and obesity. Understanding these relationships and testing them in clinical trials will help us understand whether reducing risk factors for these diseases may help with Alzheimer disease as well.

How Alzheimer Disease Is Diagnosed

Alzheimer disease can be definitively diagnosed only after death by linking clinical course with an examination of brain tissue and pathology in an autopsy. But doctors now have several methods and tools to help them determine fairly accurately whether a person who is having memory problems has "possible Alzheimer disease" (dementia may be due to another cause) or "probable Alzheimer disease" (no other cause for dementia can be found). To diagnose Alzheimer disease, doctors do the following:

- Ask questions about the person's overall health, past medical problems, ability to carry out daily activities, and changes in behavior and personality
- Conduct tests of memory, problem solving, attention, counting, and language
- Carry out medical tests, such as tests of blood, urine, or spinal fluid
- Perform brain scans, such as computerized tomography (CT) or magnetic resonance imaging (MRI)

71

These tests may be repeated to give doctors information about how the person's memory is changing over time.

Early diagnosis is beneficial for several reasons. Having an early diagnosis and starting treatment in the early stages of the disease can help preserve function for months to years, even though the underlying disease process cannot be changed. Having an early diagnosis also helps families plan for the future, make living arrangements, take care of financial and legal matters, and develop support networks.

In addition, an early diagnosis can provide greater opportunities for people to get involved in clinical trials. In a clinical trial, scientists test drugs or treatments to see which are most effective and for whom they work best.

How Alzheimer Disease Is Treated

Alzheimer disease is a complex disease, and no single "magic bullet" is likely to prevent or cure it. That's why current treatments focus on several different aspects, including helping people maintain mental function; managing behavioral symptoms; and slowing, delaying, or preventing the disease.

Helping People with Alzheimer Disease Maintain Mental Function

Four medications are approved by the U.S. Food and Drug Administration to treat Alzheimer disease. Donepezil (Aricept®), rivastigmine (Exelon®), and galantamine (Razadyne®) are used to treat mild to moderate Alzheimer disease (donepezil can be used for severe Alzheimer disease as well). Memantine (Namenda®) is used to treat moderate to severe Alzheimer disease. These drugs work by regulating neurotransmitters (the chemicals that transmit messages between neurons). They may help maintain thinking, memory, and speaking skills, and help with certain behavioral problems. However, these drugs don't change the underlying disease process and may help only for a few months to a few years.

Managing Behavioral Symptoms

Common behavioral symptoms of Alzheimer disease include sleeplessness, agitation, wandering, anxiety, anger, and depression. Scientists are learning why these symptoms occur and are studying new treatments—drug and non-drug—to manage them. Treating behavioral symptoms often makes people with Alzheimer disease more comfortable and makes their care easier for caregivers.

Slowing, Delaying, or Preventing Alzheimer Disease

Alzheimer disease research has developed to a point where scien tists can look beyond treating symptoms to think about addressing the underlying disease process. In ongoing clinical trials, scientists are looking at many possible interventions, such as cardiovascular and diabetes treatments, antioxidants, immunization therapy, cognitive training, and physical activity.

Supporting Families and Caregivers

Caring for a person with Alzheimer disease can have high physical, emotional, and financial costs. The demands of day-to-day care, changing family roles, and difficult decisions about placement in a care facility can be hard to handle. Researchers are learning a lot about Alzheimer disease caregiving, and studies are helping experts develop new ways to support caregivers.

Becoming well-informed about the disease is one important long-term strategy. Programs that teach families about the various stages of Alzheimer disease and about flexible and practical strategies for dealing with difficult caregiving situations provide vital help to those who care for people with Alzheimer disease.

Developing good coping skills and a strong support network of family and friends also are important ways that caregivers can help themselves handle the stresses of caring for a loved one with Alzheimer disease. For example, staying physically active provides physical and emotional benefits.

Some Alzheimer caregivers have found that participating in a support group is a critical lifeline. These support groups allow caregivers to find respite, express concerns, share experiences, get tips, and receive emotional comfort. The Alzheimer's Association, Alzheimer's Disease Centers, and many other organizations sponsor in-person and online support groups across the country. There are a growing number of groups for people in the early stage of Alzheimer disease and their families. Support networks can be especially valuable when caregivers face the difficult decision of whether and when to place a loved one in a nursing home or assisted living facility.

Thirty years ago, we knew very little about Alzheimer disease. Since then, scientists have made many important advances. Research supported by NIA and other organizations has expanded knowledge of brain function in healthy older people, identified ways we might lessen normal age-related declines in mental function, and deepened our understanding of the disease. Many scientists and physicians are now working together to untangle the genetic, biological, and environmental factors that, over many years, ultimately result in Alzheimer disease. This effort is bringing us closer to the day when we will be able to manage successfully or even prevent this devastating disease.

Section 8.2

Alzheimer Disease and Stress

"Stress significantly hastens progression of Alzheimer's disease,"
© 2006 University of California at Irvine. Reprinted with permission.

Stress hormones appear to rapidly exacerbate the formation of brain lesions that are the hallmarks of Alzheimer's disease, according to researchers at University of California at Irvine (UCI). The findings suggest that managing stress and reducing certain medications prescribed for the elderly could slow down the progression of this devastating disease.

In a study with genetically modified mice, Frank LaFerla, professor of neurobiology and behavior, and a team of UCI researchers found that when young animals were injected for just 7 days with dexamethasone, a glucocorticoid similar to the body's stress hormones, the levels of the protein beta-amyloid in the brain increased by 60 percent. When beta-amyloid production increases and these protein fragments aggregate, they form plaques, one of the two hallmark brain lesions of Alzheimer's disease. The scientists also found that the levels of another protein, tau, also increased. Tau accumulation eventually leads to the formation of tangles, the other signature lesion of Alzheimer's. The findings appear in [the August 2006] issue of the *Journal of Neuroscience*.

"It is remarkable that these stress hormones can have such a significant effect in such a short period of time," LaFerla said. "Although we have known for some time that higher levels of stress hormones are seen in individuals in the early stages of Alzheimer's, this is the first time we have seen how these hormones play such a direct role in exacerbating the underlying pathology of the disease."

The researchers injected 4-month-old transgenic mice with levels of dexamethasone similar to the level of hormones that would be seen in humans under stress. At this young age, there would be little formation of plaques and tangles in the brains of the mice. After 1 week, the scientists found that the level of beta-amyloid in the brains of the animals compared to what is seen in the brains of untreated 8- to 9-month-old mice, demonstrating the profound consequence of glucocorticoid exposure. When dexamethasone was given to 13-month-old mice that already had some plaque and tangle pathology, the hormone again significantly worsened the plaque lesions in the brain and led to increased accumulation of the tau protein.

"Although we expected that this drug, which, like the stress hormone cortisol, activates glucocorticoid receptors, might have some effect on plaques and tangles, it was surprising to find that such large increases were induced in relatively young mice," said James L. McGaugh, research professor of neurobiology and behavior and co-author of the paper.

The increased accumulation of beta-amyloid and tau appears to work in a "feedback loop" to hasten the progression of Alzheimer's. The researchers found that the higher levels of beta-amyloid and tau led to an increase in the levels of the stress hormones, which would come back to the brain and speed up the formation of more plaques and tangles.

According to the researchers, these findings have profound implications for how to treat the elderly who suffer from Alzheimer's disease.

"This study suggests that not only is stress management an important factor in treating Alzheimer's disease, but that physicians should pay close attention to the pharmaceutical products they prescribe for their elderly patients," said Kim Green, a postdoctoral researcher in neurobiology and behavior and first author of the paper. "Some medications prescribed for the elderly for various conditions contain glucocorticoids. These drugs may be leading to accelerated cognitive decline in patients in the early stages of Alzheimer's."

Alzheimer's disease is a progressive neurodegenerative disorder that affects 4.5 million to 5 million adults in the United States. If no effective therapies are developed, it is estimated that 13 million Americans will be afflicted with the disease by 2050.

Chapter 9

Asthma

Chapter Contents

Section 9.1

What Is Asthma?

Excerpted from "Asthma," by the National Heart, Lung,
and Blood Institute (NHLBI, www.nhlbi.nih.gov), part of the
National Institutes of Health, September 2008.

Asthma is a chronic (long-term) lung disease that inflames and narrows the airways. Asthma causes recurring periods of wheezing (a whistling sound when you breathe), chest tightness, shortness of breath, and coughing. The coughing often occurs at night or early in the morning.

Outlook

Asthma can't be cured. Even when you feel fine, you still have the disease and it can flare up at any time.

But with today's knowledge and treatments, most people who have asthma are able to manage the disease. They have few, if any, symptoms. They can live normal, active lives and sleep through the night without interruption from asthma.

For successful, comprehensive, and ongoing treatment, take an active role in managing your disease. Build strong partnerships with your doctor and other clinicians on your health care team.

Asthma Causes

The exact cause of asthma isn't known. Researchers think a combination of factors (family genes and certain environmental exposures) interact to cause asthma to develop, most often early in life. These factors include the following:

- An inherited tendency to develop allergies, called atopy

- Parents who have asthma

- Certain respiratory infections during childhood

- Contact with some airborne allergens or exposure to some viral infections in infancy or in early childhood when the immune system is developing

If asthma or atopy runs in your family, exposure to airborne allergens (for example, house dust mites, cockroaches, and possibly cat or dog dander) and irritants (for example, tobacco smoke) may make your airways more reactive to substances in the air you breathe.

Different factors may be more likely to cause asthma in some people than in others. Researchers continue to explore what causes asthma.

One theory researchers have for what causes asthma is the "hygiene hypothesis." They believe that our Western lifestyle—with its emphasis on hygiene and sanitation—has resulted in changes in our living conditions and an overall decline in infections in early childhood.

Many young children no longer experience the same types of environmental exposures and infections as children did in the past. This affects the way that the immune systems in today's young children develop during very early childhood, and it may increase their risk for atopy and asthma. This is especially true for children who have close family members with one or both of these conditions.

Asthma Risk

Asthma affects people of all ages, but it most often starts in childhood. In the United States, more than 22 million people are known to have asthma. Nearly 6 million of these people are children.

Young children who have frequent episodes of wheezing with respiratory infections, as well as certain other risk factors, are at the highest risk of developing asthma that continues beyond 6 years of age. These risk factors include having allergies, eczema (an allergic skin condition), or parents who have asthma.

Among children, more boys have asthma than girls. But among adults, more women have the disease than men. It's not clear whether or how sex and sex hormones play a role in causing asthma.

Most, but not all, people who have asthma have allergies.

Some people develop asthma because of exposure to certain chemical irritants or industrial dusts in the workplace. This is called occupational asthma.

Signs and Symptoms of Asthma

Common asthma symptoms include the following:

- **Coughing:** Coughing from asthma is often worse at night or early in the morning, making it hard to sleep.

- **Wheezing:** Wheezing is a whistling or squeaky sound that occurs when you breathe.

- **Chest tightness:** This may feel like something is squeezing or sitting on your chest.

- **Shortness of breath:** Some people who have asthma say they can't catch their breath or they feel out of breath. You may feel like you can't get air out of your lungs.

Not all people who have asthma have these symptoms. Likewise, having these symptoms doesn't always mean that you have asthma. A lung function test, done along with a medical history (including type and frequency of your symptoms) and physical exam, is the best way to diagnose asthma for certain.

The types of asthma symptoms you have, how often they occur, and how severe they are may vary over time. Sometimes your symptoms may just annoy you. Other times they may be troublesome enough to limit your daily routine.

Severe symptoms can threaten your life. It's vital to treat symptoms when you first notice them so they don't become severe.

With proper treatment, most people who have asthma can expect to have few, if any, symptoms either during the day or at night.

What causes asthma symptoms to occur?

A number of things can bring about or worsen asthma symptoms. Your doctor will help you find out which things (sometimes called triggers) may cause your asthma to flare up if you come in contact with them. Triggers may include the following:

- Allergens found in dust, animal fur, cockroaches, mold, and pollens from trees, grasses, and flowers

- Irritants such as cigarette smoke, air pollution, chemicals or dust in the workplace, compounds in home decor products, and sprays (such as hairspray)

- Certain medicines such as aspirin or other nonsteroidal anti-inflammatory drugs and nonselective beta-blockers

- Sulfites in foods and drinks

- Viral upper respiratory infections such as colds

- Exercise (physical activity)

Other health conditions—such as runny nose, sinus infections, reflux disease, psychological stress, and sleep apnea—can make asthma more difficult to manage. These conditions need treatment as part of an overall asthma care plan.

Asthma is different for each person. Some of the factors listed may not affect you. Other factors that do affect you may not be on the list. Talk to your doctor about the things that seem to make your asthma worse.

Asthma Diagnosis

Your primary care doctor will diagnose asthma based on your medical history, a physical exam, and results from tests. He or she also will figure out what your level of asthma severity is—that is, whether it's intermittent, mild, moderate, or severe. Your severity level will determine what treatment you will start on.

You may need to see an asthma specialist if the following are true:

- You need special tests to be sure you have asthma.

- You've had a life-threatening asthma attack.

- You need more than one kind of medicine or higher doses of medicine to control your asthma, or if you have overall difficulty getting your asthma well controlled.

- You're thinking about getting allergy treatments.

Asthma Treatment and Control

Asthma is a long-term disease that can't be cured. The goal of asthma treatment is to control the disease. Good asthma control will do the following:

- Prevent chronic and troublesome symptoms such as coughing and shortness of breath

- Reduce your need of quick-relief medicines

- Help you maintain good lung function

- Let you maintain your normal activity levels and sleep through the night

- Prevent asthma attacks that could result in your going to the emergency room or being admitted to the hospital for treatment

To reach this goal, you should actively partner with your doctor to manage your asthma or your child's asthma. Children aged 10 or older—and younger children who are able—also should take an active role in their asthma care.

Taking an active role to control your asthma involves working with your doctor and other clinicians on your health care team to create and follow an asthma action plan. It also means avoiding factors that can make your asthma flare up and treating other conditions that can interfere with asthma management.

An asthma action plan gives guidance on taking your medicines properly, avoiding factors that worsen you asthma, tracking your level of asthma control, responding to worsening asthma, and seeking emergency care when needed.

Asthma is treated with two types of medicines: long-term control and quick-relief medicines. Long-term control medicines help reduce airway inflammation and prevent asthma symptoms. Quick-relief, or "rescue," medicines relieve asthma symptoms that may flare up.

Your initial asthma treatment will depend on how severe your disease is. Followup asthma treatment will depend on how well your asthma action plan is working to control your symptoms and prevent you from having asthma attacks.

Your level of asthma control can vary over time and with changes in your home, school, or work environments that alter how often you are exposed to the factors that can make your asthma worse. Your doctor may need to increase your medicine if your asthma doesn't stay under control.

On the other hand, if your asthma is well controlled for several months, your doctor may be able to decrease your medicine. These adjustments either up or down to your medicine will help you maintain the best control possible with the least amount of medicine necessary.

Asthma treatment for certain groups of people, such as children, pregnant women, or those for whom exercise brings on asthma symptoms, will need to be adjusted to meet their special needs.

Emergency Care

Most people who have asthma, including many children, can safely manage their symptoms by following the steps for worsening asthma provided in the asthma action plan. However, you may need medical attention. Call your doctor for advice if the following occur:

- Your medicines don't relieve an asthma attack.
- Your peak flow is less than half of your personal best peak flow number.

Call 911 for an ambulance to take you to the emergency room of your local hospital if the you have trouble walking and talking because you're out of breath or you have blue lips or fingernails.

At the hospital, you will be closely watched and given oxygen and more medicines, as well as medicines at higher doses than you take at home. Such treatment can save your life.

Section 9.2

Stress Increases Risk of Asthma Exacerbations

Excerpted from "Expert Panel Report 3: Guidelines for the Diagnosis and Management of Asthma," by the National Heart, Lung, and Blood Institute (NHLBI, www.nhlbi.nih.gov), part of the National Institutes of Health, August 28, 2007.

Clinical trials are needed to evaluate the effect of stress and stress reduction on asthma control, but observational studies demonstrate an association between increased stress and worsening asthma.

The role of stress and psychological factors in asthma is important but not fully defined. Emerging evidence indicates that stress can play an important role in precipitating exacerbations of asthma and possibly act as a risk factor for an increase in prevalence of asthma. Chronic stressors increase the risk of asthma exacerbations, especially in children who have severely negative life events and those who have brittle asthma.

The mechanisms involved in this process have yet to be fully established and may involve enhanced generation of pro-inflammatory cytokines. In a prospective study of a birth cohort predisposed to atopy, higher caregiver stress in the first 6 months after birth was significantly associated with an increased atopic immune profile in the children (high total IgE [immunoglobulin E] level, increased production of tumor necrosis factor-alpha, and a suggested trend between higher stress and reduced interferon-gamma. Equally important are psychosocial factors that are associated with poor outcome (e.g., conflict between patients and family and the medical staff, inappropriate asthma self-care, depressive symptoms, behavioral problems, emotional problems, and disregard of perceived asthma symptoms). Asthma severity can be affected by personal or parental factors, and both should be evaluated in cases of poorly controlled asthma. For example, maternal depression is common among inner-city mothers of children who have asthma and has been associated with increased emergency department visits and poor adherence to therapy by these children. Furthermore, in a large prospective study of inner-city children who had asthma, increased exposure to violence, as reported by caretakers, predicted a higher number of symptom days in their children, with caregivers' perceived stress mediating some, although not all, of this effect. It may also be important to evaluate psychosocial and socioenvironmental factors in children who have repeated hospitalizations; however, it is not clear whether psychosocial factors affect or result from the frequent hospitalizations.

Chapter 10

Cancer and Stress

The complex relationship between physical and psychological health is not well understood. Scientists know that psychological stress can affect the immune system, the body's defense against infection and disease (including cancer); however, it is not yet known whether stress increases a person's susceptibility to disease.

What is psychological stress?

Psychological stress refers to the emotional and physiological reactions experienced when an individual confronts a situation in which the demands go beyond their coping resources. Examples of stressful situations are marital problems, death of a loved one, abuse, health problems, and financial crises.

How does stress affect the body?

The body responds to stress by releasing stress hormones, such as epinephrine (also called adrenaline) and cortisol (also called hydrocortisone). The body produces these stress hormones to help a person react to a situation with more speed and strength. Stress hormones increase blood pressure, heart rate, and blood sugar levels. Small

From "Psychological Stress and Cancer: Questions and Answers," by the National Cancer Institute (NCI, www.cancer.gov), part of the National Institutes of Health, April 29, 2008.

amounts of stress are believed to be beneficial, but chronic (persisting or progressing over a long period of time) high levels of stress are thought to be harmful.

Stress that is chronic can increase the risk of obesity, heart disease, depression, and various other illnesses. Stress also can lead to unhealthy behaviors, such as overeating, smoking, or abusing drugs or alcohol, that may affect cancer risk.

Can stress increase a person's risk of developing cancer?

Studies done over the past 30 years that examined the relationship between psychological factors, including stress, and cancer risk have produced conflicting results. Although the results of some studies have indicated a link between various psychological factors and an increased risk of developing cancer, a direct cause-and-effect relationship has not been proven.

Some studies have indicated an indirect relationship between stress and certain types of virus-related tumors. Evidence from both animal and human studies suggests that chronic stress weakens a person's immune system, which in turn may affect the incidence of virus-associated cancers, such as Kaposi sarcoma and some lymphomas.

More recent research with animal models (animals with a disease that is similar to or the same as a disease in humans) suggests that the body's neuroendocrine response (release of hormones into the blood in response to stimulation of the nervous system) can directly alter important processes in cells that help protect against the formation of cancer, such as DNA [deoxyribonucleic acid] repair and the regulation of cell growth.

Why are the study results inconsistent?

It is difficult to separate stress from other physical or emotional factors when examining cancer risk. For example, certain behaviors, such as smoking and using alcohol, and biological factors, such as growing older, becoming overweight, and having a family history of cancer, are common risk factors for cancer. Researchers may have difficulty controlling the presence of these factors in the study group or separating the effects of stress from the effects of these other factors. In some cases, the number of people in the study, length of follow-up, or analysis used is insufficient to rule out the role of chance. Also, studies may not always take into account that cancer is not a homogeneous (uniform in nature) disease.

How does stress affect people who have cancer?

Studies have indicated that stress can affect tumor growth and spread, but the precise biological mechanisms underlying these effects are not well understood. Scientists have suggested that the effects of stress on the immune system may in turn affect the growth of some tumors. However, recent research using animal models indicates that the body's release of stress hormones can affect cancer cell functions directly.

A review of studies that evaluated psychological factors and outcome in cancer patients suggests an association between certain psychological factors, such as feeling helpless or suppressing negative emotions, and the growth or spread of cancer, although this relationship was not consistently seen in all studies. In general, stronger relationships have been found between psychological factors and cancer growth and spread than between psychological factors and cancer development.

Chapter 11

Diabetes and Stress

Stress is a major contributor to diabetes, but most people don't understand what stress is or what to do about it. Here's how stress works, and some things you can do about it.

Say you're walking down the street, and you bump into a hungry, man-eating lion. (Don't you hate it when that happens?) You would sense a dangerous threat, and your body would automatically respond. Your adrenal glands would pump out a number of hormones. Chief among these is cortisol, which tells your liver and other cells to pour all their stored sugar (glucose) into your bloodstream. They do this so that your leg and arm muscles can use the glucose as fuel for running away, fighting, or maybe climbing a tree or a fire escape.

At the same time, your other cells would become "insulin-resistant." Insulin's job is to get glucose into our cells to be used as fuel. In a crisis situation, most of your cells resist insulin, so the muscles involved in fighting or fleeing will have more energy. This reaction is called "stress." In nature, the stress response is vital to survival. The antelope senses the lion (a threat) and runs. It either gets away or the lion eats it. In running, the antelope uses up the extra sugar and restores its hormonal balance. The whole thing is over in 10 minutes, and the antelope can rest.

"The Stress-Diabetes Connection: Where It Comes From—How to Deal With It" By David Spero, RN. Adapted from *Diabetes: Sugar-Coated Crisis—Who Gets It, Who Profits, and How to Stop It* by David Spero, RN (New Society Publishers, 2006). Reprinted with permission from http://www.mendosa.com/stress.htm. This article originally appeared on www.mendosa.com on December 19, 2006.

But in our society, threat isn't usually physical. When you're threatened with job loss or eviction or the breakup of your marriage or a child's drug problem or the thousands of other potential threats in modern society, you can't fight, and you can't run. You just sit there and worry. And the stress isn't over in 10 minutes either; modern stresses often act on us 24/7, week after week. Over time, insulin resistance builds up. It is a major cause of type 2 diabetes, heart disease, overweight, and many chronic illnesses.

How Does Stress Cause Illness?

Since, under stress, most of your cells become insulin-resistant, some of that extra glucose stays in the blood and causes damage to nerves and blood vessels. The rest of it gets converted to abdominal fat, and your LDL ([low-density lipoprotein] or "bad cholesterol") level goes up. Stress also raises your blood pressure and heart rate to pump blood to the leg muscles for the running away that we're not doing. This is a combination likely to cause all kinds of problems.

Stress also causes diabetes through behaviors, because the easiest way to treat stress is with food high in sugar or saturated fat. These "comfort foods" raise our levels of endorphins and serotonin, our bodies' natural "feel-good" chemicals. They make us feel more calm and more in control. But the good feelings don't last long. Our blood sugars drop again when our insulin response catches up to them, and pretty soon you feel worse than before. You need another "fix." Meanwhile, you will have added to your insulin resistance and your abdominal fat.

Another way stress hurts us is by depressing the immune system, the body's natural repair and defense program. Stress doesn't care about long-term health, because there will be no long-term unless we survive the immediate crisis. Repair can wait until the crisis is over.

But for people with less power—less money, less education, less social support, less self-confidence, lower self-esteem, a minority skin color, or disapproved body type—the crisis is never over. The economic, emotional, and sometimes physical threats are always there. The immune system stays suppressed.

So over time, chronic stress is like endlessly deferring maintenance on your car. Like your car, your body will tend to break down.

Where Does Stress Come From?

We have an image of stress as a very busy thing. The phones are ringing, we're racing around town; we've got deadlines, high noise levels, and not enough time.

All the little crises of life add up to this feeling we call "stress." But this is a mild form of stress, akin to a roller-coaster ride, a reaction that many bodies actually enjoy. Real stress is something quite different. It's a response to serious threat. Stress occurs when the threats we face exceed what we think we can control.

Now pay attention: If stress occurs when you perceive threats greater than your power to control them, then the less power you have, the more stress you will have. Let's say that hungry lion is still on the corner, but this time you're not walking; you're riding in an Abrams tank. You wouldn't be stressed at all. You might have a "cute lion" story to tell at work. When you have the power to cope, there's no stress.

Access to money, a source of power, reduces stress. Say my company is sending my job to Bangladesh. If I had a million dollars in the bank, I wouldn't worry much. It might hurt emotionally, but it wouldn't affect my health. And if I knew I could get another job easily, it would be even less stressful. But if I had 12 cents to my name, and knew getting another job would be very difficult, and had a family depending on my income, worrying about job loss might keep me up all night and keep my blood sugars up too, even if the actual move never happens. My body would be screaming, "Run! Fight! Climb a tree or something!" but I couldn't. My body would pay the price with long-term health problems.

Coping with Stress

For the mathematically minded reader, here's a useful stress formula: STRESS = (perceived) THREAT / (perceived) CONTROL.

If you want to reduce stress (and believe me, you do), this formula shows several ways to do it. We may be able to reduce the threats we face—for example, getting a roommate to help pay the rent, or moving to a safer neighborhood to avoid violence. You may be able to reduce your perception of threat—for example, realizing that if your husband yells at you, it's not the end of the world. You're still alive and you're still a good person.

We can also reduce stress by increasing our ability to control some threats. If you're a young man in a neighborhood where the police harass young men, you may be able to learn skills for avoiding the cops or dealing with them. If you have diabetes and are deathly afraid of complications, learning to control your blood sugars through diet, exercise, relaxation, and/or medications will give you more perceived and actual control and reduce stress.

Other people are a major source of power, and their support will increase your perceived control. Strengthening connections with family, friends, neighbors, your congregation, or other people who share your problems (as in a support group) will reduce your stress and help you cope.

Family relationships themselves can be a source of healing or a source of stress. If your family seems to cause you more hard feelings than good ones, perhaps you can get some help with that, through counseling or learning better communication skills. Maybe you just need to reach out to them with some honest communication.

Threat and stress can be spiritual as well as economic, emotional, or physical. We all need positive goals and reasons to live—a life without meaning or connection can be perceived as a threat to your soul. Sometimes we need to spend time figuring out what's important to us and commit to spending more energy on positive things. It's OK to get some help with this process.

Self-confidence is a major element of power and perceived control. You can build self-confidence by accomplishing small goals, by learning more skills (take a class!), or by seeing people like you accomplish something. If they can do it, you can too.

We can combine all four of these strategies by getting involved with other people in changing threatening situations—for example, organizing for more youth employment programs, cleaning up toxic pollution, or starting a neighborhood walk. You'll be reducing threat and increasing social support and sense of control at the same time.

Relaxation, meditation, and prayer are powerful ways of reducing stress. They reduce perceived threat and make you feel more in control. Perhaps you can get some relaxation tapes, go to meditation or yoga class, join a church you believe in, or just take some time every day to sit and breathe. Spending time with animals or even with plants can relax us and give us a sense of peace and connection, reducing stress.

Get Active—The Indispensable Step

The healthiest way to deal with stress is the way the animals do, with physical activity. Stress tries to help us survive the only way it knows how, by getting us to move. If you don't exercise, most of the glucose your body puts out will turn into abdominal fat. That's why stress and inactivity are a lethal combination.

So get out and run or swim or bike or walk your dog. Consider exercise that makes you stronger and tougher—kick-boxing, weight-lifting, martial arts. You'll wind up feeling more confident and therefore less stressed.

Getting active means more than just exercising. We're usually better off taking a more active role in our own lives, meaning we don't let the media and the dominant culture decide what we eat and what we do. We decide for ourselves.

When we can decide what's important to us, when we connect with other people to live in ways that are meaningful to us, we will have less stress and better blood sugar control.

Chapter 12

Erectile Dysfunction

Erectile dysfunction, sometimes called "impotence," is the repeated inability to get or keep an erection firm enough for sexual intercourse. The word "impotence" may also be used to describe other problems that interfere with sexual intercourse and reproduction, such as lack of sexual desire and problems with ejaculation or orgasm. Using the term erectile dysfunction makes it clear that those other problems are not involved.

Erectile dysfunction, or ED, can be a total inability to achieve erection, an inconsistent ability to do so, or a tendency to sustain only brief erections. These variations make defining ED and estimating its incidence difficult. Estimates range from 15 million to 30 million, depending on the definition used. According to the National Ambulatory Medical Care Survey (NAMCS), for every 1,000 men in the United States, 7.7 physician office visits were made for ED in 1985. By 1999, that rate had nearly tripled to 22.3. The increase happened gradually, presumably as treatments such as vacuum devices and injectable drugs became more widely available and discussing erectile function became accepted. Perhaps the most publicized advance was the introduction of the oral drug sildenafil citrate (Viagra) in March 1998. NAMCS data on new drugs show an estimated 2.6 million mentions

From "Erectile Dysfunction," by the National Kidney and Urologic Diseases Information Clearinghouse, a service of the National Institute of Diabetes and Digestive and Kidney Diseases (NIDDK, www.niddk.nih.gov), part of the National Institutes of Health, December 2005. Reviewed and updated by David A. Cooke, MD, FACP, November 8, 2010.

of Viagra at physician office visits in 1999, and one third of those mentions occurred during visits for a diagnosis other than ED. By 2005, more than 23 million men had been prescribed Viagra.

In older men, ED usually has a physical cause, such as disease, injury, or side effects of drugs. Any disorder that causes injury to the nerves or impairs blood flow in the penis has the potential to cause ED. Incidence increases with age: About 5 percent of 40-year-old men and between 15 and 25 percent of 65-year-old men experience ED. But it is not an inevitable part of aging.

ED is treatable at any age, and awareness of this fact has been growing. More men have been seeking help and returning to normal sexual activity because of improved, successful treatments for ED. Urologists, who specialize in problems of the urinary tract, have traditionally treated ED; however, urologists accounted for only 25 percent of Viagra mentions in 1999.

How does an erection occur?

The penis contains two chambers called the corpora cavernosa, which run the length of the organ. A spongy tissue fills the chambers. The corpora cavernosa are surrounded by a membrane, called the tunica albuginea. The spongy tissue contains smooth muscles, fibrous tissues, spaces, veins, and arteries. The urethra, which is the channel for urine and ejaculate, runs along the underside of the corpora cavernosa and is surrounded by the corpus spongiosum.

Erection begins with sensory or mental stimulation, or both. Impulses from the brain and local nerves cause the muscles of the corpora cavernosa to relax, allowing blood to flow in and fill the spaces. The blood creates pressure in the corpora cavernosa, making the penis expand. The tunica albuginea helps trap the blood in the corpora cavernosa, thereby sustaining erection. When muscles in the penis contract to stop the inflow of blood and open outflow channels, erection is reversed.

What causes erectile dysfunction (ED)?

Since an erection requires a precise sequence of events, ED can occur when any of the events is disrupted. The sequence includes nerve impulses in the brain, spinal column, and area around the penis, and response in muscles, fibrous tissues, veins, and arteries in and near the corpora cavernosa.

Damage to nerves, arteries, smooth muscles, and fibrous tissues, often as a result of disease, is the most common cause of ED. Diseases—such as diabetes, kidney disease, chronic alcoholism, multiple sclerosis, atherosclerosis, vascular disease, and neurologic disease—account for about 70 percent of ED cases. Between 35 and 50 percent of men with diabetes experience ED.

Lifestyle choices that contribute to heart disease and vascular problems also raise the risk of erectile dysfunction. Smoking, being overweight, and avoiding exercise are possible causes of ED.

Also, surgery (especially radical prostate and bladder surgery for cancer) can injure nerves and arteries near the penis, causing ED. Injury to the penis, spinal cord, prostate, bladder, and pelvis can lead to ED by harming nerves, smooth muscles, arteries, and fibrous tissues of the corpora cavernosa.

In addition, many common medicines—blood pressure drugs, antihistamines, antidepressants, tranquilizers, appetite suppressants, and cimetidine (an ulcer drug)—can produce ED as a side effect.

Experts believe that psychological factors such as stress, anxiety, guilt, depression, low self-esteem, and fear of sexual failure cause 10 to 20 percent of ED cases. Men with a physical cause for ED frequently experience the same sort of psychological reactions (stress, anxiety, guilt, depression). Other possible causes are smoking, which affects blood flow in veins and arteries, and hormonal abnormalities, such as not enough testosterone.

How is ED diagnosed?

Patient history: Medical and sexual histories help define the degree and nature of ED. A medical history can disclose diseases that lead to ED, while a simple recounting of sexual activity might distinguish among problems with sexual desire, erection, ejaculation, or orgasm.

Using certain prescription or illegal drugs can suggest a chemical cause, since drug effects account for 25 percent of ED cases. Cutting back on or substituting certain medications can often alleviate the problem.

Physical examination: A physical examination can give clues to systemic problems. For example, if the penis is not sensitive to touching, a problem in the nervous system may be the cause. Abnormal secondary sex characteristics, such as hair pattern or breast enlargement, can point to hormonal problems, which would mean that the endocrine system is involved. The examiner might discover a circulatory problem by observing decreased pulses in the wrist or ankles. And unusual characteristics of the penis itself could suggest the source of the problem—for example, a penis that bends or curves when erect could be the result of Peyronie disease.

Laboratory tests: Several laboratory tests can help diagnose ED. Tests for systemic diseases include blood counts, urinalysis, lipid profile, and measurements of creatinine and liver enzymes. Measuring the amount of free testosterone in the blood can yield information about problems with the endocrine system and is indicated especially in patients with decreased sexual desire.

Other tests: Monitoring erections that occur during sleep (nocturnal penile tumescence) can help rule out certain psychological causes of ED. Healthy men have involuntary erections during sleep. If nocturnal erections do not occur, then ED is likely to have a physical rather than psychological cause. Tests of nocturnal erections are not completely reliable, however. Scientists have not standardized such tests and have not determined when they should be applied for best results.

Psychosocial examination: A psychosocial examination, using an interview and a questionnaire, reveals psychological factors. A man's sexual partner may also be interviewed to determine expectations and perceptions during sexual intercourse.

How is ED treated?

Most physicians suggest that treatments proceed from least to most invasive. For some men, making a few healthy lifestyle changes may solve the problem. Quitting smoking, losing excess weight, and increasing physical activity may help some men regain sexual function.

Cutting back on any drugs with harmful side effects is considered next. For example, drugs for high blood pressure work in different ways. If you think a particular drug is causing problems with erection, tell your doctor and ask whether you can try a different class of blood pressure medicine.

Psychotherapy and behavior modifications in selected patients are considered next if indicated, followed by oral or locally injected drugs, vacuum devices, and surgically implanted devices. In rare cases, surgery involving veins or arteries may be considered.

Psychotherapy: Experts often treat psychologically based ED using techniques that decrease the anxiety associated with intercourse. The patient's partner can help with the techniques, which include gradual development of intimacy and stimulation. Such techniques also can help relieve anxiety when ED from physical causes is being treated.

Drug therapy: Drugs for treating ED can be taken orally, injected directly into the penis, or inserted into the urethra at the tip of the penis. In March 1998, the Food and Drug Administration (FDA) approved Viagra, the first pill to treat ED. Since that time, vardenafil hydrochloride (Levitra) and tadalafil (Cialis) have also been approved. Additional oral medicines are being tested for safety and effectiveness. At this point, there is no convincing evidence that any one of these medications is consistently superior to the others. However, it is not unusual for a patient to have a better response to one medication than another.

Viagra, Levitra, and Cialis all belong to a class of drugs called phosphodiesterase (PDE) inhibitors. Taken an hour before sexual activity, these drugs work by enhancing the effects of nitric oxide, a chemical that relaxes smooth muscles in the penis during sexual stimulation and allows increased blood flow.

While oral medicines improve the response to sexual stimulation, they do not trigger an automatic erection as injections do. The recommended dose for Viagra is 50 mg, and the physician may adjust this dose to 100 mg or 25 mg, depending on the patient. The recommended dose for either Levitra or Cialis is 10 mg, and the physician may adjust this dose to 20 mg if 10 mg is insufficient. A lower dose of 5 mg is available for patients who take other medicines or have conditions that may decrease the body's ability to use the drug. Levitra is also available in a 2.5 mg dose. Cialis is also approved for a daily dosing regimen, rather than as-needed use, at a dose of 2.5 mg to 5 mg daily.

None of these PDE inhibitors should be used more than once a day. Men who take nitrate based drugs such as nitroglycerin for heart problems should not use either drug because the combination can cause a sudden drop in blood pressure. Also, tell your doctor if you take any drugs called alpha-blockers, which are used to treat prostate enlargement or high blood pressure. Your doctor may need to adjust your ED prescription. Taking a PDE inhibitor and an alpha-blocker at the same time (within 4 hours) can cause a sudden drop in blood pressure.

Oral testosterone can reduce ED in some men with low levels of natural testosterone, but it is often ineffective and may cause liver damage. Patients also have claimed that other oral drugs—including yohimbine hydrochloride, dopamine and serotonin agonists, and trazodone—are effective, but the results of scientific studies to substantiate these claims have been inconsistent.

Improvements observed following use of these drugs may be examples of the placebo effect, that is, a change that results simply from the patient's believing that an improvement will occur.

Many men achieve stronger erections by injecting drugs into the penis, causing it to become engorged with blood. Drugs such as papaverine hydrochloride, phentolamine, and alprostadil (marketed as Caverject) widen blood vessels. These drugs may create unwanted side effects, however, including persistent erection (known as priapism) and scarring. Nitroglycerin, a muscle relaxant, can sometimes enhance erection when rubbed on the penis.

A system for inserting a pellet of alprostadil into the urethra is marketed as Muse. The system uses a prefilled applicator to deliver the pellet about an inch deep into the urethra. An erection will begin within 8 to 10 minutes and may last 30 to 60 minutes. The most common side effects are aching in the penis, testicles, and area between the penis and rectum; warmth or burning sensation in the urethra; redness from increased blood flow to the penis; and minor urethral bleeding or spotting.

Research on drugs for treating ED is expanding rapidly. Patients should ask their doctor about the latest advances.

Vacuum devices: Mechanical vacuum devices cause erection by creating a partial vacuum, which draws blood into the penis, engorging and expanding it. The devices have three components: a plastic cylinder, into which the penis is placed; a pump, which draws air out of the cylinder; and an elastic band, which is placed around the base of the penis to maintain the erection after the cylinder is removed and during intercourse by preventing blood from flowing back into the body.

One variation of the vacuum device involves a semirigid rubber sheath that is placed on the penis and remains there after erection is attained and during intercourse.

Surgery: Surgery usually has one of three goals:

- To implant a device that can cause the penis to become erect
- To reconstruct arteries to increase flow of blood to the penis
- To block off veins that allow blood to leak from the penile tissues

Implanted devices, known as prostheses, can restore erection in many men with ED. Possible problems with implants include mechanical breakdown and infection, although mechanical problems have diminished in recent years because of technological advances.

Malleable implants usually consist of paired rods, which are inserted surgically into the corpora cavernosa. The user manually adjusts the position of the penis and, therefore, the rods. Adjustment does not affect the width or length of the penis. Inflatable implants consist of paired cylinders, which are surgically inserted inside the penis and can be expanded using pressurized fluid. Tubes connect the cylinders to a fluid reservoir and a pump, which are also surgically implanted. The patient inflates the cylinders by pressing on the small pump, located under the skin in the scrotum. Inflatable implants can expand the length and width of the penis somewhat. They also leave the penis in a more natural state when not inflated.

Surgery to repair arteries can reduce ED caused by obstructions that block the flow of blood. The best candidates for such surgery are young men with discrete blockage of an artery because of an injury to the crotch or fracture of the pelvis. The procedure is almost never successful in older men with widespread blockage.

Surgery to veins that allow blood to leave the penis usually involves an opposite procedure—intentional blockage. Blocking off veins (ligation) can reduce the leakage of blood that diminishes the rigidity of the penis during erection. However, experts have raised questions about the long-term effectiveness of this procedure, and it is rarely done.

Chapter 13

Gastrointestinal Problems

Chapter Contents

Section 13.1

Irritable Bowel Syndrome

From "Irritable Bowel Syndrome," by the National Institute for
Diabetes and Digestive and Kidney Diseases (NIDDK, www.niddk
.nih.gov), part of the National Institutes of Health, September 2007.

What is irritable bowel syndrome (IBS)?

Irritable bowel syndrome is a disorder characterized most commonly by cramping, abdominal pain, bloating, constipation, and diarrhea. IBS causes a great deal of discomfort and distress, but it does
not permanently harm the intestines and does not lead to a serious
disease, such as cancer. Most people can control their symptoms with
diet, stress management, and prescribed medications. For some people,
however, IBS can be disabling. They may be unable to work, attend
social events, or even travel short distances.

As many as 20 percent of the adult population, or one in five Americans, have symptoms of IBS, making it one of the most common disorders diagnosed by doctors. It occurs more often in women than in men,
and it begins before the age of 35 in about 50 percent of people.

What are the symptoms of IBS?

Abdominal pain, bloating, and discomfort are the main symptoms of
IBS. However, symptoms can vary from person to person. Some people
have constipation, which means hard, difficult-to-pass, or infrequent
bowel movements. Often these people report straining and cramping
when trying to have a bowel movement but cannot eliminate any stool,
or they are able to eliminate only a small amount. If they are able to
have a bowel movement, there may be mucus in it, which is a fluid that
moistens and protect passages in the digestive system. Some people
with IBS experience diarrhea, which is frequent, loose, watery, stools.
People with diarrhea frequently feel an urgent and uncontrollable need
to have a bowel movement. Other people with IBS alternate between
constipation and diarrhea. Sometimes people find that their symptoms
subside for a few months and then return, while others report a constant worsening of symptoms over time.

What causes IBS?

Researchers have yet to discover any specific cause for IBS. One theory is that people who suffer from IBS have a colon, or large intestine, that is particularly sensitive and reactive to certain foods and stress. The immune system, which fights infection, may also be involved.

- Normal motility, or movement, may not be present in the colon of a person who has IBS. It can be spasmodic or can even stop working temporarily. Spasms are sudden strong muscle contractions that come and go.

- The lining of the colon called the epithelium, which is affected by the immune and nervous systems, regulates the flow of fluids in and out of the colon. In IBS, the epithelium appears to work properly. However, when the contents inside the colon move too quickly, the colon loses its ability to absorb fluids. The result is too much fluid in the stool. In other people, the movement inside the colon is too slow, which causes extra fluid to be absorbed. As a result, a person develops constipation.

- A person's colon may respond strongly to stimuli such as certain foods or stress that would not bother most people.

- Recent research has reported that serotonin is linked with normal gastrointestinal (GI) functioning. Serotonin is a neurotransmitter, or chemical, that delivers messages from one part of your body to another. Ninety-five percent of the serotonin in your body is located in the GI tract, and the other 5 percent is found in the brain. Cells that line the inside of the bowel work as transporters and carry the serotonin out of the GI tract. People with IBS, however, have diminished receptor activity, causing abnormal levels of serotonin to exist in the GI tract. As a result, they experience problems with bowel movement, motility, and sensation—having more sensitive pain receptors in their GI tract.

- Researchers have reported that IBS may be caused by a bacterial infection in the gastrointestinal tract. Studies show that people who have had gastroenteritis sometimes develop IBS, otherwise called postinfectious IBS.

- Researchers have also found very mild celiac disease in some people with symptoms similar to IBS. People with celiac disease cannot digest gluten, a substance found in wheat, rye, and barley. People with celiac disease cannot eat these foods without becoming very sick because their immune system responds by

105

damaging the small intestine. A blood test can determine whether celiac disease may be present.

How is IBS diagnosed?

If you think you have IBS, seeing your doctor is the first step. IBS is generally diagnosed on the basis of a complete medical history that includes a careful description of symptoms and a physical examination.

There is no specific test for IBS, although diagnostic tests may be performed to rule out other problems. These tests may include stool sample testing, blood tests, and x-rays. Typically, a doctor will perform a sigmoidoscopy, or colonoscopy, which allows the doctor to look inside the colon. This is done by inserting a small, flexible tube with a camera on the end of it through the anus. The camera then transfers the images of your colon onto a large screen for the doctor to see better.

If your test results are negative, the doctor may diagnose IBS based on your symptoms, including how often you have had abdominal pain or discomfort during the past year, when the pain starts and stops in relation to bowel function, and how your bowel frequency and stool consistency have changed. Many doctors refer to a list of specific symptoms that must be present to make a diagnosis of IBS.

Symptoms include the following:

- A person must have abdominal pain or discomfort for at least 12 weeks out of the previous 12 months. These 12 weeks do not have to be consecutive.
- The abdominal pain or discomfort has two of the following three features:
  - It is relieved by having a bowel movement.
  - When it starts, there is a change in how often you have a bowel movement.
  - When it starts, there is a change in the form of the stool or the way it looks.
- Certain symptoms must also be present, such as the following:
  - A change in frequency of bowel movements
  - A change in appearance of bowel movements
  - Feelings of uncontrollable urgency to have a bowel movement
  - Difficulty or inability to pass stool
  - Mucus in the stool
  - Bloating

- Bleeding, fever, weight loss, and persistent severe pain are not symptoms of IBS and may indicate other problems such as inflammation, or rarely, cancer.

The following have been associated with a worsening of IBS symptoms:

- Large meals
- Bloating from gas in the colon
- Medicines
- Wheat, rye, barley, chocolate, milk products, or alcohol
- Drinks with caffeine, such as coffee, tea, or colas
- Stress, conflict, or emotional upsets

Researchers have found that women with IBS may have more symptoms during their menstrual periods, suggesting that reproductive hormones can worsen IBS problems.

In addition, people with IBS frequently suffer from depression and anxiety, which can worsen symptoms. Similarly, the symptoms associated with IBS can cause a person to feel depressed and anxious.

What is the treatment for IBS?

Unfortunately, many people suffer from IBS for a long time before seeking medical treatment. Up to 70 percent of people suffering from IBS are not receiving medical care for their symptoms. No cure has been found for IBS, but many options are available to treat the symptoms. Your doctor will give you the best treatments for your particular symptoms and encourage you to manage stress and make changes to your diet.

Medications are an important part of relieving symptoms. Your doctor may suggest fiber supplements or laxatives for constipation or medicines to decrease diarrhea, such as Lomotil or loperamide (Imodium). An antispasmodic is commonly prescribed, which helps to control colon muscle spasms and reduce abdominal pain. Antidepressants may relieve some symptoms. However, both antispasmodics and antidepressants can worsen constipation, so some doctors will also prescribe medications that relax muscles in the bladder and intestines, such as Donnapine and Librax. These medications contain a mild sedative, which can be habit forming, so they need to be used under the guidance of a physician.

A medication available specifically to treat IBS is alosetron hydrochloride (Lotronex). Lotronex has been reapproved with significant restrictions by the U.S. Food and Drug Administration (FDA) for women with severe IBS who have not responded to conventional therapy and whose primary symptom is diarrhea. However, even in these patients, Lotronex should be used with great caution because it can have serious side effects such as severe constipation or decreased blood flow to the colon.

With any medication, even over-the-counter medications such as laxatives and fiber supplements, it is important to follow your doctor's instructions. Some people report a worsening in abdominal bloating and gas from increased fiber intake, and laxatives can be habit forming if they are used too frequently.

Medications affect people differently, and no one medication or combination of medications will work for everyone with IBS. You will need to work with your doctor to find the best combination of medicine, diet, counseling, and support to control your symptoms.

How does stress affect IBS?

Stress—feeling mentally or emotionally tense, troubled, angry, or overwhelmed—can stimulate colon spasms in people with IBS. The colon has many nerves that connect it to the brain. Like the heart and the lungs, the colon is partly controlled by the autonomic nervous system, which responds to stress. These nerves control the normal contractions of the colon and cause abdominal discomfort at stressful times. People often experience cramps or "butterflies" when they are nervous or upset. In people with IBS, the colon can be overly responsive to even slight conflict or stress. Stress makes the mind more aware of the sensations that arise in the colon, making the person perceive these sensations as unpleasant.

Some evidence suggests that IBS is affected by the immune system, which fights infection in the body. The immune system is affected by stress. For all these reasons, stress management is an important part of treatment for IBS. Stress management options include the following:

- Stress reduction (relaxation) training and relaxation therapies such as meditation
- Counseling and support
- Regular exercise such as walking or yoga
- Changes to the stressful situations in your life
- Adequate sleep

What does the colon do?

The colon, which is about 5 feet long, connects the small intestine to the rectum and anus. The major function of the colon is to absorb water, nutrients, and salts from the partially digested food that enters from the small intestine. Two pints of liquid matter enter the colon from the small intestine each day. Stool volume is a third of a pint. The difference between the amount of fluid entering the colon from the small intestine and the amount of stool in the colon is what the colon absorbs each day.

Colon motility—the contraction of the colon muscles and the movement of its contents—is controlled by nerves, hormones, and impulses in the colon muscles. These contractions move the contents inside the colon toward the rectum. During this passage, water and nutrients are absorbed into the body, and what is left over is stool. A few times each day contractions push the stool down the colon, resulting in a bowel movement. However, if the muscles of the colon, sphincters, and pelvis do not contract in the right way, the contents inside the colon do not move correctly, resulting in abdominal pain, cramps, constipation, a sense of incomplete stool movement, or diarrhea.

Can changes in diet help IBS?

For many people, careful eating reduces IBS symptoms. Before changing your diet, keep a journal noting the foods that seem to cause distress. Then discuss your findings with your doctor. You may want to consult a registered dietitian who can help you make changes to your diet. For instance, if dairy products cause your symptoms to flare up, you can try eating less of those foods. You might be able to tolerate yogurt better than other dairy products because it contains bacteria that supply the enzyme needed to digest lactose, the sugar found in milk products. Dairy products are an important source of calcium and other nutrients. If you need to avoid dairy products, be sure to get adequate nutrients in the foods you substitute, or take supplements.

In many cases, dietary fiber may lessen IBS symptoms, particularly constipation. However, it may not help with lowering pain or decreasing diarrhea. Whole grain breads and cereals, fruits, and vegetables are good sources of fiber. High-fiber diets keep the colon mildly distended, which may help prevent spasms. Some forms of fiber keep water in the stool, thereby preventing hard stools that are difficult to pass. Doctors usually recommend a diet with enough fiber to produce soft, painless bowel movements. High-fiber diets may cause gas and bloating, although some people report that these symptoms go away within a few weeks. Increasing fiber intake by 2 to 3 grams per day will help reduce the risk of increased gas and bloating.

Drinking six to eight glasses of plain water a day is important, especially if you have diarrhea. Drinking carbonated beverages, such as sodas, may result in gas and cause discomfort. Chewing gum and eating too quickly can lead to swallowing air, which also leads to gas.

Large meals can cause cramping and diarrhea, so eating smaller meals more often, or eating smaller portions, may help IBS symptoms. Eating meals that are low in fat and high in carbohydrates such as pasta, rice, whole-grain breads and cereals (unless you have celiac disease), fruits, and vegetables may help.

Is IBS linked to other health problems?

As its name indicates, IBS is a syndrome—a combination of signs and symptoms. IBS has not been shown to lead to a serious disease, including cancer. Through the years, IBS has been called by many names, among them colitis, mucous colitis, spastic colon, or spastic bowel. However, no link has been established between IBS and inflammatory bowel diseases such as Crohn disease or ulcerative colitis.

Section 13.2

Peptic Ulcers

Excerpted from "What I Need to Know about Peptic Ulcers," by the National Institute of Diabetes and Digestive and Kidney Diseases (NIDDK, www.niddk.nih.gov), part of the National Institutes of Health, September 2009.

What is a peptic ulcer?

A peptic ulcer is a sore in the lining of your stomach or duodenum. The duodenum is the first part of your small intestine. A peptic ulcer in the stomach is called a gastric ulcer. One that is in the duodenum is called a duodenal ulcer. A peptic ulcer also may develop just above your stomach in the esophagus, the tube that connects the mouth to the stomach. But most peptic ulcers develop in the stomach or duodenum.

Many people have peptic ulcers. You can have both gastric and duodenal ulcers at the same time and you also can have more than one ulcer in your lifetime.

Peptic ulcers can be treated successfully. Seeing your doctor is the first step.

What causes peptic ulcers?

Most peptic ulcers are caused by the following:

• *Helicobacter pylori* (*H. pylori*), a germ that causes infection

• Nonsteroidal anti-inflammatory drugs (NSAIDs), such as aspirin and ibuprofen

H. pylori is the most common cause of peptic ulcers. Doctors think *H. pylori* may be spread through unclean food or water or by mouth-to-mouth contact, such as kissing. Even though many people have an *H. pylori* infection, most of them never develop an ulcer.

Use of NSAIDs is the second most common cause of peptic ulcers. But not everyone who takes NSAIDs gets a peptic ulcer. Ulcers caused by NSAIDs are more often found in people who have the following characteristics:

- Are age 60 or older
- Are female
- Have taken NSAIDs for a long time
- Have had an ulcer before

Other causes of peptic ulcers are rare. One rare cause is Zollinger-Ellison syndrome—a disease that makes the body produce too much stomach acid, which harms the lining of the stomach or duodenum.

Stress or spicy food does not cause peptic ulcers, but either can make ulcer symptoms worse.

What are the symptoms of peptic ulcers?

A dull or burning pain in your stomach is the most common symptom of peptic ulcers. You may feel the pain anywhere between your belly button and breastbone. The pain often:

- starts between meals or during the night;
- briefly stops if you eat or take antacids;
- lasts for minutes to hours;
- comes and goes for several days or weeks.

Other symptoms of peptic ulcers may include the following:

- Weight loss
- Poor appetite
- Bloating
- Burping
- Vomiting
- Feeling sick to your stomach

Even if your symptoms are mild, you may have peptic ulcers. You should see your doctor to talk about your symptoms. Peptic ulcers can get worse if they aren't treated.

Call your doctor right away if you have the following:

- Sudden sharp stomach pain that doesn't go away
- Black or bloody stools
- Bloody vomit or vomit that looks like coffee grounds

These symptoms could be signs an ulcer has:

- broken a blood vessel;

- gone through, or perforated, your stomach or duodenal wall;

- stopped food from moving from your stomach into the duodenum.

These symptoms must be treated quickly. You may need surgery.

How are peptic ulcers diagnosed?

Tell your doctor about your symptoms and which medicines you take. Be sure to mention those you get without a prescription, such as Bayer, Motrin, Advil, or Aleve. These medicines are all NSAIDs.

To see if you have an *H. pylori* infection, your doctor will test your blood, breath, or stool. About half of all people who develop an ulcer from NSAIDs also have an *H. pylori* infection.

Your doctor also may want to look inside your stomach and duodenum by doing an endoscopy or an upper gastrointestinal (GI) series—a type of x-ray. Both procedures are painless.

For an endoscopy, you will be given medicine to relax you. Then the doctor will pass an endoscope—a thin, lighted tube with a tiny camera—through your mouth to your stomach and duodenum. Your doctor also may take a small piece of tissue—no bigger than a match head—to look at through a microscope. This process is called a biopsy.

For an upper GI series, you will drink a liquid called barium. The barium will make your stomach and duodenum show up clearly on the x-rays.

How are peptic ulcers treated?

If you have peptic ulcers, they can be cured. Depending on what caused your ulcers, your doctor may prescribe one or more of the following medicines:

- A proton pump inhibitor (PPI) or histamine receptor blocker (H2 blocker) to reduce stomach acid and protect the lining of your stomach and duodenum

- One or more antibiotics to kill an *H. pylori* infection

- A medicine that contains bismuth subsalicylate, such as Pepto-Bismol, to coat the ulcers and protect them from stomach acid

These medicines will stop the pain and help heal the ulcers.

If an NSAID caused your peptic ulcers, your doctor may tell you to do the following:

- Stop taking the NSAID.

- Reduce how much of the NSAID you take.

- Take a PPI or H2 blocker with the NSAID.

- Switch to another medicine that won't cause ulcers.

You should take only the medicines your doctor tells you to take and all medicines exactly as your doctor tells you to, even if your pain stops.

Tell your doctor if the medicines make you feel sick or dizzy or cause diarrhea or headaches. Your doctor can change your medicines.

And if you smoke, quit. You also should avoid alcohol. Smoking and drinking alcohol slow the healing of ulcers and can make them worse.

Can antacids or milk help peptic ulcers heal?

Neither antacids—such as Tums—nor milk can heal peptic ulcers, although each may make you feel better briefly. Check with your doctor before taking antacids or drinking milk while your ulcers are healing.

Some of the antibiotics used for *H. pylori* infection may not work as well if you take antacids. And while antacids may make ulcer pain go away for a while, they won't kill the *H. pylori* germ. Only antibiotics can do that.

Many people used to think that drinking milk helped peptic ulcers heal. But doctors know now that while milk may make ulcers feel better briefly, it also increases stomach acid. Too much stomach acid makes ulcers worse.

What if peptic ulcers don't heal?

In many cases, medicines heal ulcers. If an *H. pylori* infection caused your ulcers, you must finish all antibiotics and take any other medicines your doctor prescribes. The infection and ulcers will only heal if you take all medicines as prescribed.

When you have finished your medicines, your doctor will do a breath or stool test to be sure the *H. pylori* infection is gone. Sometimes, the *H. pylori* germ is still there, even after a person has taken all the medicines correctly. If that happens, your doctor will prescribe different antibiotics to get rid of the infection and cure your ulcers.

Rarely, surgery is needed to help ulcers heal. You may need surgery if your ulcers:

- don't heal;
- keep coming back;
- bleed;
- perforate the stomach or duodenal wall;
- block food from moving out of the stomach.

Surgery can remove the ulcers or reduce the amount of acid in your stomach.

Can peptic ulcers come back?

Yes. If you smoke or take NSAIDs, your ulcers may come back. If you need to take an NSAID, your doctor may switch you to a different medicine or add medicines to help prevent ulcers.

What can I do to prevent peptic ulcers?

To help prevent ulcers caused by *H. pylori*, do the following:

- Wash your hands with soap and water after using the bathroom and before eating.
- Eat food that has been washed well and cooked properly.
- Drink water from a clean, safe source.

To help prevent ulcers caused by NSAIDs, do the following:

- Stop using NSAIDs, if possible.
- Take NSAIDs with a meal, if you still need NSAIDs.
- Use a lower dose of NSAIDs.
- Ask your doctor about medicines to protect your stomach and duodenum while taking NSAIDs.
- Ask your doctor about switching to a medicine that won't cause ulcers.

Section 13.3

Stress Gastritis

Excerpted from "Gastritis," by the National Institute of Diabetes and Digestive and Kidney Diseases (NIDDK, www.niddk.nih.gov), part of the National Institutes of Health, January 2010.

Gastritis is a condition in which the stomach lining—known as the mucosa—is inflamed. The stomach lining contains special cells that produce acid and enzymes, which help break down food for digestion, and mucus, which protects the stomach lining from acid. When the stomach lining is inflamed, it produces less acid, enzymes, and mucus.

Gastritis may be acute or chronic. Sudden, severe inflammation of the stomach lining is called acute gastritis. Inflammation that lasts for a long time is called chronic gastritis. If chronic gastritis is not treated, it may last for years or even a lifetime.

Erosive gastritis is a type of gastritis that often does not cause significant inflammation but can wear away the stomach lining. Erosive gastritis can cause bleeding, erosions, or ulcers. Erosive gastritis may be acute or chronic.

The relationship between gastritis and symptoms is not clear. The term gastritis refers specifically to abnormal inflammation in the stomach lining. People who have gastritis may experience pain or discomfort in the upper abdomen, but many people with gastritis do not have any symptoms.

The term gastritis is sometimes mistakenly used to describe any symptoms of pain or discomfort in the upper abdomen. Many diseases and disorders can cause these symptoms. Most people who have upper abdominal symptoms do not have gastritis.

What causes gastritis?

Helicobacter pylori (H. pylori) infection causes most cases of chronic nonerosive gastritis. *H. pylori* are bacteria that infect the stomach lining. *H. pylori* are primarily transmitted from person to person. In areas with poor sanitation, *H. pylori* may be transmitted through contaminated food or water.

In industrialized countries like the United States, 20 to 50 percent of the population may be infected with *H. pylori*. Rates of *H. pylori* infection are higher in areas with poor sanitation and higher population density. Infection rates may be higher than 80 percent in some developing countries.

The most common cause of erosive gastritis—acute and chronic—is prolonged use of nonsteroidal anti-inflammatory drugs (NSAIDs) such as aspirin and ibuprofen. Other agents that can cause erosive gastritis include alcohol, cocaine, and radiation.

Traumatic injuries, critical illness, severe burns, and major surgery can also cause acute erosive gastritis. This type of gastritis is called stress gastritis.

Less common causes of erosive and nonerosive gastritis include the following:

- Autoimmune disorders in which the immune system attacks healthy cells in the stomach lining
- Some digestive diseases and disorders, such as Crohn disease and pernicious anemia
- Viruses, parasites, fungi, and bacteria other than *H. pylori*

What are the symptoms of gastritis?

Many people with gastritis do not have any symptoms, but some people experience symptoms such as the following:

- Upper abdominal discomfort or pain
- Nausea
- Vomiting

These symptoms are also called dyspepsia.

Erosive gastritis may cause ulcers or erosions in the stomach lining that can bleed. Signs of bleeding in the stomach include the following:

- Blood in vomit
- Black, tarry stools
- Red blood in the stool

What are the complications of gastritis?

Most forms of chronic nonspecific gastritis do not cause symptoms. However, chronic gastritis is a risk factor for peptic ulcer disease, gastric polyps, and benign and malignant gastric tumors.

Some people with chronic *H. pylori* gastritis or autoimmune gastritis develop atrophic gastritis. Atrophic gastritis destroys the cells in the stomach lining that produce digestive acids and enzymes.

Atrophic gastritis can lead to two types of cancer: gastric cancer and gastric mucosa-associated lymphoid tissue (MALT) lymphoma.

How is gastritis diagnosed?

The most common diagnostic test for gastritis is endoscopy with a biopsy of the stomach. The doctor will usually give the patient medicine to reduce discomfort and anxiety before beginning the endoscopy procedure. The doctor then inserts an endoscope, a thin tube with a tiny camera on the end, through the patient's mouth or nose and into the stomach. The doctor uses the endoscope to examine the lining of the esophagus, stomach, and first portion of the small intestine. If necessary, the doctor will use the endoscope to perform a biopsy, which involves collecting tiny samples of tissue for examination with a microscope.

Other tests used to identify the cause of gastritis or any complications include the following:

- **Upper gastrointestinal (GI) series:** The patient swallows barium, a liquid contrast material that makes the digestive tract visible in an x-ray. X-ray images may show changes in the stomach lining, such as erosions or ulcers.

- **Blood test:** The doctor may check for anemia, a condition in which the blood's iron-rich substance, hemoglobin, is diminished. Anemia may be a sign of chronic bleeding in the stomach.

- **Stool test:** This test checks for the presence of blood in the stool, another sign of bleeding in the stomach.

- **Tests for *H. pylori* infection:** The doctor may test a patient's breath, blood, or stool for signs of infection. *H. pylori* infection can also be confirmed with biopsies taken from the stomach during endoscopy.

How is gastritis treated?

Medications that reduce the amount of acid in the stomach can relieve symptoms that may accompany gastritis and promote healing of the stomach lining. These medications include the following:

- **Antacids**, such as Alka-Seltzer, Maalox, Mylanta, Rolaids, and Rio-pan, may help gastritis. Many brands on the market use different combinations of three basic salts—magnesium, calcium, and aluminum—with hydroxide or bicarbonate ions to neutralize the acid in the stomach. These drugs may produce side effects such as diarrhea or constipation.

- **Histamine 2 (H2) blockers**, such as famotidine (Pepcid AC) and ranitidine (Zantac 75), are used to treat gastritis. H2 blockers decrease acid production. They are available both over the counter and by prescription.

- **Proton pump inhibitors (PPIs)**, such as omeprazole (Prilosec, Zegerid), lansoprazole (Prevacid), pantoprazole (Protonix), rabeprazole (AcipHex), esomeprazole (Nexium), and dexlansoprazole (Kapidex), are another type of gastritis treatment. All of these drugs are available by prescription, and some are also available over the counter. PPIs decrease acid production more effectively than H2 blockers.

Depending on the cause of the gastritis, additional measures or treatments may be needed. For example, if gastritis is caused by prolonged use of NSAIDs, a doctor may advise a person to stop taking NSAIDs, reduce the dose of NSAIDs, or switch to another class of medications for pain. PPIs may be used to prevent stress gastritis in critically ill patients.

Treating *H. pylori* infections is important, even if a person is not experiencing symptoms from the infection. Untreated *H. pylori* gastritis may lead to cancer or the development of ulcers in the stomach or small intestine. The most common treatment is a triple therapy that combines a PPI and two antibiotics—usually amoxicillin and clarithromycin—to kill the bacteria. Treatment may also include bismuth subsalicylate (Pepto-Bismol) to help kill bacteria.

After treatment, the doctor may use a breath or stool test to make sure the *H. pylori* infection is gone. Curing the infection can be expected to cure the gastritis and decrease the risk of other gastrointestinal diseases associated with gastritis, such as peptic ulcer disease, gastric cancer, and MALT lymphoma.

Chapter 14

Headache and Its Link to Stress

You're sitting at your desk, working on a difficult task, when it suddenly feels as if a belt or vice is being tightened around the top of your head. Or you have periodic headaches that occur with nausea and increased sensitivity to light or sound. Maybe you are involved in a routine, non-stressful task when you're struck by head or neck pain.

Sound familiar? If so, you've suffered one of the many types of headache that can occur on its own or as part of another disease or health condition.

Anyone can experience a headache. Nearly two out of three children will have a headache by age 15. More than nine in 10 adults will experience a headache sometime in their life. Headache is our most common form of pain and a major reason cited for days missed at work or school as well as visits to the doctor. Without proper treatment, headaches can be severe and interfere with daily activities.

Certain types of headache run in families. Episodes of headache may ease or even disappear for a time and recur later in life. It's possible to have more than one type of headache at the same time.

Primary headaches occur independently and are not caused by another medical condition. It's uncertain what sets the process of a primary headache in motion. A cascade of events that affect blood vessels and nerves inside and outside the head causes pain signals to be sent to the brain. Brain chemicals called neurotransmitters are involved in

Excerpted from "Headache: Hope Through Research," by the National Institute of Neurological Disorders and Stroke (NINDS, www.ninds.nih.gov), part of the National Institutes of Health, November 2010.

creating head pain, as are changes in nerve cell activity (called cortical spreading depression). Migraine, cluster, and tension-type headache are the more familiar types of primary headache.

Secondary headaches are symptoms of another health disorder that causes pain-sensitive nerve endings to be pressed on or pulled or pushed out of place. They may result from underlying conditions including fever, infection, medication overuse, stress or emotional conflict, high blood pressure, psychiatric disorders, head injury or trauma, stroke, tumors, and nerve disorders (particularly trigeminal neuralgia, a chronic pain condition that typically affects a major nerve on one side of the jaw or cheek).

Headaches can range in frequency and severity of pain. Some individuals may experience headaches once or twice a year, whereas others may experience headaches more than 15 days a month. Some headaches may recur or last for weeks at a time. Pain can range from mild to disabling and may be accompanied by symptoms such as nausea or increased sensitivity to noise or light, depending on the type of headache.

Why Headaches Hurt

Information about touch, pain, temperature, and vibration in the head and neck is sent to the brain by the trigeminal nerve, one of 12 pairs of cranial nerves that start at the base of the brain.

The nerve has three branches that conduct sensations from the scalp, the blood vessels inside and outside of the skull, the lining around the brain (the meninges), and the face, mouth, neck, ears, eyes, and throat.

Brain tissue itself lacks pain-sensitive nerves and does not feel pain. Headaches occur when pain-sensitive nerve endings called nociceptors react to headache triggers (such as stress, certain foods or odors, or use of medicines) and send messages through the trigeminal nerve to the thalamus, the brain's "relay station" for pain sensation from all over the body. The thalamus controls the body's sensitivity to light and noise and sends messages to parts of the brain that manage awareness of pain and emotional response to it. Other parts of the brain may also be part of the process, causing nausea, vomiting, diarrhea, trouble concentrating, and other neurological symptoms.

When to See a Doctor

Not all headaches require a physician's attention. But headaches can signal a more serious disorder that requires prompt medical care.

Immediately call or see a physician if you or someone you're with experience any of these symptoms:

- Sudden, severe headache that may be accompanied by a stiff neck

- Severe headache accompanied by fever, nausea, or vomiting that is not related to another illness

- "First" or "worst" headache, often accompanied by confusion, weakness, double vision, or loss of consciousness

- Headache that worsens over days or weeks or has changed in pattern or behavior

- Recurring headache in children

- Headache following a head injury

- Headache and a loss of sensation or weakness in any part of the body, which could be a sign of a stroke

- Headache associated with convulsions

- Headache associated with shortness of breath

- Two or more headaches a week

- Persistent headache in someone who has been previously headache-free, particularly in someone over age 50

- New headaches in someone with a history of cancer or HIV/AIDS [human immunodeficiency virus/acquired immunodeficiency syndrome]

Diagnosing Your Headache

How and under what circumstances a person experiences a headache can be key to diagnosing its cause. Keeping a headache journal can help a physician better diagnose your type of headache and determine the best treatment. After each headache, note the time of day when it occurred; its intensity and duration; any sensitivity to light, odors, or sound; activity immediately prior to the headache; use of prescription and nonprescription medicines; amount of sleep the previous night; any stressful or emotional conditions; any influence from weather or daily activity; foods and fluids consumed in the past 24 hours; and any known health conditions at that time. Women should record the days of their menstrual cycles. Include notes about other family members who have a history of headache or other disorder. A pattern may emerge that can be helpful to reducing or preventing headaches.

Once your doctor has reviewed your medical and headache history and conducted a physical and neurological exam, lab screening and diagnostic tests may be ordered to either rule out or identify conditions that might be the cause of your headaches. Blood tests and urinalysis can help diagnose brain or spinal cord infections, blood vessel damage, and toxins that affect the nervous system.

Testing a sample of the fluid that surrounds the brain and spinal cord can detect infections, bleeding in the brain (called a brain hemorrhage), and measure any buildup of pressure within the skull. Diagnostic imaging, such as with computed tomography (CT) and magnetic resonance imaging (MRI), can detect irregularities in blood vessels and bones, certain brain tumors and cysts, brain damage from head injury, brain hemorrhage, inflammation, infection, and other disorders. Neuroimaging also gives doctors a way to see what's happening in the brain during headache attacks. An electroencephalogram (EEG) measures brain wave activity and can help diagnose brain tumors, seizures, head injury, and inflammation that may lead to headaches.

Headache Types and Their Treatment

The *International Classification of Headache Disorders,* published by the International Headache Society, is used to classify more than 150 types of primary and secondary headache disorders.

Primary headache disorders are divided into four main groups: Migraine, tension-type headache, trigeminal autonomic cephalgias (a group of short-lasting but severe headaches), and a miscellaneous group.

Migraine

If you suffer from migraine headaches, you're not alone. About 12 percent of the U.S. population experience migraines, one form of vascular headaches. Vascular headaches are characterized by throbbing and pulsating pain caused by the activation of nerve fibers that reside within the wall of brain blood vessels traveling within the meninges. Blood vessels narrow, temporarily, which decreases the flow of blood and oxygen to the brain. This causes other blood vessels to open wider and increase blood flow.

Migraines involve recurrent attacks of moderate to severe pain that is throbbing or pulsing and often strikes one side of the head.

Untreated attacks last from 4 to 72 hours. Other common symptoms are increased sensitivity to light, noise, and odors; and nausea and vomiting. Routine physical activity, movement, or even coughing or sneezing can worsen the headache pain.

Migraines occur most frequently in the morning, especially upon waking. Some people have migraines at predictable times, such as before menstruation or on weekends following a stressful week of work. Many people feel exhausted or weak following a migraine but are usually symptom-free between attacks.

A number of different factors can increase your risk of having a migraine. These factors, which trigger the headache process, vary from person to person and include sudden changes in weather or environment, too much or not enough sleep, strong odors or fumes, emotion, stress, overexertion, loud or sudden noises, motion sickness, low blood sugar, skipped meals, tobacco, depression, anxiety, head trauma, hangover, some medications, hormonal changes, and bright or flashing lights. Medication overuse or missed doses may also cause headaches. In some 50 percent of migraine sufferers, foods or ingredients can trigger headaches. These include aspartame, caffeine (or caffeine withdrawal), wine and other types of alcohol, chocolate, aged cheeses, monosodium glutamate, some fruits and nuts, fermented or pickled goods, yeast, and cured or processed meats. Keeping a diet journal will help identify food triggers.

Migraines occur in both children and adults, but affect adult women three times more often than men. There is evidence that migraines are genetic, with most migraine sufferers having a family history of the disorder. They also frequently occur in people who have other medical conditions. Depression, anxiety, bipolar disorder, sleep disorders, and epilepsy are more common in individuals with migraine than in the general population. Migraine sufferers—in particular those individuals who have pre-migraine symptoms referred to as aura—have a slightly increased risk of having a stroke.

Migraine in women often relates to changes in hormones. The headaches may begin at the start of the first menstrual cycle or during pregnancy. Most women see improvement after menopause, although surgical removal of the ovaries usually worsens migraines. Women with migraine who take oral contraceptives may experience changes in the frequency and severity of attacks, whereas women who do not suffer from headaches may develop migraines as a side effect of oral contraceptives.

Migraine is divided into four phases, all of which may be present during the attack:

- Premonitory symptoms: These occur up to 24 hours prior to developing a migraine. These include food cravings, unexplained mood changes (depression or euphoria), uncontrollable yawning, fluid retention, or increased urination.

- Aura: Some people will see flashing or bright lights or what looks like heat waves immediately prior to or during the migraine, whereas others may experience muscle weakness or the sensation of being touched or grabbed.

- Headache: A migraine usually starts gradually and builds in intensity. It is possible to have migraine without a headache.

- Postdrome (following the headache): Individuals are often exhausted or confused following a migraine. The postdrome period may last up to a day before people feel healthy.

The two major types of migraine are the following:

- Migraine with aura, previously called classic migraine, includes visual disturbances and other neurological symptoms that appear about 10 to 60 minutes before the actual headache and usually last no more than an hour. Individuals may temporarily lose part or all of their vision. The aura may occur without headache pain, which can strike at any time. Other classic symptoms include trouble speaking; an abnormal sensation, numbness, or muscle weakness on one side of the body; a tingling sensation in the hands or face, and confusion. Nausea, loss of appetite, and increased sensitivity to light, sound, or noise may precede the headache.

- Migraine without aura, or common migraine, is the more frequent form of migraine. Symptoms include headache pain that occurs without warning and is usually felt on one side of the head, along with nausea, confusion, blurred vision, mood changes, fatigue, and increased sensitivity to light, sound, or noise.

Other types of migraine include the following:

- Abdominal migraine mostly affects young children and involves moderate to severe pain in the middle of the abdomen lasting 1 to 72 hours, with little or no headache. Additional symptoms include nausea, vomiting, and loss of appetite. Many children who develop abdominal migraine will have migraine headaches later in life.

- Basilar-type migraine mainly affects children and adolescents. It occurs most often in teenage girls and may be associated with their menstrual cycle. Symptoms include partial or total loss of vision or double vision, dizziness and loss of balance, poor muscle coordination, slurred speech, a ringing in the ears, and fainting. The throbbing pain may come on suddenly and is felt on both sides at the back of the head.

- Hemiplegic migraine is a rare but severe form of migraine that causes temporary paralysis—sometimes lasting several days—on one side of the body prior to or during a headache. Symptoms such as vertigo, a pricking or stabbing sensation, and problems seeing, speaking, or swallowing may begin prior to the headache pain and usually stop shortly thereafter. When it runs in families the disorder is called familial hemiplegic migraine (FHM). Though rare, at least three distinct genetic forms of FHM have been identified. These genetic mutations make the brain more sensitive or excitable, most likely by increasing brain levels of a chemical called glutamate.

- Menstrually related migraine affects women around the time of their period, although most women with menstrually related migraine also have migraines at other times of the month. Symptoms may include migraine without aura (which is much more common during menses than migraine with aura), pulsing pain on one side of the head, nausea, vomiting, and increased sensitivity to sound and light.

- Migraine without headache is characterized by visual problems or other aura symptoms, nausea, vomiting, and constipation, but without head pain. Headache specialists have suggested that fever, dizziness, and/or unexplained pain in a particular part of the body could also be possible types of headache-free migraine.

- Ophthalmoplegic migraine is an uncommon form of migraine with head pain, along with a droopy eyelid, large pupil, and double vision that may last for weeks, long after the pain is gone.

- Retinal migraine is a condition characterized by attacks of visual loss or disturbances in one eye. These attacks, like the more common visual auras, are usually associated with migraine headaches.

- Status migrainosus is a rare and severe type of acute migraine in which disabling pain and nausea can last 72 hours or longer. The pain and nausea may be so intense that sufferers need to be hospitalized.

Migraine treatment is aimed at relieving symptoms and preventing additional attacks. Quick steps to ease symptoms may include napping or resting with eyes closed in a quiet, darkened room; placing a cool cloth or ice pack on the forehead, and drinking lots of fluid, particularly if the migraine is accompanied by vomiting. Small amounts of caffeine may help relieve symptoms during a migraine's early stages.

Drug therapy for migraine is divided into acute and preventive treatment. Acute or "abortive" medications are taken as soon as symptoms occur to relieve pain and restore function. Preventive treatment involves taking medicines daily to reduce the severity of future attacks or keep them from happening. The U.S. Food and Drug Administration (FDA) has approved a variety of drugs for these treatment methods. Headache drug use should be monitored by a physician, since some drugs may cause side effects.

Acute treatment for migraine may include any of the following drugs.

- Triptan drugs increase levels of the neurotransmitter serotonin in the brain. Serotonin causes blood vessels to constrict and lowers the pain threshold. Triptans—the preferred treatment for migraine—ease moderate to severe migraine pain and are available as tablets, nasal sprays, and injections.

- Ergot derivative drugs bind to serotonin receptors on nerve cells and decrease the transmission of pain messages along nerve fibers. They are most effective during the early stages of migraine and are available as nasal sprays and injections.

- Non-prescription analgesics or over-the-counter drugs such as ibuprofen, aspirin, or acetaminophen can ease the pain of less severe migraine headache.

- Combination analgesics involve a mix of drugs such as acetaminophen plus caffeine and/or a narcotic for migraine that may be resistant to simple analgesics.

- Nonsteroidal anti-inflammatory drugs can reduce inflammation and alleviate pain.

- Nausea relief drugs can ease queasiness brought on by various types of headache.

- Narcotics are prescribed briefly to relieve pain. These drugs should not be used to treat chronic headaches.

Taking headache relief drugs more than three times a week may lead to medication overuse headache (previously called rebound headache), in which the initial headache is relieved temporarily but reappears as the drug wears off. Taking more of the drug to treat the new headache leads to progressively shorter periods of pain relief and results in a pattern of recurrent chronic headache.

Headache pain ranges from moderate to severe and may occur with nausea or irritability. It may take weeks for these headaches to end once the drug is stopped.

Everyone with migraine needs effective treatment at the time of the headaches. Some people with frequent and severe migraine need preventive medications. In general, prevention should be considered if migraines occur one or more times weekly, or if migraines are less frequent but disabling. Preventive medicines are also recommended for individuals who take symptomatic headache treatment more than three times a week. Physicians will also recommend that a migraine sufferer take one or more preventive medications 2 to 3 months to assess drug effectiveness, unless intolerable side effects occur.

Several preventive medicines for migraine were initially marketed for conditions other than migraine.

- Anticonvulsants may be helpful for people with other types of headaches in addition to migraine. Although they were originally developed for treating epilepsy, these drugs increase levels of certain neurotransmitters and dampen pain impulses.

- Beta blockers are drugs for treating high blood pressure that are often effective for migraine.

- Calcium channel blockers are medications that are also used to treat high blood pressure treatment and help to stabilize blood vessel walls. These drugs appear to work by preventing the blood vessels from either narrowing or widening, which affects blood flow to the brain.

- Antidepressants are drugs that work on different chemicals in the brain; their effectiveness in treating migraine is not directly related to their effect on mood. Antidepressants may be helpful for individuals with other types of headaches because they increase the production of serotonin and may also affect levels of other chemicals, such as norepinephrine and dopamine. The types of antidepressants used for migraine treatment include selective serotonin reuptake inhibitors, serotonin and norepinephrine reuptake inhibitors, and tricyclic antidepressants (which are also used to treat tension-type headaches).

Natural treatments for migraine include riboflavin (vitamin B2), magnesium, coenzyme Q10, and butterbur.

Non-drug therapy for migraine includes biofeedback and relaxation training, both of which help individuals cope with or control the development of pain and the body's response to stress.

Lifestyle changes that reduce or prevent migraine attacks in some individuals include exercising, avoiding food and beverages that trigger headaches, eating regularly scheduled meals with adequate hydration, stopping certain medications, and establishing a consistent sleep schedule. Obesity increases the risk of developing chronic daily headache, so a weight loss program is recommended for obese individuals.

Tension-Type

Tension-type headache, previously called muscle contraction headache, is the most common type of headache. Its name indicates the role of stress and mental or emotional conflict in triggering the pain and contracting muscles in the neck, face, scalp, and jaw. Tension-type headaches may also be caused by jaw clenching, intense work, missed meals, depression, anxiety, or too little sleep. Sleep apnea may also cause tension-type headaches, especially in the morning. The pain is usually mild to moderate and feels as if constant pressure is being applied to the front of the face or to the head or neck. It also may feel as if a belt is being tightened around the head. Most often the pain is felt on both sides of the head. People who suffer tension-type headaches may also feel overly sensitive to light and sound but there is no pre-headache aura as with migraine. Typically, tension-type headaches usually disappear once the period of stress or related cause has ended.

Tension-type headaches affect women slightly more often than men. The headaches usually begin in adolescence and reach peak activity in the 30s. They have not been linked to hormones and do not have a strong hereditary connection.

There are two forms of tension-type headache: Episodic tension-type headaches occur between 10 and 15 days per month, with each attack lasting from 30 minutes to several days. Although the pain is not disabling, the severity of pain typically increases with the frequency of attacks. Chronic tension-type attacks usually occur more than 15 days per month over a 3-month period. The pain, which can be constant over a period of days or months, strikes both sides of the head and is more severe and disabling than episodic headache pain. Chronic tension headaches can cause sore scalps—even combing your hair can be painful. Most individuals will have had some form of episodic tension-type headache prior to onset of chronic tension-type headache.

Depression and anxiety can cause tension-type headaches. Headaches may appear in the early morning or evening, when conflicts in the office or at home are anticipated. Other causes include physical postures that strain head and neck muscles (such as holding your chin down while reading or holding a phone between your shoulder and ear), degenerative arthritis of the neck, and temporomandibular joint dysfunction (a disorder of the joints between the temporal bone located above the ear and the mandible, or lower jaw bone).

The first step in caring for a tension-type headache involves treating any specific disorder or disease that may be causing it. For example, arthritis of the neck is treated with anti-inflammatory medication and temporomandibular joint dysfunction may be helped by corrective devices for the mouth and jaw. A sleep study may be needed to detect sleep apnea and should be considered when there is a history of snoring, daytime sleepiness, or obesity.

A physician may suggest using analgesics, nonsteroidal anti-inflammatory drugs, or antidepressants to treat a tension-type headache that is not associated with a disease. Triptan drugs, barbiturates (drugs that have a relaxing or sedative effect), and ergot derivatives may provide relief to people who suffer from both migraine and tension-type headache.

Alternative therapies for chronic tension-type headaches include biofeedback, relaxation training, meditation, and cognitive-behavioral therapy to reduce stress. A hot shower or moist heat applied to the back of the neck may ease symptoms of infrequent tension headaches. Physical therapy, massage, and gentle exercise of the neck may also be helpful.

Trigeminal Autonomic Cephalgias

Some primary headaches are characterized by severe pain in or around the eye on one side of the face and autonomic (or involuntary) features on the same side, such as red and teary eye, drooping eyelid, and runny nose. These disorders, called trigeminal autonomic cephalgias (cephalgia meaning head pain), differ in attack duration and frequency, and have episodic and chronic forms. Episodic attacks occur on a daily or near-daily basis for weeks or months with pain-free remissions. Chronic attacks occur on a daily or near-daily basis for a year or more with only brief remissions.

Cluster headache—the most severe form of primary headache—involves sudden, extremely painful headaches that occur in "clusters," usually at the same time of the day and night for several weeks. They strike one side of the head, often behind or around one eye, and may be preceded by a migraine-like aura and nausea. The pain usually peaks 5 to 10 minutes after onset and continues at that intensity for up to 3 hours. The nose and the eye on the affected side of the face may get red, swollen, and teary. Some people will experience restlessness and agitation, changes in heart rate and blood pressure, and sensitivity to light, sound, or smell. Cluster headaches often wake people from sleep.

Cluster headaches generally begin between the ages of 20 and 50 but may start at any age, occur more often in men than in women, and are more common in smokers than in nonsmokers. The attacks are usually less frequent and shorter than migraines. It's common to have one to three cluster headaches a day with two cluster periods a year, separated by months of freedom from symptoms. The cluster periods often appear seasonally, usually in the spring and fall, and may be mistaken for allergies. A small group of people develop a chronic form of the disorder, which is characterized by bouts of headaches that can go on for years with only brief periods (1 month or less) of remission. Cluster headaches occur more often at night than during the day, suggesting they could be caused by irregularities in the body's sleep-wake cycle. Alcohol (especially red wine) and smoking can provoke attacks. Studies show a connection between cluster headache and prior head trauma. An increased familial risk of these headaches suggests that there may be a genetic cause.

Treatment options include oxygen therapy—in which pure oxygen is breathed through a mask to reduce blood flow to the brain—and triptan drugs. Certain antipsychotic drugs, calcium-channel blockers, and anticonvulsants can reduce pain severity and frequency of attacks. In extreme cases, electrical stimulation of the occipital nerve to prevent nerve signaling or surgical procedures that destroy or cut certain facial nerves may provide relief.

Paroxysmal hemicrania is a rare form of primary headache that usually begins in adulthood. Pain and related symptoms may be similar to those felt in cluster headaches, but with shorter duration. Attacks typically occur 5 to 40 times per day, with each attack lasting 2 to 45 minutes. Severe throbbing, claw-like, or piercing pain is felt on one side of the face—in, around, or behind the eye and occasionally reaching to the back of the neck. Other symptoms may include red and watery eyes, a drooping or swollen eyelid on the affected side of the face, and nasal congestion. Individuals may also feel dull pain, soreness, or tenderness between attacks or increased sensitivity to light on the affected side of the face. Paroxysmal hemicrania has two forms: Chronic, in which individuals experience attacks on a daily basis for a year or more, and episodic, in which the headaches may stop for months or years before recurring.

Certain movements of the head or neck, external pressure to the neck, and alcohol use may trigger these headaches. Attacks occur more often in women than in men and have no familial pattern.

The nonsteroidal anti-inflammatory drug indomethacin can quickly halt the pain and related symptoms of paroxysmal hemicrania, but symptoms recur once the drug treatment is stopped. Non-prescription analgesics and calcium-channel blockers can ease discomfort, particularly if taken when symptoms first appear.

SUNCT (short-lasting, unilateral, neuralgiform headache attacks with conjunctival injection and tearing) is a very rare type of headache with bursts of moderate to severe burning, piercing, or throbbing pain that is usually felt in the forehead, eye, or temple on one side of the head. The pain usually peaks within seconds of onset and may follow a pattern of increasing and decreasing intensity. Attacks typically occur during the day and last from 5 seconds to 4 minutes per episode. Individuals generally have five to six attacks per hour and are pain-free between attacks. This primary headache is slightly more common in men than in women, with onset usually after age 50. SUNCT may be episodic, occurring once or twice annually with headaches that remit and recur, or chronic, lasting more than 1year.

Symptoms include reddish or bloodshot eyes (conjunctival injection), watery eyes, stuffy or runny nose, sweaty forehead, puffy eyelids, increased pressure within the eye on the affected side of the head, and increased blood pressure. SUNCT is very difficult to treat. Anticonvulsants may relieve some of the symptoms, whereas anesthetics and corticosteroid drugs can treat some of the severe pain felt during these headaches. Surgery and glycerol injections to block nerve signaling along the trigeminal nerve have poor outcomes and provide only temporary relief in severe cases. Doctors are beginning to use deep brain stimulation (involving a surgically implanted battery-powered electrode that emits pulses of energy to surrounding brain tissue) to reduce the frequency of attacks in severely affected individuals.

Miscellaneous Primary Headaches

Other headaches that are not caused by other disorders include: Chronic daily headache refers to a group of headache disorders that occur at least 15 days a month during a 3-month period. In addition to chronic tension-type headache, chronic migraine, and medication overuse headache (discussed in the preceding text), these headaches include hemicrania continua and new daily persistent headache. Individuals feel constant, mostly moderate pain throughout the day on the sides or top of the head. They may also experience other types of headache. Adolescents and adults may experience chronic daily headaches. In children, stress from school and family activities may contribute to these headaches.

Hemicrania continua is marked by continuous, fluctuating pain that always occurs on the same side of the face and head. The headache may last from minutes to days and is associated with symptoms including tearing, red and irritated eyes, sweating, stuffy or runny nose, and swollen and drooping eyelids. The pain may get worse as the headache progresses. Migraine-like symptoms include nausea, vomiting, and sensitivity to light and sound.

Physical exertion and alcohol use may increase headache severity. The disorder is more common in women than in men and its cause is unknown. Hemicrania continua has two forms: Chronic, with daily headaches, and remitting or episodic, in which headaches may occur over a period of 6 months and are followed by a pain-free period of weeks to months before recurring. Most individuals have attacks of increased pain three to five times per 24-hour cycle. The nonsteroidal anti-inflammatory drug indomethacin usually provides rapid relief from symptoms. Corticosteroids may also provide temporary relief from some symptoms.

New daily persistent headache (NDPH), previously called chronic benign daily headache, is known for its constant daily pain that ranges from mild to severe. Individuals can often recount the exact date and time that the headache began. Daily headaches can occur for more than 3 months (and sometimes years) without lessening or ending. Symptoms include an abnormal sensitivity to light or sound, nausea, lightheadedness, and a pressing, throbbing, or tightening pain felt on both sides of the head. NDPH occurs more often in women than in men. Most sufferers do not have a prior history of headache. NDPH may occur spontaneously or following infection, medication use, trauma, high spinal fluid pressure, or other condition. The disorder has two forms: One that usually ends on its own within several months and does not require treatment, and a longer-lasting form that is difficult to treat. Muscle relaxants, antidepressants, and anticonvulsants may provide some relief.

Primary stabbing headache, also known as "ice pick" or "jabs and jolts" headache, is characterized by intense piercing pain that strikes without warning and generally lasts 1 to 10 seconds. The stabbing pain usually occurs around the eye but may be felt in multiple sites along the trigeminal nerve. Onset typically occurs between 45 and 50 years of age. Some individuals may have only one headache per year whereas others may have multiple headaches daily. Most attacks are spontaneous but headaches may be triggered by sudden movement, bright lights, or emotional stress. Primary stabbing headache occurs most often in people who have migraine, hemicrania continua, tension-type, or cluster headaches. The disorder is hard to treat, because each attack is extremely short. Indomethacin and other headache preventive medications can relieve pain in people who have multiple episodes of primary stabbing headache.

Primary exertional headache may be brought on by fits of coughing or sneezing or intense physical activity such as running, basketball, lifting weights, or sexual activity. The headache begins at the onset of activity. Pain rarely lasts more than several minutes but can last up to 2 days. Symptoms may include nausea and vomiting. This type of headache is typically seen in individuals who have a family history of migraine. Warm-up exercises prior to the physical activity can help prevent the headache and indomethacin can relieve the headache pain.

Hypnic headache, previously called "alarm-clock" headache, awakens people mostly at night. Onset is usually after age 50. Hypnic headache may occur 15 or more times per month, with no known trigger. Bouts of mild to moderate throbbing pain usually last from 15 minutes to 3 hours after waking and are most often felt on both sides of the head. Other symptoms include nausea or increased sensitivity to sound or light. Hypnic headache may be a disorder of rapid eye movement (REM) sleep as the attacks occur most often during dreaming. Both men and women are affected by this disorder, which is usually treated with caffeine, indomethacin, or lithium.

If you've ever eaten or inhaled a cold substance very fast, you may have had what's called an ice cream headache (sometimes called "brain freeze"). This headache happens when cold materials such as cold drinks or ice cream hit the warm roof of your mouth. Local blood vessels constrict to reduce the loss of body heat and then relax and allow the blood flow to increase. The resulting burst of pain lasts for about 5 minutes. Ice cream headache is more common in individuals who have migraine. The pain stops once the body adapts to the temperature change.

Coping with Headache

Headache treatment is a partnership between you and your doctor, and honest communication is essential. Finding a quick fix to your headache may not be possible. It may take some time for your doctor or specialist to determine the best course of treatment. Avoid using over-the-counter medicines more than twice a week, as they may actually worsen headache pain and the frequency of attacks.

Visit a local headache support group meeting (if available) to learn how others with headache cope with their pain and discomfort. Relax whenever possible to ease stress and related symptoms, get enough sleep, regularly perform aerobic exercises, and eat a regularly scheduled and healthy diet that avoids food triggers. Gaining more control over your headache, stress, and emotions will make you feel better and let you embrace daily activities as much as possible.

Chapter 15

Heart and Cardiovascular Problems

Chapter Contents

Section 15.1

Stress and Heart Disease

Excerpted from "Your Guide to Living Well with Heart Disease," by the
National Heart, Lung, and Blood Institute (NHLBI, www.nhlbi.nih.gov),
part of the National Institutes of Health, 2006.

Stress is linked to heart disease in a number of ways. Research
shows that the most commonly reported trigger for a heart attack is
an emotionally upsetting event, particularly one involving anger. In
addition, some common ways of coping with stress, such as overeating,
heavy drinking, and smoking, are clearly bad for your heart.

The good news is that sensible health habits can have a protective
effect. For people with heart disease, regular physical activity not only
relieves stress but also can directly lower the risk of heart disease
complications. Participating in a stress management program can help
to prevent recurrent heart attacks and repeat heart procedures. Good
relationships count, too. Developing strong personal ties can help to
improve recovery after a heart attack.

Much remains to be learned about the connections between stress
and heart disease, but a few things are clear. Staying physically active,
developing a wide circle of supportive people in your life, and sharing
your feelings and concerns with them can help you to be happier and
live longer.

Section 15.2

Stress and Blood Pressure

Does stress increase my blood pressure?

In today's fast-paced world filled with increasing demands, it's important to manage your stress level. Some people cope with stress by overeating or eating unhealthy foods, smoking, drinking, and other activities that raise their risk for heart attack, stroke, and high blood pressure.

What happens to the body during stress?

Stress is not a confirmed risk factor for either high blood pressure or heart disease. Scientists continue to study how stress relates to our health, but it has not been proven to cause heart disease. And while blood pressure may increase temporarily when you're stressed, stress has not been proven to cause diagnosable high blood pressure.

How much stress do you live with and what is the cost to your health?

Stress definitely affects our bodies. In addition to the emotional discomfort we feel when faced with a stressful situation, our bodies react by releasing stress hormones (adrenaline and cortisol) into the blood.

These hormones prepare the body for the "fight or flight response" by making the heart beat faster and constricting blood vessels to get more blood to the core of the body instead of the extremities. Constriction of blood vessels and increase in heart rate does raise blood pressure, but only temporarily; when the stress reaction goes away, blood pressure returns to its pre-stress level. This is called situational stress, and its effects are generally short-lived and disappear when the stressful event is over.

"Fight or flight" is a valuable response when we are faced with an imminent threat that we can handle by confronting or fleeing. However, our modern world contains many stressful events that we can't handle with those options. Chronic (constant) stress causes our bodies to go into high gear on and off for days or weeks at a time. The links between chronic stress and blood pressure are not clear.

This kind of stress is a difficult concept to pin down and measure, which is one of the problems researchers run into when trying to answer the question about stress and high blood pressure. Without a universal definition of chronic stress, stress levels are hard to measure and responses to stress vary from person to person. Stress, even chronic stress, does not cause high blood pressure. The fact is that experts don't know what causes high blood pressure, but contributing factors include being overweight, eating a diet high in sodium, being physically inactive, and drinking too much alcohol. And people who are under stress may be more likely to eat too much, drink too much alcohol, and be less active.

Section 15.3

Stress and Cholesterol Levels

There is good evidence to show that stress can increase a person's heart rate, lower the immune system's ability to fight colds, and increase certain inflammatory markers but can stress also raise a person's cholesterol? It appears so for some people, according to a new study that examines how reactions to stress over a period of time can raise a person's lipid levels.

This finding is reported in the November [2005] issue of *Health Psychology,* published by the American Psychological Association (APA). In a sample of 199 healthy middle-aged men and women, researchers Andrew Steptoe, DSc, and Lena Brydon, PhD, of University College London examined how individuals react to stress and whether this reaction can increase cholesterol and heighten cardiovascular risk in the future. Changes in total cholesterol, including low-density lipoprotein (LDL) and high-density lipoprotein (HDL), were assessed in the participants before and 3 years after completing two stress tasks.

Our study found that individuals vary in their cholesterol responses to stress, said Dr. Steptoe. "Some of the participants show large increases even in the short term, while others show very little response. The cholesterol responses that we measured in the lab probably reflect the way people react to challenges in everyday life as well. So the larger cholesterol responders to stress tasks will be large responders to emotional situations in their lives. It is these responses in everyday life that accumulate and lead to an increase in fasting cholesterol or lipid levels 3 years later. It appears that a person's reaction to stress is one mechanism through which higher lipid levels may develop."

The stress testing session involved examining the participants' cardiovascular, inflammatory, and hemostatic functions before and after their responses to performance on moderately stressful behavioral tasks. The stress tasks used were computerized color-word interference and mirror tracing. The color-word task involved flashing a series of target color words in incongruous colors on a computer screen (for example, yellow letters spelling the color blue). At the bottom of the computer screen, four names of colors were displayed in incorrect colors. The object of the task was to match the name of the color to the target word. The other task used was mirror tracing, which required the participant to trace a star seen in a mirror image. The participants were told to focus more on accuracy than on speed in both tasks.

At the follow up 3 years later, cholesterol levels in all the participants in the study had gone up, as might be expected through passage of time. However, individuals with larger initial stress responses had substantially greater rises in cholesterol than those with small stress responses. The people in the top third of stress responders were three times more likely to have a level of 'bad' (low-density lipoprotein) cholesterol above clinical thresholds than were people in the bottom third of stress responders. These differences were independent of their baseline levels of cholesterol levels, gender, age, hormone replacement, body mass index, smoking, or alcohol consumption.

The authors found no sex differences among the participants in their cholesterol levels and response to stress. Steptoe and Brydon speculate on the reasons why acute stress responses may raise fasting serum lipids. One possibility may be that stress encourages the body to produce more energy in the form of metabolic fuels—fatty acids and glucose. These substances require the liver to produce and secrete more LDL, which is the principal carrier of cholesterol in the blood. Another reason may be that stress interferes with lipid clearance and a third possibility could be that stress increases production of a number of inflammatory processes like interleukin 6, tumor necrosis factor, and C-reactive protein that also increase lipid production.

Even though these lipid responses to stress were not large, said Dr. Steptoe, "the levels are something to be concerned about. It does give us an opportunity to know whose cholesterol may rise in response to stress and give us warning for those who may be more at risk for coronary heart disease."

Source: "Associations Between Acute Lipid Stress Responses and Fasting Lipid Levels 3 Years Later," Andrew Steptoe, DSc, and Lena Brydon, PhD, University College London; *Health Psychology,* Vol. 24, No. 6 [November 2005].

Section 15.4

Stress and Stroke

Are you stressed out? There is a growing body of research connecting chronic stress with an increased risk of stroke, particularly ischemic stroke. In a study of more than 13,000 people, men reporting chronic stress over a 20-year period had double the risk of stroke as men without chronic stress (the increased risk was not significant in women).

Did yelling at my spouse give me a stroke?

No. While chronic elevated blood pressure increases the risk of a stroke, a brief increase in blood pressure due to emotions or exercise does not. On the other hand, chronic stress—emotional or physical stress that continues for some time—does contribute to stroke risk. This is especially true if you have other stroke risk factors.

For example, in a Danish study of more than 12,000 adults, those who reported experiencing stress at least weekly were nearly 50% more likely to die of a stroke over a 13-year period than those who said they never or hardly ever felt stress. Participants who often felt stress also tended to have other stroke risk factors such as smoking, a diagnosis of hypertension, or little physical activity.

If you feel chronically stressed—or are constantly yelling at your spouse—consider some therapy or lifestyle changes. Counseling can help with emotional and relationship issues, and stress-reduction courses, offered at many hospitals and clinics, can teach you specific techniques for coping with stress. Lifestyle practices such as exercise, yoga, tai chi, and meditation can also help lower stress and blood pressure.

Chapter 16

Infertility and Stress

The idea that stress causes infertility is an old one. Couples struggling to conceive hear it all the time: "Just relax!" "Have a glass of wine!" "Take the pressure off by adopting a child, and you'll get pregnant in no time!"

Today's researchers, however, believe that psychological factors—while important—are secondary to biological ones. They know that the interaction between factors is complex. And while some studies support the idea that stress-reducing interventions boost pregnancy, the jury is still out.

The Impact of Stress

A 1993 study by Alice D. Domar, PhD, and co-authors reveals just how distressing infertility can be. The *Journal of Psychosomatic Obstetrics and Gynecology* (Vol. 14, Suppl., 45–52) article reported that infertile women's anxiety and depression levels equaled those of women with conditions such as cancer, HIV [human immunodeficiency virus], and chronic pain.

But does infertility cause stress or does stress cause infertility? Answers to that question have shifted over time, says Annette L. Stanton, PhD, a psychiatry professor at the University of California, Los Angeles School of Medicine.

Clay, Rebecca A. "Does stress hinder conception?" *Monitor on Psychology,* September 2006, 37(8), 46–47. http://www.apa.org/monitor/sept06/stress.aspx. Copyright © 2006 by the American Psychological Association. Reproduced with permission. No further reproduction or distribution is permitted without written permission from the American Psychological Association.

In a 2002 article in the *Journal of Consulting and Clinical Psychology*(Vol. 70, No. 3, 751–770), Stanton and her co-authors explain that researchers under the sway of psychoanalytic theory once believed that infertility was the result of women's unconscious conflict. Now researchers have confirmed that biomedical causes account for most fertility problems, with psychological factors playing a much more limited role.

Jacky Boivin, PhD, a senior lecturer at the School of Psychology at Cardiff University in Wales, exemplifies that more nuanced approach. Citing converging evidence from many different areas, Boivin believes stress and fertility are related. But it's not a simple causal relationship, she emphasizes. Stress can cause individuals to smoke or indulge in other fertility-harming habits, she says, or can cause them to drop out of fertility treatment prematurely. Highly stressed individuals may be ambivalent about having children and therefore avoid sex. And because of variation in people's responses to stress, a population-wide relationship between stress and infertility doesn't necessarily mean stress will impair an individual's fertility.

That complexity—and the difficulty of researching it—makes Boivin reluctant to even say there's a link between stress and fertility.

"The second you say to women that there's a connection, they think 'I'm so stressed at work, I've probably shut down my ovaries and will never get pregnant!'" she says. "Stress could disrupt fertility, but it very rarely—if ever—causes people never to conceive."

While animals shut down reproductive functioning in times of scarce resources and other stresses, Boivin explains, humans have ways of overcoming that adaptive mechanism. After all, she points out, women continue to bear children during wars, famines, and other situations far more extreme than anything modern Americans endure.

Psychological Interventions

Can treating stress improve pregnancy rates?

Domar thinks so. In a widely cited 2000 study in *Health Psychology* (Vol. 19, No. 6, 568–575), Domar and her co-authors randomly assigned 184 nondepressed women to cognitive-behavioral therapy, a support group, and a control group. Those in the intervention groups not only saw significant psychological improvement but also had significantly higher pregnancy rates than the control group.

"Both intervention groups had almost triple the take-home baby rate of the control," says Domar, executive director of the Domar Center for Complementary Health Care in Waltham, Massachusetts, and an assistant professor of obstetrics/gynecology and reproductive biology at Harvard Medical School.

However, Domar and her co-authors admit that the study had some methodological problems. For one thing, many of the participants—especially those in the control group—dropped out. Some left the study because they got pregnant, others because they needed more psychological support. These and other limitations make definitive recommendations about psychological treatment impossible, the authors note.

And not all studies are as positive as Domar's, says Boivin. In a 2003 article in *Social Science and Medicine* (Vol. 57, No. 12, 2,325–2,341), Boivin reviewed the literature on psychosocial interventions for infertile patients. When it came to improving pregnancy rates, the results were mixed. Only eight of the 25 studies she analyzed examined interventions' effects on pregnancy rates, with three showing a positive effect and five showing no effect.

What the analysis did show was that interventions—especially group interventions emphasizing education about infertility and relaxation or coping training—reduced patients' anxiety, depression, and so called infertility specific stress. Future studies could evaluate yoga, meditation, and other such ways of achieving relaxation, adds Boivin, because what works best may vary from woman to woman.

"If people are thinking of using some kind of intervention—and you can go on the internet and find a million things claiming they'll get you pregnant—they should be motivated to use them to improve their quality of life rather than to increase their pregnancy rates," says Boivin. "That's where, chances are, it's going to work."

Rebecca A. Clay is a writer in Washington, DC.

Chapter 17

Multiple Sclerosis and Stress

Chapter Contents

Section 17.1

Does Multiple Sclerosis Worsen Stress?

A close friend of mine is planning her wedding. At dinner a few nights ago, while describing the preparations, she became increasingly distraught. Finally she stopped, looked up at me sadly, and sighed, "I guess I just don't handle stress very well."

My first thought was, who does? Whether getting married, starting a new job or leaving an old one, or dealing with the loss of a loved one, life can sometimes seem overwhelming. And being told we need to reduce our stress often makes us feel even more pressured: Taking yoga classes or practicing deep breathing are just more things to add to our to-do list.

Ironically, even though everyone experiences it, stress is difficult to define objectively. "Different people really mean different things when they talk about stress," said Nicholas LaRocca, PhD, the director of Health Care Delivery and Policy Research for the National Multiple Sclerosis Society. "Not just the general public, but scientists, too."

There are many kinds of potentially stressful situations, and each person has his or her own response. One person may be devastated by the loss of a job, while another may find working full time stressful. There's everyday stress, like being stuck in traffic, or there's traumatic stress, such as divorce or loss of a child. There are even general stresses brought on by war or terrorism.

Multiple sclerosis brings its own kinds of stress. New York City paramedic Maggie Staiger was diagnosed in August 2001, and a month later she worked as a paramedic at the World Trade Center site. "All these things are happening—you have to give yourself shots, your whole life changes—and then everyone tells you to try not to get stressed out. How in the world are you not supposed to get stressed out?" she said.

Stressing over Stress

Dr. LaRocca calls it "stress related to worrying about stress." If you think that stress could cause an exacerbation—which has never been definitively proven—then you may stress over managing your stress.

Rosalind Kalb, PhD, director of the Society's Professional Resource Center, agreed. "People can be so worried about anything making their disease worse that it becomes another stress in and of itself." In addition, friends or family members may feel responsible or guilty for causing stress, thinking that they may be worsening a person's MS.

"Issues that need to be discussed sometimes don't come up because a family member is afraid to bring them up," Dr. Kalb said. "Rather than being brought out into the open and resolved, they get swept under the carpet because the person doesn't want to bring up something that might upset the loved one with MS."

"One idea I find incredibly offensive is the idea that I wouldn't have MS if I'd managed my stress better," Staiger said. "There's the implication that if you can affect it with your mind then it was caused by your mind." She adds, "When I first got diagnosed, and then there was the World Trade Center, I was reading all this stuff about MS that emphasized 'try to avoid stress, try to avoid stress.' I thought, this is horrible! But I realized that, while I can't really avoid stress, I can change my reaction to stress."

The Missing Link

The first thing to know is that while stress can make us feel worse, whether upsetting our stomachs or knotting our neck muscles, no research group has been able to prove any direct cause-and-effect relationship between MS and stress. Many have tried.

"There's no doubt that there is a link in a general sense between stress and other things that happen to the human body," Dr. LaRocca said. "But what they are and how they operate in each case is not so clear." He added, "People get caught up in this question: Is stress making MS worse? I think we need to focus deeper than that and try to define stress in a scientifically rigorous way and then relate it to what's happening to the immune system."

Dr. Kalb agreed. "If people say they feel worse, I believe them, but we just don't know what the mechanism is." It's difficult to separate out the general effects of stress—such as making people feel more tired or jittery—from what actually happens to the immune system when it is under stress. The immune system is made up of many different elements working together, almost like a web. It is a mistake to point to a single factor, like stress, and blame it for everything.

"It's important for people with MS to know that there have been a lot of studies, but we still don't have conclusive evidence that stress causes exacerbations. I personally doubt that it causes them alone," said David Mohr, PhD, an associate professor in the department of Psychiatry and Neurology at the University of California, San Francisco.

Dr. Mohr recently conducted a "metastudy" of 14 studies on MS and stress, which was published in the March 19, 2004, issue of the *British Medical Journal.* While the data from that study shows an association between stress and exacerbations, Mohr is careful to point out many variables, such as medications, or a viral or bacterial infection. Time is also a major factor, in more ways than one.

When people remember a stressful event, they do so through hindsight. Since memory is often kind, small details tend to get erased and large details can become linked in a way they weren't in reality. "Life is full of stress," Dr. LaRocca said. "You can always find some sort of stressful situation in your life." He pointed out that one of the dilemmas scientists face is that it's "very difficult to go back and retrospectively look at this before people developed MS."

What Is Known about Stress?

Stress initially acts to protect you, releasing chemicals that make your reactions sharper and your mind move faster. Interestingly, the main hormone released during stress, cortisol, is anti-inflammatory, and derivatives of cortisol, such as prednisone, are often used to treat exacerbations. Dr. Mohr said that one possibility is that it's not stress itself that helps cause problems, but rather the resolution of stress, when levels of anti-inflammatory cortisol drop.

Dr. Mohr also points out that exacerbations may originate before stressful events. "Processes are going on that may occur over months, and your body is trying to manage those," he said. "Sometimes those processes get shut down, and sometimes they go on to become fullblown exacerbations." If you are stressed when no exacerbation is developing, then nothing may happen. However, if you are stressed when an exacerbation is developing, Dr. Mohr said, "it may increase the risk a little bit." In other words, stress alone will not cause an exacerbation, but it might be one factor in a complex set of factors that lead to an exacerbation.

"Saying that stress causes exacerbations is certainly premature," Dr. Mohr said. He is currently enrolling people with MS in the San

Francisco Bay and Seattle areas in a study designed to track whether learning stress management techniques can reduce development of new brain lesions or occurrences of new exacerbations. For information about participating, call 800-923-1033 or visit www.ucsf.edu/bmrc.

Eliminating Stress?

Getting rid of stress is not the same as cutting out french fries. "People with MS have at times been told to quit their jobs to avoid job-related stress," Dr. LaRocca said. "However, people find that if they withdraw from significant life activities, it can actually make their stress worse." Instead, he said, the key is to learn how to deal with stress, not try to escape it.

"I think people have to start by acknowledging that stress is normal in everyday life and that families—with or without MS—have issues that they have to work on and resolve as a family," Dr. Kalb said. She suggests family meetings, family counseling, and individual therapy for figuring out "stress triggers" and managing stress. A stress trigger could be external (noise, disturbing news, caffeine) or internal (depression, anxieties about money, etc.). And no two people are affected the same way by any particular event or thought pattern.

Managing Stress the Healthy Way

After Maggie Staiger was diagnosed, she decided to try hypnosis to help control the pain caused by her MS-related nerve damage. "I was so skeptical because nothing was working," she said, "so why would hypnosis work?" After two sessions, she was convinced—so convinced that she decided to study hypnosis herself and offer hypnosis to other people.

"Through hypnosis you still have all those stresses around you, but you're not responding in a way that is destructive to you," Staiger said. "The stressor of chronic pain is really debilitating, and relieving that stress of always feeling uncomfortable and never getting proper rest was a huge load off me—that made me feel better."

Other people turn to exercise, meditation, prayer groups, or psychotherapy to help with stressful situations, but everyone agrees that whatever you do—or don't do—no one should ever feel guilty about feeling stressed. For better or worse, stress is a normal part of life, and everyone goes through it differently. The person you admire for traveling alone to Tibet may be the person who is barricaded behind the bedroom door during a family picnic.

The relationship between stress and MS is still so tenuous and little understood, that, as Dr. Kalb said, "Until we can explain it, all we can do is encourage people to try to figure out how to handle stresses that are part of their lives"—which, for anyone, can only be a win-win situation.

Health Reference Series *Medical Advisor's Notes and Updates*

Data suggesting a link between stress and multiple sclerosis continues to accumulate. The best evidence so far pertains to acute, severe stressors; it is less clear whether more chronic forms of stress have the same effects.

A number of MS patients in Israel and Lebanon were subject to rocket bombardments and wartime conditions during the 2006 Hezbollah-Israeli war. Several studies have examined the impacts of these exposures on their MS disease activity. A 2008 study in *Annals of Neurology* found a sharp increase in the number of MS exacerbations among Israeli patients exposed to rocket attacks during the war. A 2010 study in the *Journal of Neurological Science* of Lebanese MS patients in the war zone also found significant increases in clinical relapses as well as brain lesions by MRI [magnetic resonance imaging].

Interestingly, a 2010 follow-up study on the Israeli patient group found that patients who employed more effective coping strategies had fewer MS exacerbations. This supports the idea that the effects of stress on MS can be mitigated, but further research into this area is needed.

Section 17.2

Taming Stress in Multiple Sclerosis

Excerpted from "Taming Stress in Multiple Sclerosis: Staying Well," By Frederick Foley, PhD, with Jane Sarnoff. © 2010 National Multiple Sclerosis Society (www.nationalmssociety.org). Reprinted with permission.

Causes of Stress

Brought to You by Evolution

When our ancestors were taking a morning stroll and met a tiger, they could run or fight. Either action demanded that their bodies adjust rapidly to meet the emergency, and they experienced stress as part of the process.

Without stress, we would not be able to act in times of danger. In fact, without some stress to get us to focus on a problem we might do almost nothing. Many people perform best while under stress. Other times, however, people are immobilized by the pressure that stress creates and prevents people from doing what needs to be done.

Today's Tigers

Stress can be caused by both pleasant and unpleasant demands and changes. In other words, people can be just as stressed by getting a promotion as by not getting one.

Stress usually begins with alarm, the modern equivalent of noticing a tiger. However, our options are rarely as simple as running away or fighting. For example, most people are very stressed at the prospect of having to use a cane or wheelchair. Many eventually experience relief or accept the benefits of the aid once the stressor—the idea of using a cane or other assistive device—has been sufficiently worked through.

Stress and MS

Having any chronic illness increases stress. MS is no exception. In fact, there are many stressful situations that are common with MS:

- diagnostic uncertainties (before the definite MS diagnosis);

- the unpredictability of MS;

- the invisibility of some symptoms (which can cause people with MS to feel misunderstood by others);

- the visibility of the symptoms, particularly newly emerging ones (to which others may react before the person has had time to adjust);

- the need to adjust and readjust to changing abilities;

- financial stress and concerns about employment;

- the presence—or possibility—of cognitive impairment;

- loss of control (e.g., coming and going of unpredictable symptoms);

- the need to make decisions about disease-modifying treatment and adjusting to the treatment if it is chosen.

Does Stress Increase the Risk of Attacks or Affect the Long-Term Course of MS?

Many people with MS feel that there is a definite connection between stress and MS. Some believe that controlling stress can have a beneficial impact on MS. And still others believe that neither stress nor controlling stress has any effect on MS. Scientifically speaking, the jury is still out. A relationship between stress and the onset of MS or MS relapses is considered possible, but hasn't been powerfully demonstrated in studies. Can a stressful event cause nerve damage or lesions? Can nerve damage or lesions increase someone's experience of stress? More research is needed to answer these questions.

Can Stress Make MS Symptoms Feel Worse?

Many people with MS say "yes." They experience more symptoms during stressful times. When the stress abates, their symptoms seem less troubling or less severe. This could be understood by looking at the stress and coping process.

During times of stress, more energy is required to think, problem-solve, and handle daily life. For example, one's ability to be patient with family members often wanes after a tough day. At stressful or demanding times, symptoms may be experienced more strongly because the energy to deal with them and get on with life has been drained.

We all have finite reservoirs of our ability to cope. At demanding times, our supply may temporarily run dry. Any difficulty, including MS symptoms, is more challenging at these moments.

Stress can't be—and shouldn't be—totally avoided. The challenge is to learn to reduce its intensity and use it to work for, not against, us.

Signs of Stress

Emotional Signs

- Chronic irritability or resentment
- Feeling down in the dumps, demoralized
- Continual boredom
- Excessive nervousness or anxiety
- Feeling overwhelmed
- Nightmares

Thought-Related Signs

- Worrying every day
- Distractibility
- Expecting the worst to happen much of the time
- Difficulty making everyday decisions

Physical Signs

- Clammy hands or sweating
- Constipation/diarrhea
- Dry mouth
- Headache
- Heart palpitations
- Stomachaches, knots, cramps, or nausea
- Muscle spasms or tightness
- Lump in throat
- Faintness
- Fatigue/weariness
- Sleeping too much/too little

- Short and shallow breathing

Recognizing Stress

Common signs of stress include changes in breathing, tight muscles, cold sweaty hands, and clenched teeth. But different people show their stress in different ways. In people with MS, some of the common signs of stress—fatigue and muscle tightness, for example—may also be symptoms of the disease. Understanding your stress responses and learning to separate them from your MS symptoms may help you recognize when you are stressed.

Knowing what causes or increases your stress can be the first step in taming it. What daily events or concerns stress you most? You may find it helpful to make a list of the things that have caused you the most stress in the last 2 weeks.

You may want to ask those nearest to you to help you recognize your stressors. But don't be overly influenced by what others think should stress you—just take note of what they think has caused you stress. A situation isn't stressful unless you react to it with stress.

Taming Stress in Your Mind

Stress often evolves from the way we interpret situations—and the way we relate to the world around us. So much in life could lead to stress: Lost buttons, long lines, irritating people, unreasonable requests, insurance forms, voice mail.

Take a look at your stress producers. In what ways can you reinterpret situations so that they don't cause you so much stress? How can you relate differently to people to avoid stress?

If personal thinking patterns create or increase stress, new thinking patterns can be learned. Here are some examples of thinking that increases stress:

- You think: "Total failure" whenever you're short of absolute perfection. (Alternative: "I did a pretty good job—I'll do it better next time.")

- You think: You are responsible for everything: "I wonder what I did to make him feel like that?" (Alternative: "I am not the center of everyone's world.")

- You think: "Should" about everything: "I should be treated fairly." (Alternative: "I'd like to be treated fairly, but . . . ")

- You think: "I probably won't be able to do that . . . no use trying." (Alternative: "I think I'll give it a try and see how far I can go.")

- You think· One thing is everything: "I messed that up, I'll mess up everything." (Alternative: "I am not very good at that, but I'm good at many other things.")

Can You Cut Stress down to Size?

Some very ordinary events—combined with negative thinking habits—can produce major stress. Other events are stressful to even the most optimistic or resilient people.

When you examine your stress producers, review the pressures that may have been part of your life for so long you may not immediately identify them as stressors. Examples include a declining relationship with your partner; declining job performance; an ongoing effort to hide your symptoms; or financial problems such as battles with insurance companies or entitlement programs.

Doing this may help start the process of identifying resources. You may want to consider a marriage counselor, job coach, financial planner, patient advocate, or accommodation at work. Regardless of the stressor, stress is never trivial.

Talk Your Way out of Stress

Sharing your thoughts and feelings can relieve stress. Building a support network of people who know about your illness and the difficulties you face is one way to gain a wider range of opinions.

Talking with others can sometimes help you see the things that cause you stress in a new light. There are more than 1,600 self-help groups affiliated with the National MS Society. Call 800-344-4867 for a list of groups that are near you or can be reached by telephone. There may be one that's right for you. You might also find the online MS-specific chat rooms offered by our collaborative partner, MS World (msworld.org) to be very helpful.

Talking with friends and family often means educating them so that they will better understand your experience. Some people can do this on their own; other people prefer the help of a social worker or other counselor to help them communicate with the important people in their lives. Your Society chapter can give you referrals.

Expressing Anger

Letting your anger out can relieve stress—and it is most effective when done without blaming others. You might say "I'm so angry" instead of "You make me so angry." After expressing your anger, you may want to do a few cycles of deep breathing to help you regain your calm. When calm, make a plan to face the underlying situation that made you so angry. Expressing anger may relieve stress, but it doesn't change the situation.

Reopening the Issues

Every time we meet someone new, or start a new job, we have to find out where we can assert ourselves and where we need to make changes or compromises. People with MS often negotiate and renegotiate as symptoms come and go, particularly if their abilities have been altered. In telling others how you feel, always mention that MS is changeable and that flexibility in expectations (yours and theirs) is key. Leave the door open.

This Is More Than Just Stress

Depression is a common disorder that is generally related to a chemical imbalance. According to the *Archives of General Psychology,* major depressive disorder affects approximately 14.8 million American adults, or about 6.7 percent of the population age 18 and older, in a given year. There is evidence that people with MS have an even greater incidence of depression than the general population. In MS, depression may be associated with the biology of the disease. Although depression is a serious illness, it can be treated effectively. Diagnosis and treatment require a professional therapist who is experienced with MS patients or one who is willing to work with your MS professional.

Special Problems with Stress, Depression, and MS

Some of the symptoms of stress are remarkably similar to symptoms of depression and some mimic or overlap symptoms of multiple sclerosis. Depression is very common in MS. The research shows that more than 50 percent of people with MS will experience significant depression at some point along the way. In addition, some studies suggest that people who are taking an interferon beta medication (Avonex®, Betaseron®, Extavia® or Rebif®) may be at even greater risk for depression.

Depression causes people to lose interest in their usual activities. In addition, they often experience five or more of the symptoms listed, to some degree. (Notice that symptoms such as fatigue or inability to concentrate can also be symptoms of MS.)

If you, or those close to you, think that you have become depressed or if you have had five or more of these symptoms continue for more than 2 weeks, talk to your physician or to a mental health professional.

Each of the interferon medications used to treat multiple sclerosis carries a warning that the medication should be used with caution by persons who have a history of depression. If you are taking an interferon medication for your MS, have a history of depression, or experience significant changes in mood, please talk with your doctor.

Signs of Depression

- Sleeping too much or too little

- Marked changes in appetite, or weight gain or loss

- Agitation and anxiety or a slowing down of mental and physical activity

- Decreased energy and increased fatigue

- Feelings of worthlessness, guilt, and self-reproach

- Indecisiveness, memory loss, difficulty in concentrating

- Feeling "blue" or "down in the dumps" most of the day, nearly every day

- Loss of interest in doing things that normally would interest you; difficulty feeling pleasure when things happen that would normally be pleasurable

- Thoughts of death or suicide or of harming yourself or others

Cognition and Stress

Not long ago, cognitive changes were thought to be rare in MS. Today MS-related cognitive changes are known to occur in about half the people with MS. As with all other symptoms of MS, the type and the extent of cognitive problems differ widely from person to person. Many of these changes are minimal. Only 10 percent of people with MS have severe cognitive problems.

The most common problems are in the areas of recall or recent memory, speed of thinking or information processing, and the ability to focus and sustain attention. Changes in planning and problem-solving abilities are also relatively common.

These cognitive changes are a consequence of MS lesions in the brain—not caused by stress, depression, medication, or fatigue. But stress can also affect thinking. In times of great stress it is common for anyone to forget things, or have difficulty concentrating or making decisions—changes that can be confusing and worrisome to a person with MS.

These sorts of stress-related lapses are temporary and improve when the stressful time passes. If you notice cognitive symptoms, no matter what you think might be the cause, it is important to talk with your physician about what you are experiencing. Having problems with cognition can cause or exacerbate stress. The loss of any ability is stressful—and so is the fear of that loss.

The National MS Society has published a helpful booklet on this subject. *Solving Cognitive Problems,* by Dr. Nicholas LaRocca, explains cognitive problems in detail—and what can be done about them. People with MS-related cognitive problems may find it helpful to develop or concentrate on these strategies to reduce stress due to cognitive problems.

For example:

- Keep a daily diary or a notebook for lists to reduce the stress of trying to recall a day's activities.

- Ask for written information and instructions to reduce the need for remembering details.

- Share concerns and responsibilities with others to lighten your load practically and emotionally.

- Discuss cognitive rehabilitation techniques—designed to improve performance—with your MS professional.

- Practice some form of stress management on a daily basis.

- Ask your National MS Society chapter for information and assistance.

Techniques and Strategies for Taming Stress

Everyday Strategies

See if you can get everyday stress under control:

- Simplify your life. Relax a few standards. Let the grass grow. Ask yourself if you want to do a particular task, if it needs to be done perfectly, or not at all.

- Plan ahead in situations that could cause stress. Take a book with you if waiting may be necessary. Make plans for where to meet or call if plans go awry.

- Get extra sleep before family gatherings or important events.
- Learn to say no. You don't have to do anything if you don't have the time, energy or desire.
- Make your requests for help as specific as possible: "Would you please help me by . . . "
- If old interests and activities become more difficult or too time consuming, replace them with new ones that fit your current needs.
- Get very practical:
  - Make an extra set of keys.
  - Update your telephone/address directory.
  - Keep the car and other important appliances in good working order.
  - If small things you need don't work, get new ones: Shoelaces, alarm clock, can opener.
  - Keep a good supply of small items you use all the time: Toilet paper, batteries, stamps, change for the bus.
  - Investigate and use gadgets, aids, and devices that save time or effort.
- Do the unpleasant things early in the day so that you don't have to worry about them.
- Carry a notebook to write yourself—and others—notes for the day, the week, the month.
- If you find that you are breathing in a short, shallow pattern, it's time to take a break. That kind of breathing often accompanies stress. To break the pattern, sit down for a minute. Take deep, slow breaths and relax all your muscles.
- Don't try to answer the phone on the first ring. Let it ring. Consider buying an answering machine.
- Make a 3/4 rule: Fill the gas tank when it is 3/4 empty; order more medication when it is 3/4 gone; replace juice when the quart is 3/4 gone.
- When you find a task difficult or stress producing, try to find a better way of doing it. If you can't think of an easier way, ask a friend to help you look at the problem. Once you have found a solution,

you might want to make a note of it to remind yourself of good choices you have made that might be adapted for other problems.

- If the morning rush is stressful:

  - Get up 15 minutes earlier.

  - Ask someone else to take on a morning task.

  - Do some of the preparation the night before.

  - Make sure that all your morning tasks are absolutely necessary.

- Make equal exchanges in your life. Do you find it too stressful to travel to see your family and friends? Give yourself permission to use the same money to make regular phone visits.

- Use your imagination to get yourself used to an event you are not looking forward to. You need to visit a new doctor? Imagine what you are going to wear, what questions you want to ask, what questions will be asked of you. Think about the visit the way you would like it to be. Then imagine the worst thing that could happen and how you would deal with it.

- Remind yourself that you are a person—not a "multiple sclerosis patient."

- Drive 10 miles an hour slower. And try a new route from time to time. If long car rides cause you stress, listen to audiotapes of books or pleasant music.

- Schedule rest periods. (You may want to set an alarm to tell you that it's time to rest.) Knowing that you are going to rest on a regular basis can stop you from feeling guilty about doing it.

- Try to do something you enjoy each day.

- Sit quietly for a minute or two before starting your meal. Say grace if you wish, or just notice—really notice—where you are, what you are eating, who you are with.

- Take a shower at the end of the day. Let water carry cares down the drain.

- Spend as much time as possible with people who aren't worriers.

- Learn to revise time schedules. If you told a friend you would meet at noon, and you are running late, is there any reason the appointment can't be changed to 1:00?

- Do one thing at a time. Don't think about the next task before you have finished the one you are working on. Let yourself feel a sense of accomplishment before moving on.

- Boredom can be stressful: Take a course, join a club, learn a new skill.

- Eat regular, balanced meals. Keep prepared foods in the house for times when you don't feel like cooking or shopping.

- Reduce reliance on cigarettes, caffeine, and alcohol. Ask your doctor for help if necessary.

- Work toward the "Best Sense of Humor" award; don't try for "Gets the Most Done."

- Ask for help when you need it.

- Use support and education services. Let the experiences of others help you solve problems—and your experiences to help others.

Relaxation

One of the most unhelpful things that you can be asked is "Why don't you just relax?"

Relaxation isn't something you just decide to do. People have to learn to relax. You can discover what works for you, and then practice.

There is no one right way to relax. Some people find that reading, listening to music, meditation, or prayer in a quiet room relaxes them. Others garden, paint, cook, or do puzzles.

Many people use one or more of the relaxation techniques described in the following text. Read through the descriptions and consider which might be best for you. Give one a try for a month or so. If it doesn't work, try another. And try again. Different methods of managing stress through relaxation may work better at different times.

To make relaxation easier, give yourself permission to take time for yourself. Don't feel guilty about shutting a door and telling everyone to give you some alone time.

Deep Breathing

Deep breathing can help reduce tension and allow your mind and body to feel more comfortable. The exercise takes only a few minutes and can be done almost anywhere at any time. Try deep breathing to start the day and then repeat it several times throughout the day.

Deep breathing can also help you relax just before an event that might be stressful.

NOTE: You may want to make a tape of these instructions to play while you are learning the exercises.

1. Sit with your back straight and your shoulders comfortably back.

2. Put your hand on your belly, below the waist, so that you can feel your breathing.

3. Inhale through your nose slowly and deeply. The air will feel cool. Concentrate on the feeling of the air as it moves into all parts of your body.

4. As the air reaches your belly, let your belly expand. Some people tend to tighten their bellies as they breathe in. Your hands on your belly will let you feel the movement.

5. Draw in as much air as you can. Then, hold your breath for a few seconds—four or five is fine. You don't need to distract yourself by counting unless it makes you more comfortable.

6. Begin to exhale. Shape your lips as if you were going to whistle and slowly breathe out between your lips. Use your lips to control how fast you exhale.

7. Concentrate on the feeling of the air leaving all parts of your body. The air coming out should feel warm.

8. Your hands will let you feel the breath leave your body. Your belly will deflate and as it does, the large muscle under your ribs—the diaphragm—will get larger.

9. When you feel your lungs empty, sit quietly for a moment and then repeat the inhale/exhale cycle. Repeat the cycle four or five times.

10. Sit quietly for a minute or two.

Clear Your Mind

The "Clear Your Mind" exercise is an enjoyable relaxation exercise for many. However, it takes practice to do it well, and may seem deceptively easy. This exercise may be frustrating or require more practice if there are difficulties with attention and concentration.

1. Choose a time when you have about 10 minutes available in a place that is relatively free of noise and distraction and where you will not be interrupted.

2. Loosen tight clothing, remove your shoes, and sit in a position that is comfortable.

3. Close your eyes and do two inhale/exhale cycles of deep breathing.

4. With your eyes still closed, picture in your mind a pleasant, restful place. Try to visualize as many details as possible: What objects are present, the color of the sky, who is present, etc. Concentrate on that place. Watch the wind blow on the trees or the water. Notice how the leaves turn slowly. Imagine your other senses experiencing the scene. Feel the gentle cool breeze on your skin. Breathe deeply and slowly, and imagine the smells associated with your scene, perhaps the fresh salty air of the ocean, or the clean woodsy smell of the country. Imagine hearing the sounds associated with your scene, perhaps the sound of the breeze moving softly through the trees or the call of birds.

5. Some people have difficulty visualizing or creating a "picture" in their mind's eye. If this is the case, you may find this exercise is not for you. An alternative approach is to follow steps 1 through 3 above. Instead of visualizing a relaxing scene in step 4, concentrate on a word—"calm"—or a thought —"I am loved."

6 Don't worry if other thoughts or images break in—it isn't easy to clear your mind. When you notice your mind has drifted, gently return your thoughts to your image or word. If you have trouble, do another cycle of deep breathing and try again. It may take considerable practice to learn to clear your mind. As you do so, the relaxation will become deeper and you will feel refreshed and more energetic.

7. End the mind clearing by stretching—to reawaken your body to the world around you—and exhaling.

Meditation

You may want to continue on to deeper meditation once you have learned to clear your mind. Many people find that meditation greatly decreases the stress in their lives. It takes about 15 minutes once or twice a day. Try to meditate at the same times each day.

1. Sit as you would for mind clearing in a quiet place, free from distractions. Unplug the phone and close the door. Tell everyone you are going to be busy for 15 minutes.

2. Do two or three cycles of deep breathing.

3. Pick a word or phrase that makes you feel calm. Although any word will do, many people find that words that end in an m or n sound are most helpful—words like "calm," "home," "noon," or "one."

4. Close your eyes and repeat the word or phrase over and over either in your mind or out loud. Concentrate on the way the word sounds inside your head. Try not to think about what you are doing or how you are feeling.

5. If you have trouble relaxing or concentrating on the word, stop, do a cycle of deep breathing, and try again.

6. End the exercise by gently stretching and exhaling.

7. Although 15 minutes may be the ultimate goal of the meditation period, the actual time isn't really important.

Be realistic. Don't worry if you only are able to concentrate for a few minutes at first. Just sit quietly for the rest of the time period. (Just sitting quietly will do you good.) With practice, the time and the depth of relaxation will increase.

Visualization

Visualization is a combination of meditation, clearing your mind, imagination, and deep breathing. With visualization you do more than just see an appealing scene. You move yourself—in your mind—into the picture. You watch yourself reaching your hand out to pick a flower or to trail your fingers through a sunlit stream. You go to the beach and let the sand sift through your hand onto your leg.

Start the exercise by doing three or four cycles of deep breathing, and end the exercise by stretching and exhaling. If you can't enter the picture at first, do a cycle or two of deep breathing and try again. As with the "Clear Your Mind" exercise, try to experience the scene with as many of your senses as possible. Hear the sound the rushing stream makes, and how the sound changes as you change the position of your hand. Smell the cool fresh scent of the stream, and feel the water on your fingers. The entire exercise can take as little as 5 and as long as 15 minutes.

Progressive Muscle Relaxation

Progressive muscle relaxation is often used as an aid to stress management. And, done in bed before you go to sleep, it can be an aid to a sound night's sleep.

Going through your body's entire group of muscles—tensing, relaxing, and focusing on the changes—will take about 12 to 15 minutes. If it takes less than that, you are moving at a non-relaxing speed. These exercises will provide the most benefit if you do them twice a day. If there are some muscle groups that you cannot work with comfortably, skip them.

If you have significant spasticity in some muscles, strongly tensing those muscle groups could trigger a spasm. You may want to speak with a physical therapist or other MS health professional about ways to work in a more comfortable way.

Many people, especially those with cognitive problems, find that the exercises are easier to do along with a prerecorded tape. You can prepare the tape yourself or ask someone with a relaxing voice to do it for you.

You will work with each of 17 muscle groups in a specific order. Tense, but don't strain each muscle group. Hold the tense position for the slow count of five, paying attention to the way those muscles feel. Relax the muscles—letting them go totally limp. Focus for a count of five on how the muscles feel when relaxed.

To prepare for the exercise, wear comfortable, loose-fitting clothing, remove glasses or contact lenses, and sit up in a chair without crossing your legs or arms. You may also do this lying down in bed.

1. Clench both hands. Focus on how your hands feel and how the tension moves into the forearms. Relax. Notice what the muscles in your hands and forearms feel like now.

2. Touch your fingers to your shoulders. Raise your arms level with your shoulders. Focus on the tension in your biceps and upper arms. Relax and focus on the change in feeling.

3. Shrug your shoulders, raising them as high as possible. Focus on the tension in your shoulders. Relax and focus on the change.

4. Wrinkle your forehead. Notice where tension occurs—around your eyes and forehead. Relax and focus on the change.

5. Close your eyes tightly. Focus on the tension. Relax and focus on the change.

6. Clench your teeth. Focus on the tension in your jaw, mouth, and chin. Relax and focus on the change.

7. Press as much of your tongue as possible onto the roof of your mouth. Focus on the tension in your mouth and throat. Relax and focus on the change.

8. Move your head slowly backwards as far as you comfortably can, keeping your shoulders level. Focus on the tension in your neck and upper back. Relax and focus on the change.

9. Pull your head forward, down onto your chest. Focus on the tension in your neck, shoulders, and upper back. Relax and focus on the change. NOTE: If you experience Lhermitte's sign—an electrical-like shock—in your spine when you tip your neck forward, skip this step.

10. Move away from the back of your chair, arch your back, and push your arms upward. Focus on the tension in your back and shoulders. Relax and focus on the change.

11. Fill your lungs with air and hold the breath. Focus on the tension in your chest and back. Exhale all the way, relax, and focus on the change.

12. Pull your stomach as far back toward your spine as you can. Focus on the tension in your stomach muscles and changes in your breathing. Relax and focus on the change.

13. Without pulling your stomach in, tense your stomach muscles. Focus on the tension. Relax and focus on the change.

14. Tense the muscles in your buttocks. Focus on the tension. Relax and focus on the change.

15. Flex your thigh muscles by straightening your legs or tensing the muscles. Focus on the tension. Relax and focus on the change.

16. Lift your feet off of the ground. Point your toes up, your heels down. Focus on the tension in your feet, ankles, and calves. Lower your feet, relax, and focus on the change.

17. Lift your feet slightly and curl your toes all the way down. Focus on the tension on the top of your feet and in your arches. Lower your feet, relax, and focus on the change.

After you have learned to be aware of tension in all 17 muscle groups, you may want to focus only on those groups that give you the most trouble. Tense and relax those groups—often the jaw, neck, and stomach—several times during the day. Check your "high tension" muscle groups from time to time to judge how relaxed you are.

Yoga

Yoga involves breathing exercises and a range of stretches that revolve around the spine. Yoga increases the body's flexibility and releases tension. Many community centers have courses in yoga. Some of the movements may be easy for you. Other movements may need practice or adaptation. And still others may need to be omitted. Discuss your plans with your physician or physical therapist before you begin.

Tai Chi

Tai chi involves deep breathing, slow gentle movements, and relaxation. As a conditioning regime, it is considered more gentle than yoga. Many of the positions can be done while sitting. Discuss your plans with your physician or physical therapist and ask your Society chapter about "adapted" tai chi classes in your area.

Traditional Exercise Programs

Any physical activity done on a regular basis has been found to reduce stress and improve physical and mental health. Walking, swimming, or gardening can all relieve stress. Speak with your physician or physical therapist about developing a program to suit your needs and abilities.

There Is No "Right Way"

It is important to remember that there is no "right way" to cope with stress. Even within the same family, some members may handle the MS situation by wanting to talk about it, read about it, and participate in support groups; others may ignore it much of the time. If an approach is working for you, you may be tempted to conclude it is the right way for your loved ones.

Dr. Nicholas LaRocca, an expert on coping and MS, advises people to recognize that no one method is inherently better or worse than any other. Family members and professionals should refrain from passing judgment on what is "healthy" or "right" for others. Respect is a stress reducer by itself.

Chapter 18

Obesity, Cortisol, and Stress

Does stress affect eating, weight, and where fat is distributed on the body? This is a question that has begged an answer from experts for many years. The body makes cortisol to help us handle stress. When stress goes up, cortisol levels go up. And it's often repeated that obese people have higher cortisol levels than lean people.

Cortisol is a hormone in a group of steroids commonly referred to as glucocorticoids. Cortisol is a hormone produced by the adrenal gland as a part of your daily hormonal cycle. However, it is also a key hormone involved in the body's response to stress, both physical and emotional. Cortisol increases blood sugar levels, increases blood pressure, and suppresses the immune system, which is part of the body's fight-or-flight response that is essential for survival. Your hypothalamus, via the pituitary gland, directs the adrenal glands to secrete both cortisol and adrenaline.

Adrenaline production increases your alertness and energy level, also increasing your metabolism by helping fat cells to release energy. Cortisol has widespread actions which help restore homeostasis after stress, including increasing production of glucose from protein to quickly increase the body's energy during stressful times.

However, cortisol has a two-fold effect on fat. When the stress first occurs, fat is broken down to supply the body with a rapid source of energy. When we experience something stressful, our brains release a

"Cortisol and Weight," © 2007 ProjectAware (www.project-aware.org). Reprinted with permission.

substance known as corticotropin-releasing hormone (CRH), which puts the body on alert and sends it into "fight or flight" mode. As the body gears up for battle, the pupils dilate, thinking improves, and the lungs take in more oxygen. But something else happens as well: Our appetite is suppressed, and the digestive system shuts off temporarily. CRH also triggers the release of the hormones adrenaline and cortisol, which help mobilize carbohydrate and fat for quick energy. When the immediate stress is over, the adrenaline dissipates, but the cortisol lingers to help bring the body back into balance. And one of the ways it gets things back to normal is to increase our appetites so we can replace the carbohydrate and fat we should have burned while fleeing or fighting.

"But when was the last time you responded to stress with such physicality?" asks Dr. Pamela Peeke, author of *Fight Fat After Forty* and an assistant clinical professor of medicine at the University of Maryland School of Medicine. Your body assumes you have just physically exerted yourself, for example running from a lion, and need to restock your reserves by eating a lot of carbohydrates or fatty food that can easily be stored as fat. In reality, you are probably still sitting in your car or at your desk, still fuming and stressed out. Dr. Peeke notes that, "In today's modern world, this elegant survival mechanism may be an anachronism that causes the body to refuel when it doesn't need to. Sustained stress keeps up cortisol, that cursed hunger promoter, elevated and that keeps appetite up, too."

This is where the potential second effect of cortisol comes into play. Experts now believe that the problem for many of us is being in a constant state of stress. Exposure to cortisol over the long term can lead to weight gain, as your appetite and insulin levels are continuously increased. If stress and cortisol levels stay high, so will insulin levels, says Robert M. Sapolsky, PhD, a professor of biological sciences and neuroscience at Stanford University. Continual stress leads to a constant state of excess cortisol production, which stimulates glucose production. This excess glucose then typically is converted into fat, ending up as stored fat. According to Dr. Sapolsky, "The net effect of this will be increased fat deposition in a certain part of the body." Furthermore, according to the authors of the book *The Cortisol Connection,* stress and the resulting chronic overload of cortisol, make you feel tired and listless. So you overeat to renew your energy and comfort yourself, with the end result of accumulated extra inches around the middle.[1]

It is generally suggested that stress-induced cortisol weight is usually gained around the waistline, because fat cells in that area are more sensitive to cortisol. The fat cells in your abdomen are richer in stress hormone receptors, are particularly sensitive to high insulin, and are very effective at storing energy—more so than fat cells you would find in other areas of the body. This is the most dangerous place to gain weight, as it can lead to metabolic syndrome, diabetes, and heart disease.

A recent study conducted by researchers at Yale University compared women who stored fat primarily in their abdomens with women who stored it mostly in their hips. They found that the women with belly fat reported feeling more threatened by stressful tasks and having more stressful lives. They also produced higher levels of cortisol than the women with fat on their hips. And that, the authors reasoned, suggests that cortisol causes fat to be stored in the center of the body.[2]

However, some researchers believe that cortisol's connection to obesity may be more unsubstantiated than first thought and that cortisol levels may not be the sole, major factor involved in obesity and fat distribution. There are questions as to whether cortisol may rise prior to weight gain or if its increase is an impact of the weight itself.

One area of research involves mutations in a gene called the proopiomelanocortin (POMC) gene, which may cause obesity but simultaneously decreases glucocorticoid levels. This research shows that cortisol alone may not be the major culprit in weight gain, and suggests that glucocorticoids are merely part of a chain of hormonal and neuronal signals associated with obesity.[3]

"The message has gotten across that glucocorticoids are involved in all obesity. And there is a lot of common talk about the role of stress in increasing glucocorticoids," says Malcolm Low, MD, PhD, a senior scientist and associate director in the OHSU [Oregon Health Sciences University] Center for the Study of Weight Regulation and Associated Disorders. "It seems to make sense: There is a lot of stress today, and obesity is up. But when you look at the facts, it is not as clear." Low notes, "There are multiple controls in our body that regulate body weight and appetite. Glucocorticoids are clearly involved in control of body weight. But it is not the only hormone involved. There are multiple systems involved in the brain and outside the brain that regulate how much fat we are going to have and how much appetite. There is no simple answer to treating obesity."

Marci Gluck, PhD, of the New York Obesity Research Center at St. Luke's-Roosevelt Hospital and Columbia University, studies the complicated relationship between cortisol, stress, and weight gain. "Most scientists agree that it is not a simple one-to-one relationship between cortisol and weight gain," she says. "There are so many different peptides and hormones involved. Cortisol might not be the primary one."

Based on a review of literature addressing obesity and cortisol status, the two most integral lab parameters to assess systemic cortisol status and its relationship to obesity is measurement of daily cortisol production rate (CPR) and measurement of 24-hour mean plasma cortisol concentrations.[4–7] Thus far, few studies have utilized these parameters for measurement of cortisol concentration in obesity, and of the studies that have been done using these parameters, none of these publications has reported elevated plasma cortisol concentrations in obese individuals.[7, 9–11]

However, recent reports have suggested that a state of elevated cortisol levels in fat tissue cells without elevated cortisol levels in the blood may exist in obesity.[4] Yet, these findings are inconsistent. It is possible that high levels of cortisol within the cells, such as in fat cells, may play a causative role in obesity, but this possibility requires further investigation.

If we do accept that chronic stress and elevated cortisol may be factors in weight problems, what can you do if you want to reduce cortisol? First, focus on becoming stress resistant. One of the best things to reduce stress and improve insulin sensitivity, for example, is getting regular exercise, even a daily brisk walk. Exercise not only helps promote weight loss by burning calories, but is also beneficial because it helps neutralize stress and its effects, which in turn helps you keep weight off. Just a daily brisk walk can help to distract yourself from what is causing stress in your life, allowing your body time to move and awaken.

Second, practice stress reduction techniques such as meditation, yoga, and breathing exercises. Improving time management can also be essential to reducing stress in one's hectic lifestyle. These activities or similar techniques, as well as getting adequate sleep, can help reduce your body's physiological response to daily stressors.

Third, how a person perceives stressful situations is also important. One individual may feel major stress from a particular situation, whereas another person will handle it better by using the event as an opportunity to learn. Hence, stress makes life difficult, but our reaction to it is important as well.

References

1. Talbot S, Kramer W. *The Cortisol Connection. 1st ed.* Berkeley, CA: Publishers Group West, 2002.

2. Epel ES, McEwen B, Seeman T, Matthews K, Castellazzo G, Brownell KD, Bell J, Ickovics JR. Stress and body shape:

Stress-induced cortisol secretion is consistently greater among women with central fat. *Psychosom Med.* 2000 Sep-Oct;62(5):623–32.

3. Smart JL, Tolle V, Low MJ. Glucocorticoids exacerbate obesity and insulin resistance in neuron-specific proopiomelanocortin-deficient mice. *J Clin Invest.* 2006 Feb;116(2):495–505. Epub 2006 Jan 26. Erratum in: *J Clin Invest.* 2006 Mar;116(3):842.

4. Salehi M, Ferenczi A, Zmoff B. Obesity and Cortisol Status. *Horm Metab Res* 2005;37:193–197.

5. Prezio JA, Carreon G, Clerkin E, Meloni CR, Kyle LH, Canary JJ. Influence of body composition on adrenal function in obesity. *J Clin Endocrinol Metab* 1964;24:481–485.

6. Streeten DH, Stevenson CT, Dalakos TG, Nicholas JJ, Dennick LG, Fellerman H. The diagnosis of hypercortisolism: Biochemical criteria differentiating patients from lean and obese normal subjects and from female on oral contraceptives. *J Clin Endocrinol Metab* 1969;29:1191–211.

7. Jessop DS, Dallman MF, Flaming D, Lightman SL. Resistance to glucocorticoid feedback in obesity. *J Clin Endocrinol Metab* 2001;86:4109–4114.

8. Hellman L, Nakada F, Curti J Et al. Cortisol is secreted episodically by normal man. *J Clin Endocrinol Metab* 1970;30:411–422.

9. Chalew SA, Nagel H, Burt D, Edwards CR. The integrated concentration of cortisone is reduced in obese children. *J Pediatr Endocrinal Metab* 1997; 10: 287–290.

10. Chalew SA, Lozano RA, Armour KM, Zadik Z, Kowarski AA. Reduction of plasma cortisol levels in childhood obesity. *J Pediatr* 1991; 119: 778–780.

11. Strain GW, Zumoff B, Kream J, Strain JJ, Levin J, Fukushia D. Sex difference in the influence of obesity on the 24 hr mean plasma concentration of cortisol. *Metabolism* 1982: 31: 209–212.

Chapter 19

Pain

Chapter Contents

Section 19.1

Chronic Pain and Stress-Related Disorders

From "Chronic Pain and PTSD: A Guide for Patients," by the
National Center for PTSD (www.ptsd.va.gov), part of the Veterans
Administration, June 15, 2010.

What is chronic pain?

Chronic pain is when a person suffers from pain in a particular area of the body (for example, in the back or the neck) for at least 3 to 6 months. It may be as bad as, or even worse than, short-term pain, but it can feel like more of a problem because it lasts a longer time. Chronic pain lasts beyond the normal amount of time that an injury takes to heal.

Chronic pain can come from many things. Some people get chronic pain from normal wear and tear of the body or from ageing. Others have chronic pain from various types of cancer, or other chronic medical illnesses. In some cases the chronic pain may be from an injury that happened during an accident or an assault. Some chronic pain has no explanation.

How common is chronic pain?

Approximately one in three Americans suffer from some kind of chronic pain in their lifetimes, and about one quarter of them are not able to do day-to-day activities because of their chronic pain. Between 80% and 90% of Americans experience chronic problems in the neck or lower back.

How do health care providers evaluate pain?

Care providers generally assess chronic pain during a physical exam, but how much pain someone is in is hard to determine. Every person is different and perceives and experiences pain in different ways. There is often very little consistency when different doctors try to measure a patient's pain. Sometimes the care provider may not believe the patient, or might minimize the amount of pain. All of these things can be frustrating for the person in pain. Additionally, this kind of experience often makes patients feel helplessness and hopeless, which in turn increases tension and pain and makes the person more upset. Conversation between the doctor and patient is important, including sharing information about treatment options. If no progress is made, get a second opinion.

What is the experience of chronic pain like physically?

There are many forms of chronic pain, including pain felt in the low back (most common); the neck; the mouth, face, and jaw (TMJ); the pelvis; or the head (e.g., tension and migraine headaches). Of course, each type of condition results in different experiences of pain.

People with chronic pain are less able to function well in daily life than those who do not suffer from chronic pain. They may have trouble with things such as walking, standing, sitting, lifting light objects, doing paperwork, standing in line at a grocery store, going shopping, or working. Many patients with chronic pain cannot work because of their pain or physical limitations.

What is the experience of chronic pain like psychologically?

Research has shown that many patients who experience chronic pain (up to 100% of these patients) tend to also be diagnosed with depression. Because the pain and disability are always there and that may even become worse over time, many of them think suicide is the only way to end their pain and frustration. They think they have no control over their life. This frustration may also lead the person to use drugs or have unneeded surgery.

What is the relationship between chronic pain and PTSD?

Some people's chronic pain stems from a traumatic event, such as a physical or sexual assault, a motor vehicle accident, or some type of disaster. Under these circumstances the person may experience both chronic pain and PTSD. The person in pain may not even realize the connection between their pain and a traumatic event. Approximately 15% to 35% of patients with chronic pain also have PTSD. Only 2% of people who do not have chronic pain have PTSD. One study found that 51% of patients with chronic low back pain had PTSD symptoms. For people with chronic pain, the pain may actually serve as a reminder of the traumatic event, which will tend to make the PTSD even worse. Survivors of physical, psychological, or sexual abuse tend to be more at risk for developing certain types of chronic pain later in their lives.

Section 19.2

Back Pain and Stress

Could the day be coming when a person who complains of back pain be given a psychological assessment in addition to a physical one?

The list of potential triggers of back pain is a long one, including such factors as genetic predisposition, congenital malformations, and traumatic injuries. A growing number of studies affirm that the mind-body connection also plays a role in back pain, both in setting off an initial "back pain attack" and in contributing to ongoing chronic pain.

In several recent studies, psychological distress proved to increase the risk both of developing back pain and of experiencing a slow recovery. For instance, in a Swedish study, anxiety and the practice of "catastrophizing"—assuming the worst in any given situation—were found to increase the risk of developing back pain. And in a study conducted in this country, people who reported higher levels of anger and psychological distress also reported higher levels of chronic back pain. These and other findings underscore the need for a multidimensional view of back pain and the recognition that back pain can involve much more than just the muscles and bones of our backs.

Understanding the Connection between Stress and Your Back

By now, most of us are familiar with the "fight-or-flight" response. When confronted by a threat—whether physical or emotional, concrete or imagined—the hypothalamus releases noradrenaline and adrenaline. These and other related hormones trigger a complex cascade of actions, leading to a state of physiological and psychological hyperalertness.

The difficulty comes when this state of hyperalertness becomes our default setting. Stress is an inescapable fact of modern life. We now know that if we're hyperaware of the multitude of stressors we face on a daily level, we are predisposed to develop a number of diseases, including depression and heart disease.

On the musculoskeletal level, the fight-or-flight response causes muscles to tense in preparation for action—and if this response is not deactivated, muscles can go into painful spasms and severe back pain can result.

Breaking the Cycle That Leads to Back Pain

While stress-relaxation techniques can't make a stressful situation disappear, they can help you consciously release any muscle tension you may have accumulated in anticipation of or in response to the situation. Here are some techniques to consider to help relieve your back pain:

- **Breathing exercises:** One breathing technique that can quiet the fight-or-flight response is known as 2:1 breathing. Try a pattern of inhaling to the count of three and exhaling to the count of six. Repeat several times.

- **Body scan:** Begin by either lying or sitting down. Do several cycles of 2:1 breathing. Once you are fully relaxed, conduct a full mental sweep of your body, as though you were undergoing a deliberate and complete X-ray. Go slowly but steadily, noting any areas of tightness or tension. Once you've finished the scan, return to those tight or tense areas and let your attention linger there. Consciously "breathe into" those areas for several breathing cycles and imagine the muscles relaxing. The body scan takes time—but if it is done on a regular basis, it can help you become aware of the early warning signs of an impending back pain attack. In particular, it can help you become aware of your individual "signal spots," those places that hurt when your back first begins acting up but before a full-blown attack is already under way. You can then take action, pacing yourself appropriately.

- **Meditation:** This has been found to reduce stress and counteract the fight-or-flight response. One meditation technique is known as "taking the one chair." Imagine yourself in a room in which there is only a single chair. Sit down on the chair and observe your thoughts and emotions pass in front of you. Remember that you are occupying the only chair in the room, so your thoughts have no place to rest. Watch them pass on out of the room.

- **Exercise:** Exercise—particularly meditative exercise such as yoga, walking, or swimming—is a potent stress reducer. Be sure to ask your physician for guidelines relevant to your individual condition, just in case you should steer clear of a particular type of exercise.

Chapter 20

Pregnancy and Stress

Pregnancy is a time of many changes for a woman: in her body, in her emotions and in the life of her family. As welcome as these changes may be, they often add new stresses to the lives of busy pregnant women who already face many demands at home and at work.

Too much stress can be uncomfortable for anyone. In the short term, a high level of stress can cause fatigue, sleeplessness, anxiety, poor appetite or overeating, headaches, and backaches. When a high level of stress continues for a long period, it may contribute to potentially serious health problems, such as lowered resistance to infections, high blood pressure, and heart disease. High levels of stress also may pose some special risks for pregnant women.

Most women cope well with the emotional and physical changes of pregnancy and other stresses in their lives. A pregnant woman who feels she is coping well with stress (taking good care of herself, feeling energized rather than drained, and functioning well at home and work) probably does not face health risks from stress.

Pregnant women who are concerned about the level of stress in their lives should discuss their feelings with their partner, family, or friends. These individuals can often provide support, which can help reduce stress. A pregnant woman who is having trouble coping with stress also can ask her health care provider to refer her to resources in her community that can help her take steps to reduce and cope with stress.

What types of stress may affect pregnancy outcome?

Routine stresses, such as work deadlines and traffic delays, probably don't contribute much to pregnancy complications. Stress is not all bad. When managed properly, a little stress can provide us with the drive to meet new challenges.

But certain types of severe or long-lasting stress may pose a risk in pregnancy. Some studies suggest that women who experience negative life events, such as divorce, death in the family, serious illness, or loss of a job, may be at increased risk of having a premature (born before 37 completed weeks of pregnancy) and/or low birthweight (less than 5 1/2 pounds) baby.[1,2] However, most women who experience negative life events do not have adverse pregnancy outcomes. A recent study found that maternal characteristics including depression, panic disorder, drug use, domestic violence, and having two or more medical conditions were associated with high levels of stress during pregnancy.[3]

Women who experience a catastrophic event during pregnancy also may be at increased risk of having a premature and/or low-birthweight baby. One study found that pregnant women who worked within 2 miles of the World Trade Center in New York on September 11, 2001, had significantly shorter gestations and significantly smaller babies than women who worked farther from the site.[1,4] Another study found that pregnant women who experienced a major earthquake had shorter gestations than women who did not experience the event.[5] The timing of the event may influence pregnancy outcome. Studies suggest that women who experienced the World Trade Center attack or an earthquake in the first trimester of pregnancy tended to deliver earlier than women who experienced these catastrophic events later in pregnancy.[1,4,5]

Chronic stress may play a role in adverse pregnancy outcomes. A recent study found that low-income women with chronic stress (resulting from difficulty obtaining food, caring for a child with a chronic illness, or being unemployed) were at increased risk of having a low-birthweight baby.[6]

Racism is another form of chronic stress that may contribute to pregnancy problems. African-American women may experience stress from racism throughout their lifetime. This may help explain why African-American women are more likely to deliver premature and low-birthweight babies than women from other racial/ethnic groups.[1]

Some women may experience serious chronic stress over the pregnancy itself, possibly increasing their risk of adverse pregnancy outcomes.[1,2] These women may be especially worried about the health of their baby or about how they will cope with labor and delivery. They should discuss their concerns with their health care provider, who can refer them to a mental health professional, if needed.

Most women who experience severe stress in pregnancy have healthy, full-term babies. Some women may be more vulnerable than others to the effects of stress in pregnancy due to physical or other risk factors.[2]

What are the risks of high stress levels in pregnancy?

A number of studies suggest that high levels of stress in pregnancy may contribute to premature birth and low birthweight.[1,2] Babies born too small and too soon are at increased risk for health problems during the newborn period, lasting disabilities (such as mental retardation and cerebral palsy), and even death.

How may stress contribute to adverse pregnancy outcomes?

Researchers do not completely understand how stress may contribute to adverse pregnancy outcomes. However, certain stress-related hormones may play a role. For example, stress may contribute to preterm labor by triggering the release of a hormone called corticotropin-releasing hormone (CRH). CRH, which is produced by the brain and the placenta, is closely tied to labor. It prompts the body to release chemicals called prostaglandins, which help trigger uterine contractions.

Severe or prolonged stress may interfere with the functioning of the immune system. This could cause a pregnant woman to be more susceptible to infections involving the uterus. Uterine infections are an important cause of premature birth, especially those occurring at less than 28 weeks of pregnancy.[1]

Stress may affect a woman's behavior. Some women react to stress by smoking cigarettes, drinking alcohol, or taking illicit drugs, all of which have been linked to premature birth, low birthweight, and other pregnancy complications.[1] Use of alcohol and certain illicit drugs increases the risk of birth defects.

Does a high level of stress in pregnancy have long-term effects on the baby (besides any caused by prematurity and low birthweight)?

Some studies suggest that high levels of stress in pregnancy may affect a child's mental and emotional development.[7,8] Maternal stress may contribute to learning problems, such as difficulty paying attention, and to increased anxiety and fearfulness.[7,8] It is not known how maternal stress may cause these problems. However, some studies suggest that stress-related hormones in the mother's blood may cross the placenta and affect the fetus's developing brain.[8]

How can a pregnant woman reduce stress?

Each pregnant woman needs to identify the personal and work-related sources of stress in her life and develop effective ways to deal with them. If she feels overwhelmed by stress, she should consult her health care provider.

Pregnancy-related discomforts (such as nausea, fatigue, frequent urination, swelling, and backache) can be stressful, especially if a pregnant woman tries to do all the activities she did before pregnancy. She can help reduce her stress by recognizing that these symptoms are temporary and by asking her health care provider how to cope with them. A woman also can consider cutting back on unnecessary activities when she is uncomfortable.

Many pregnant women experience mood swings during pregnancy. These are caused by hormonal changes and are normal. However, mood swings may make it difficult for a pregnant woman to cope with stress.

A pregnant woman can cope better with the stresses in her life if she is healthy and fit. She should eat healthy foods; get plenty of sleep; avoid alcohol, cigarettes, and drugs; and exercise regularly (with her health care provider's OK). Exercise helps keep pregnant women fit, helps prevent some common discomforts of pregnancy (such as backache, fatigue, and constipation), and relieves stress.

Having a good support network, including the pregnant woman's partner, extended family, and friends can help a pregnant woman relieve stress. A pregnant woman should ask for and accept help from people who are close to her. For example, they can help her with routine chores and childcare, talk with her about her feelings and concerns, or go with her to prenatal visits. Some studies suggest that having a good support network reduces a woman's risk of having a low-birthweight baby.[1]

A number of stress-reduction techniques can be helpful for pregnant women. These include yoga classes for pregnant women, biofeedback, meditation, and guided mental imagery. A health care provider may be able to refer a pregnant woman to local classes or experts. Childbirth education classes teach relaxation techniques and help reduce anxiety by educating parents-to-be about what to expect during labor and delivery.

Does post-traumatic stress disorder affect pregnancy?

Some individuals who experience or witness a traumatic event, such as rape, combat, a natural disaster, terrorist attacks (such as the September 11 attack on the World Trade Center), or death of a loved one, develop post-traumatic stress disorder (PTSD). Affected individuals may experience severe anxiety, flashbacks of the event, nightmares, intense physical reactions to reminders of the event (such as palpitations and sweating), and other problems, such as startling easily.

Post-traumatic stress disorder is common during pregnancy. One study found that almost 8 percent of pregnant women are affected.[9] Women with PTSD may be at increased risk for a number of pregnancy complications, including miscarriage, hyperemesis gravidarum (a severe form of pregnancy-related vomiting), and preterm labor.[9] Affected women also are more likely to have risky health behaviors, such as smoking, drinking alcohol, or drug use, that can contribute to pregnancy complications.[10] Women who suspect that they have PTSD should discuss their symptoms with their health care provider or a mental health professional. There are a number of effective treatments, including talk therapies, that can ease symptoms.

Does the March of Dimes support research on stress in pregnancy?

March of Dimes grantees are studying the connection between stress reactions and adverse pregnancy outcomes.

A number of recent grantees have been seeking to determine how stress-related factors in a pregnant woman's environment (including home and neighborhood conditions, racism, occupation, income, and major life events) may contribute to her risk for preterm labor. These studies may improve understanding of the causes of preterm labor, and lead to new ways to prevent and treat it.

Another grantee is evaluating the cognitive and behavioral functioning of 11-year-old children who were in utero at the time of a natural disaster (Quebec ice storm of 1998). This study could lead to better recommendations for how to prevent or limit potential harm of intense stress to pregnant women and their developing babies.

References

1. Institute of Medicine Committee on Understanding Premature Birth and Assuring Healthy Outcomes, Board on Health Sciences Policy, Behrman, R.E., and Butler, A.S. (eds.). *Preterm*

Birth: Causes, Consequences, and Prevention. Washington, DC, The National Academies Press, 2006.

2. American College of Obstetricians and Gynecologists (ACOG). Psychosocial Risk Factors: Perinatal Screening and Intervention. ACOG Committee Opinion, number 343, August 2006.

3. Woods, S.M., Melville, J.L., Guo, Y., Fan, M.-Y. & Gavin, A. Psychosocial Stress During Pregnancy. *American Journal of Obstetrics and Gynecology,* volume 202, number 1, pages 61.e1-61.e7, January 2010.

4. Lederman, S.A., et al. The Effects of the World Trade Center Event on Birth Outcomes among Term Deliveries at Three Lower Manhattan Hospitals. *Environmental Health Perspectives,* volume 112, number 17, December 2004, pages 1772–1778.

5. Glynn, L.M., et al. When Stress Happens Matters: Effects of Earthquake Timing on Stress Responsivity in Pregnancy. *American Journal of Obstetrics and Gynecology,* volume 184, number 4, March 2001, pages 637–642.

6. Borders, A.E.B., et al. Chronic Stress and Low Birthweight Neonates in a Low-Income Population of Women. *Obstetrics and Gynecology,* volume 109, number 2, part 1, February 2007, pages 331–338.

7. Bergman, K., et al. Maternal Stress During Pregnancy Predicts Cognitive Ability and Fearfulness in Infancy. *Journal of the American Academy of Child and Adolescent Psychiatry,* volume 46, number 11, November 2007, pages 1454–1463.

8. Talge, N.M., et al. Antenatal Maternal Stress and Long-Term Effects on Child Neurodevelopment: How and Why? *Journal of Child Psychol Psychiatry,* volume 48, number 3-4, March-April 2007, pages 245–261.

9. Cook, C.A.L., et al. Posttraumatic Stress Disorder in Pregnancy: Prevalence, Risk Factors, and Treatment. *Obstetrics and Gynecology,* volume 103, 2004, pages 710–717.

10. Morland, L., et al. Posttraumatic Stress Disorder and Pregnancy Health: Preliminary Update and Implications. *Psychosomatics,* volume 48, number 4, July-August 2007, pages 304–308.

Chapter 21

Skin Problems

Chapter Contents

Section 21.1

What Is Psoriasis?

Excerpted from "Questions and Answers about Psoriasis," by the National Institute of Arthritis and Musculoskeletal and Skin Diseases (NIAMS, www.niams.nih.gov), part of the National Institutes of Health, April 2009.

Psoriasis is a chronic (long-lasting) skin disease of scaling and inflammation that affects greater than 3 percent of the United States population, or more than 5 million adults. Although the disease occurs in all age groups, it primarily affects adults. It appears about equally in males and females.

Psoriasis occurs when skin cells quickly rise from their origin below the surface of the skin and pile up on the surface before they have a chance to mature. Usually this movement (also called turnover) takes about a month, but in psoriasis it may occur in only a few days.

In its typical form, psoriasis results in patches of thick, red (inflamed) skin covered with silvery scales. These patches, which are sometimes referred to as plaques, usually itch or feel sore. They most often occur on the elbows, knees, other parts of the legs, scalp, lower back, face, palms, and soles of the feet, but they can occur on skin anywhere on the body. The disease may also affect the fingernails, the toenails, and the soft tissues of the genitals, and inside the mouth. Although it is not unusual for the skin around affected joints to crack, about 30 percent of those with psoriasis experience joint inflammation that produces symptoms of arthritis. This condition is called psoriatic arthritis.

Psoriasis and Quality of Life

Individuals with psoriasis may experience significant physical discomfort and some disability. Itching and pain can interfere with basic functions, such as self-care, walking, and sleep. Plaques on hands and feet can prevent individuals from working at certain occupations, playing some sports, and caring for family members or a home. The frequency of medical care is costly and can interfere with an employment or school schedule. People with moderate to severe psoriasis may feel self-conscious about their appearance and have a poor self-image that stems from fear of public rejection and psychosexual concerns. Psychological distress can lead to significant depression and social isolation.

Causes of Psoriasis

Psoriasis is a skin disorder driven by the immune system, especially involving a type of white blood cell called a T cell. Normally, T cells help protect the body against infection and disease. In the case of psoriasis, T cells are put into action by mistake and become so active that they trigger other immune responses, which lead to inflammation and to rapid turnover of skin cells.

In many cases, there is a family history of psoriasis. Researchers have studied a large number of families affected by psoriasis and identified genes linked to the disease. Genes govern every bodily function and determine the inherited traits passed from parent to child.

People with psoriasis may notice that there are times when their skin worsens, called flares, then improves. Conditions that may cause flares include infections, stress, and changes in climate that dry the skin. Also, certain medicines, including beta-blockers, which are prescribed for high blood pressure, and lithium may trigger an outbreak or worsen the disease.

Psoriasis Diagnosis

Occasionally, doctors may find it difficult to diagnose psoriasis, because it often looks like other skin diseases. It may be necessary to confirm a diagnosis by examining a small skin sample under a microscope.

There are several forms of psoriasis. Some of these include the following:

- **Plaque psoriasis:** Skin lesions are red at the base and covered by silvery scales.

- **Guttate psoriasis:** Small, drop-shaped lesions appear on the trunk, limbs, and scalp. Guttate psoriasis is most often triggered by upper respiratory infections (for example, a sore throat caused by streptococcal bacteria).

- **Pustular psoriasis:** Blisters of noninfectious pus appear on the skin. Attacks of pustular psoriasis may be triggered by medications, infections, stress, or exposure to certain chemicals.

- **Inverse psoriasis:** Smooth, red patches occur in the folds of the skin near the genitals, under the breasts, or in the armpits. The symptoms may be worsened by friction and sweating.

- **Erythrodermic psoriasis:** Widespread reddening and scaling of the skin may be a reaction to severe sunburn or to taking corticosteroids (cortisone) or other medications. It can also be caused by a prolonged period of increased activity of psoriasis that is poorly controlled.

Another condition in which people may experience psoriasis is psoriatic arthritis. This is a form of arthritis that produces the joint inflammation common in arthritis and the lesions common in psoriasis. The joint inflammation and the skin lesions don't necessarily have to occur at the same time.

Treatment of Psoriasis

Doctors generally treat psoriasis in steps based on the severity of the disease, size of the areas involved, type of psoriasis, and the patient's response to initial treatments. This is sometimes called the "1-2-3" approach. In step 1, medicines are applied to the skin (topical treatment). Step 2 uses light treatments (phototherapy). Step 3 involves taking medicines by mouth or injections that treat the whole immune system (called systemic therapy).

Over time, affected skin can become resistant to treatment, especially when topical corticosteroids are used. Also, a treatment that works very well in one person may have little effect in another. Thus, doctors often use a trial-and-error approach to find a treatment that works, and they may switch treatments periodically (for example, every 12 to 24 months) if a treatment does not work or if adverse reactions occur.

Topical Treatment

Treatments applied directly to the skin may improve its condition. Doctors find that some patients respond well to ointment or cream forms of corticosteroids, vitamin D3, retinoids, coal tar, or anthralin. Bath solutions and lubricants may be soothing, but they are seldom strong enough to improve the condition of the skin. Therefore, they usually are combined with stronger remedies.

- **Corticosteroids:** These drugs reduce inflammation and the turnover of skin cells, and they suppress the immune system. Available in different strengths, topical corticosteroids are usually applied to the skin twice a day. Short-term treatment is often effective in improving, but not completely eliminating, psoriasis. Long-term use or overuse of highly potent (strong) corticosteroids can cause thinning of the skin, internal side effects, and resistance to the treatment's benefits. If less than 10 percent of the skin is involved, some doctors will prescribe a high-potency corticosteroid ointment. High-potency corticosteroids may also be prescribed for plaques that don't improve with other treatment, particularly those on the hands or feet. In situations where the objective of treatment is comfort, medium-potency corticosteroids may be prescribed for the broader skin areas of the torso or limbs. Low-potency preparations are used on delicate skin areas.

- **Calcipotriene:** This drug is a synthetic form of vitamin D3 that can be applied to the skin. Applying calcipotriene ointment twice a day controls the speed of turnover of skin cells. Because calcipotriene can irritate the skin, however, it is not recommended for use on the face or genitals. It is sometimes combined with topical corticosteroids to reduce irritation. Use of more than 100 grams of calcipotriene per week may raise the amount of calcium in the body to unhealthy levels.

- **Retinoid:** Topical retinoids are synthetic forms of vitamin A. The retinoid tazarotene is available as a gel or cream that is applied to the skin. If used alone, this preparation does not act as quickly as topical corticosteroids, but it does not cause thinning of the skin or other side effects associated with steroids. However, it can irritate the skin, particularly in skin folds and the normal skin surrounding a patch of psoriasis. It is less irritating and sometimes more effective when combined with a corticosteroid. Because of the risk of birth defects, women of childbearing age must take measures to prevent pregnancy when using tazarotene.

- **Coal tar:** Preparations containing coal tar (gels and ointments) may be applied directly to the skin, added (as a liquid) to the bath, or used on the scalp as a shampoo. Coal tar products are available in different strengths, and many are sold over the counter (not requiring a prescription). Coal tar is less effective than corticosteroids and many other treatments and, therefore, is sometimes combined with ultraviolet B (UVB) phototherapy for a better result. The most potent form of coal tar may irritate the skin, is messy, has a strong odor, and may stain the skin or clothing. Thus, it is not popular with many patients.

- **Anthralin:** Anthralin reduces the increase in skin cells and inflammation. Doctors sometimes prescribe a 15- to 30-minute application of anthralin ointment, cream, or paste once each day to treat chronic psoriasis lesions. Afterward, anthralin must be washed off the skin to prevent irritation. This treatment often fails to adequately improve the skin, and it stains skin, bathtub, sink, and clothing brown or purple. In addition, the risk of skin irritation makes anthralin unsuitable for acute or actively inflamed eruptions.

- **Salicylic acid:** This peeling agent, which is available in many forms such as ointments, creams, gels, and shampoos, can be applied to reduce scaling of the skin or scalp. Often, it is more effective when combined with topical corticosteroids, anthralin, or coal tar.

- **Clobetasol propionate:** This is a foam topical medication, which has been approved for the treatment of scalp and body psoriasis. The foam penetrates the skin very well, is easy to use, and is not as messy as many other topical medications.

- **Bath solutions:** People with psoriasis may find that adding oil when bathing, then applying a lubricant, soothes their skin. Also, individuals can remove scales and reduce itching by soaking for 15 minutes in water containing a coal tar solution, oiled oatmeal, Epsom salts, or Dead Sea salts.

- **Lubricants:** When applied regularly over a long period, lubricants have a soothing effect. Preparations that are thick and greasy usually work best because they seal water in the skin, reducing scaling and itching.

Light Therapy

Natural ultraviolet light from the sun and controlled delivery of artificial ultraviolet light are used in treating psoriasis. It is important that light therapy be administered by a doctor, since spending time in the sun or a tanning bed can cause skin damage and can increase the risk of skin cancer.

- **Sunlight:** Much of sunlight is composed of bands of different wavelengths of ultraviolet (UV) light. When absorbed into the skin, UV light suppresses the process leading to disease, causing activated T cells in the skin to die. This process reduces inflammation and slows the turnover of skin cells that causes scaling.

196

Daily, short, nonburning exposure to sunlight clears or improves psoriasis in many people. Therefore, exposing affected skin to sunlight is one initial treatment for the disease.

- **Ultraviolet B (UVB) phototherapy:** UVB is light with a short wavelength that is absorbed in the skin's epidermis. An artificial source can be used to treat mild and moderate psoriasis. Some physicians will start treating patients with UVB instead of topical agents. A UVB phototherapy, called broadband UVB, can be used for a few small lesions, to treat widespread psoriasis, or for lesions that resist topical treatment. This type of phototherapy is normally given in a doctor's office by using a light panel or light box. Some patients use UVB light boxes at home under a doctor's guidance. A newer type of UVB, called narrowband UVB, emits the part of the ultraviolet light spectrum band that is most helpful for psoriasis. Narrowband UVB treatment is superior to broadband UVB, but it is less effective than PUVA treatment (see next paragraph). It is gaining in popularity because it does help and is more convenient than PUVA. At first, patients may require several treatments of narrowband UVB spaced close together to improve their skin. Once the skin has shown improvement, a maintenance treatment once each week may be all that is necessary. However, narrowband UVB treatment is not without risk. It can cause more severe and longer lasting burns than broadband treatment.

- **Psoralen and ultraviolet A phototherapy (PUVA):** This treatment combines oral or topical administration of a medicine called psoralen with exposure to ultraviolet A (UVA) light. UVA has a long wavelength that penetrates deeper into the skin than UVB. Psoralen makes the skin more sensitive to this light. PUVA is normally used when more than 10 percent of the skin is affected or when the disease interferes with a person's occupation (for example, when a teacher's face or a salesperson's hands are involved). Compared with broadband UVB treatment, PUVA treatment taken two to three times a week clears psoriasis more consistently and in fewer treatments. However, it is associated with more short-term side effects, including nausea, headache, fatigue, burning, and itching. Care must be taken to avoid sunlight after ingesting psoralen to avoid severe sunburns, and the eyes must be protected for 1 to 2 days with UVA-absorbing glasses. Long-term treatment is associated with an increased risk of squamous cell and, possibly, melanoma skin cancers.

Simultaneous use of drugs that suppress the immune system, such as cyclosporine, have little beneficial effect and increase the risk of cancer.

- **Light therapy combined with other therapies:** Studies have shown that combining ultraviolet light treatment and a retinoid, like acitretin, adds to the effectiveness of UV light for psoriasis. For this reason, if patients are not responding to light therapy, retinoids may be added. UVB phototherapy, for example, may be combined with retinoids and other treatments. One combined therapy program, referred to as the Ingram regimen, involves a coal tar bath, UVB phototherapy, and application of an anthralin-salicylic acid paste that is left on the skin for 6 to 24 hours. A similar regimen, the Goeckerman treatment, combines coal tar ointment with UVB phototherapy. Also, PUVA can be combined with some oral medications (such as retinoids) to increase its effectiveness.

Systemic Treatment

For more severe forms of psoriasis, doctors sometimes prescribe medicines that are taken internally by pill or injection. This is called systemic treatment.

- **Methotrexate:** Like cyclosporine, methotrexate slows cell turnover by suppressing the immune system. It can be taken by pill or injection. Patients taking methotrexate must be closely monitored because it can cause liver damage and/or decrease the production of oxygen-carrying red blood cells, infection-fighting white blood cells, and clot-enhancing platelets. As a precaution, doctors do not prescribe the drug for people who have had liver disease or anemia (an illness characterized by weakness or tiredness due to a reduction in the number or volume of red blood cells that carry oxygen to the tissues). It is sometimes combined with PUVA or UVB treatments. Methotrexate should not be used by pregnant women, or by women who are planning to get pregnant, because it may cause birth defects.

- **Retinoids:** A retinoid, such as acitretin, is a compound with vitamin A-like properties that may be prescribed for severe cases of psoriasis that do not respond to other therapies. Because this treatment also may cause birth defects, women must protect themselves from pregnancy beginning 1 month before through 3 years after treatment with acitretin. Most patients experience a recurrence of psoriasis after these products are discontinued.

- **Cyclosporine:** Taken orally, cyclosporine acts by suppressing the immune system to slow the rapid turnover of skin cells. It may provide quick relief of symptoms, but the improvement stops when treatment is discontinued. The best candidates for this therapy are those with severe psoriasis who have not responded to, or cannot tolerate, other systemic therapies. Its rapid onset of action is helpful in avoiding hospitalization of patients whose psoriasis is rapidly progressing. Cyclosporine may impair kidney function or cause high blood pressure (hypertension). Therefore, patients must be carefully monitored by a doctor. Also, cyclosporine is not recommended for patients who have a weak immune system or those who have had skin cancers as a result of PUVA treatments in the past. It should not be given with phototherapy.

- **6-Thioguanine:** This drug is nearly as effective as methotrexate and cyclosporine. It has fewer side effects, but there is a greater likelihood of anemia. This drug must also be avoided by pregnant women and by women who are planning to become pregnant, because it may cause birth defects.

- **Hydroxyurea:** Compared with methotrexate and cyclosporine, hydroxyurea is somewhat less effective. It is sometimes combined with PUVA or UVB treatments. Possible side effects include anemia and a decrease in white blood cells and platelets. Like methotrexate and retinoids, hydroxyurea must be avoided by pregnant women or those who are planning to become pregnant, because it may cause birth defects.

- **Biologic response modifiers:** Recently, attention has been given to a group of drugs called biologics, which are made from proteins produced by living cells instead of chemicals. They interfere with specific immune system processes which cause the overproduction of skin cells and inflammation. These drugs are injected (sometimes by the patient). Patients taking these treatments need to be monitored carefully by a doctor. Because these drugs suppress the immune system response, patients taking these drugs have an increased risk of infection, and the drugs may also interfere with patients taking vaccines. Also, some of these drugs have been associated with other diseases (like central nervous system disorders, blood diseases, cancer, and lymphoma) although their role in the development of or contribution to these diseases is not yet understood. Some are approved for adults only, and their effects on pregnant or nursing women are not known.

- **Antibiotics:** These medications are not indicated in routine treatment of psoriasis. However, antibiotics may be employed when an infection, such as that caused by the bacteria Streptococcus, triggers an outbreak of psoriasis, as in certain cases of guttate psoriasis.

Combination Therapy

Combining various topical, light, and systemic treatments often permits lower doses of each and can result in increased effectiveness. There are many approaches for treating psoriasis. Therefore, doctors are paying more attention to combination therapy.

Psychological Support

Some individuals with moderate to severe psoriasis may benefit from counseling or participation in a support group to reduce self-consciousness about their appearance or relieve psychological distress resulting from fear of social rejection.

Promising Areas of Psoriasis Research

Significant progress has been made in understanding the inheritance of psoriasis. A number of genes involved in psoriasis are already known or suspected. In a multifactor disease (involving genes, environment, and other factors), variations in one or more genes may produce a greater likelihood of getting the disease. Researchers are continuing to study the genetic aspects of psoriasis.

Since discovering that inflammation in psoriasis is triggered by T cells, researchers have been studying new treatments that quiet immune system reactions in the skin. Among these are treatments that block the activity of T cells or block cytokines (proteins that promote inflammation).

Recent research has suggested that psoriasis patients may be at greater risk of cardiovascular problems, especially if the psoriasis is severe, as well as obesity, high blood pressure, and diabetes. Researchers are trying to determine the reasons for these associations and how best to treat patients.

Section 21.2

The Psoriasis-Stress Link

No one knows exactly what causes psoriasis. However, it is understood that the immune system and genetics play major roles in its development. Most researchers agree that the immune system is somehow mistakenly triggered, which causes a series of events, including acceleration of skin cell growth. A normal skin cell matures and falls off the body in 28 to 30 days. A skin cell in a patient with psoriasis takes only 3 to 4 days to mature and instead of falling off (shedding), the cells pile up on the surface of the skin, forming psoriasis lesions.

Scientists believe that at least 10 percent of the general population inherits one or more of the genes that create a predisposition to psoriasis. However, only 2 percent to 3 percent of the population develops the disease. Researchers believe that for a person to develop psoriasis, the individual must have a combination of the genes that cause psoriasis and be exposed to specific external factors known as "triggers."

Psoriasis Triggers

Psoriasis triggers are not universal. What may cause one person's psoriasis to become active, may not affect another. Established psoriasis triggers include the following.

Stress

Stress can cause psoriasis to flare for the first time or aggravate existing psoriasis. Relaxation and stress reduction may help prevent stress from impacting psoriasis.

Injury to Skin

Psoriasis can appear in areas of the skin that have been injured or traumatized. This is called the Koebner [KEB-ner] phenomenon.

Vaccinations, sunburns, and scratches can all trigger a Koebner response. The Koebner response can be treated if it is caught early enough.

Medications

Certain medications are associated with triggering psoriasis, including the following:

- **Lithium:** Used to treat manic depression and other psychiatric disorders. Lithium aggravates psoriasis in about half of those with psoriasis who take it.

- **Antimalarials:** Plaquenil, Quinacrine, chloroquine, and hydroxychloroquine may cause a flare of psoriasis, usually 2 to 3 weeks after the drug is taken. Hydroxychloroquine has the lowest incidence of side effects.

- **Inderal:** This high blood pressure medication worsens psoriasis in about 25 percent to 30 percent of patients with psoriasis who take it. It is not known if all high blood pressure (beta blocker) medications worsen psoriasis, but they may have that potential.

- **Quinidine:** This heart medication has been reported to worsen some cases of psoriasis.

- **Indomethacin:** This is a nonsteroidal anti-inflammatory drug used to treat arthritis. It has worsened some cases of psoriasis. Other anti-inflammatories usually can be substituted. Indomethacin's negative effects are usually minimal when it is taken properly. Its side effects are usually outweighed by its benefits in psoriatic arthritis.

Other Triggers

Although scientifically unproven, some people with psoriasis suspect that allergies, diet, and weather trigger their psoriasis. Strep infection is known to trigger guttate psoriasis.

Section 21.3

Is Acne Linked to Stress?

"Link Found Between Teens' Stress Levels and Acne Severity,"
March 6, 2007. © 2007 Wake Forest University Baptist Medical Center.
Reprinted with permission.

The largest study ever conducted on acne and stress reveals that teenagers who were under high levels of stress were 23 percent more likely to have increased acne severity, according to researchers from Wake Forest University School of Medicine and colleagues.

"Acne significantly affects physical and psychosocial well-being, so it is important to understand the interplay between the factors that exacerbate acne," said Gil Yosipovitch, MD, lead author and a professor of dermatology. "Our study suggests a significant association between stress and severity of acne."

The results of the study, which involved 94 adolescents from Singapore, were reported in the March 6, 2007 issue of *Acta Derm Venereol,* a Swedish medical journal.

While psychological stress had been identified among many factors that can worsen acne, there has been little research to understand the mechanisms behind this relationship. The study looked at whether levels of sebum, the oily substance that coats the skin and protects the hair, increase in times of stress and are related to acne severity. Hormone levels, sebum production, and bacteria are all known to play major roles in acne.

The study involved secondary school students in Singapore with a mean age of 14.9 years. The students' self-reported stress levels and acne severity were measured at two different times—just before mid-year exams and during summer break. Students' long-term career prospects are influenced by the results of the examinations and they are known to induce psychological stress.

Stress levels were measured using the Perceived Stress Scale, a 14-item, self-questionnaire that is widely used in stress research. Acne severity was measured using a system that classifies acne based on type and number of lesions. Ninety-two percent of the girls and 95 percent of the boys reported having acne.

Acne is an inflammatory disease of the skin caused by changes in the hair follicle and the sebaceous glands of the skin that produce sebum. The oily substance plugs the pores, resulting in whiteheads or blackheads (acne comedonica) and pimples (acne papulopustulosa).

The researchers suspected that stress increases the quantity of sebum, which leads to increased acne severity. However, the results showed that sebum production didn't differ significantly between the high-stress and low-stress conditions.

The researchers did find that students reporting high stress were 23 percent more likely to have increased severity of acne papulopustulosa. Levels of stress were not linked to severity of acne comedonica.

"Our research suggests that acne severity associated with stress may result from factors others than sebum quantity," said Yosipovitch. "It's possible that inflammation may be involved."

Singapore was selected as the study location because sebum production is known to fluctuate with variations in temperature and humidity. In Singapore's tropical climate, temperature and humidity are consistent throughout the year.

The research was funded by the National Medical Research Council of Singapore. Co-researchers were Aerlyn Dawn, MD, from Wake Forest, Mark Tang, MD, Chee Leok Goh, MD, and Yiong Hauk Chan, PhD, all from National Skin Center and National University of Singapore, and Lim Fong Seng, MD, from National Healthcare Group Polyclinics, Singapore.

Chapter 22

Sleep

Chapter Contents

Section 22.1

Stress, Behavior, and Sleep

Excerpted from "The Human Brain: Sleep and Stress," © 2004 The Franklin Institute (www.fi.edu). Reprinted with permission. Reviewed by David A. Cooke, MD, FACP, November 8, 2010.

Every animal sleeps, but why the brain needs sleep has remained a mystery. Neuroscientists now believe sleep is not only crucial to brain development, but is also necessary to help consolidate the effects of waking experience—by converting memory into more permanent and/or enhanced forms.

Sleeping problems are almost always involved in mental disorders, including depression, schizophrenia, Alzheimer's disease, stroke, as well as head injury. And symptoms are strongly influenced by the amount of sleep a person gets. Difficulties may arise from the drugs used to control symptoms of a disorder, or from changes in the brain regions and neurotransmitters that control sleep.

Stress, Behavior and Sleep

Many of us know what it is like to go without sleep and how it can affect our mood and stress level. Here you will find important information about why you may be losing sleep and intriguing studies about sleep deprivation. You may be surprised.

The Effects of Sleep Deprivation

Adequate sleep is crucial to proper brain function—no less so than air, water, and food—but stress can modify sleep-wakefulness cycles.

Any amount of sleep deprivation will diminish mental performance, cautions Mark Mahowald, a professor of neurology at the University of Minnesota Medical School. "One complete night of sleep deprivation is as impairing in simulated driving tests as a legally intoxicating blood-alcohol level."

At the American Diabetes Association's annual meeting in June 2001, Eve Van Cauter, PhD, reported that people who regularly do not get enough sleep can become less sensitive to insulin. This increases their risk for diabetes and high blood pressure—both serious threats to the brain.

Previous work by Dr. Van Cauter, a professor of medicine at the University of Chicago, found that "metabolic and endocrine changes resulting from a significant sleep debt mimic many of the hallmarks of aging. We suspect that chronic sleep loss may not only hasten the onset but could also increase the severity of age-related ailments such as diabetes, hypertension, obesity, and memory loss."

Stress Hormones and Insomnia Study

That stress can affect proper sleep seems obvious, but researchers at Pennsylvania State University College of Medicine have found another reason why middle-aged men may be losing sleep. It's not just because of what they worry about. Rather, it's due to "increased vulnerability of sleep to stress hormones," according to Dr. Alexandros N. Vgontzas.

As men age, it appears they become more sensitive to the stimulating effects of corticotropin-releasing hormone (CRH). When both young and middle-aged men were administered CRH, the older men remained awake longer and slept less deeply. (People who don't get enough of this "slow-wave" sleep may be more prone to depression.)

"The increased prevalence of insomnia in middle age may, in fact, be the result of deteriorating sleep mechanisms associated with increased sensitivity to arousal-producing stress hormones, such as CRH and cortisol," Vgontzas and colleagues suggest.

In another study, the researchers compared patients with insomnia to those without sleep disturbances. They found that "insomniacs with the highest degree of sleep disturbance secreted the highest amount of cortisol, particularly in the evening and nighttime hours," suggesting that chronic insomnia is a disorder of sustained hyperarousal of the body's stress response system.

Stress and Sleep Patterns Study

Why do some people lose sleep during periods of stress, while others seem to "sleep like a baby"? Research suggests that the difference may be explained by the ways people cope.

At Tel Aviv University, Dr. Avi Sadeh conducted a study of students. He found that those "who tended to focus on their emotions and anxiety during the high-stress period were more likely to shorten their sleep, while those who tended to ignore emotions and focus on tasks extended their sleep and shut themselves off from stress."

During a routine week of studies, and again during a highly stressful month, sleep patterns of 36 students (aged 22 to 32) were documented. Sleep quality improved or remained the same for students who directed their focus away from their emotions, but diminished for those who fretted and brooded as a way to cope with stress.

Almost titling his paper, "If you can't cope with it, sleep on it," Sadeh said "sometimes sleep can help you regulate your nervousness and offer you an escape from stress, particularly when there's nothing you can do about it."

Children's Sleep Patterns Related to Behavior Study

A Northwestern University study of 500 preschoolers found that those who slept less than 10 hours in a 24-hour period (including daytime naps) were 25% more likely to misbehave. They were consistently at greatest risk for "acting out" behavioral problems, such as aggression and oppositional or noncompliant behavior.

Research shows that sleep disturbances in children are not only associated with medical problems (allergies, ear infections, hearing problems), but also with psychiatric and social issues. Children who were aggressive, anxious, or depressed had more trouble falling and staying asleep. Although sleep problems usually decline as children get older, these early patterns are the best indicator of future sleep troubles.

Section 22.2

Insomnia

From "Insomnia," by the National Heart, Lung, and Blood
Institute (NHLBI, www.nhlbi.nih.gov), part of the National
Institutes of Health, March 2009.

What Is Insomnia?

Insomnia is a common condition in which you have trouble falling or
staying asleep. This condition can range from mild to severe, depending
on how often it occurs and for how long.

Insomnia can be chronic (ongoing) or acute (short-term). Chronic
insomnia means having symptoms at least 3 nights a week for more
than a month. Acute insomnia lasts for less time.

Some people who have insomnia may have trouble falling asleep.
Other people may fall asleep easily but wake up too soon. Others may
have trouble with both falling asleep and staying asleep.

As a result, insomnia may cause you to get too little sleep or have
poor-quality sleep. You may not feel refreshed when you wake up.

Overview

There are two types of insomnia. The most common type is called
secondary or comorbid insomnia. This type of insomnia is a symptom
or side effect of some other problem.

More than eight out of 10 people who have insomnia are believed to
have secondary insomnia. Certain medical conditions, medicines, sleep
disorders, and substances can cause secondary insomnia.

In contrast, primary insomnia isn't due to a medical problem, medicines, or other substances. It is its own disorder. A number of life
changes can trigger primary insomnia, including long-lasting stress
and emotional upset.

Insomnia can cause excessive daytime sleepiness and a lack of energy.
It also can make you feel anxious, depressed, or irritable. You may have
trouble focusing on tasks, paying attention, learning, and remembering.
This can prevent you from doing your best at work or school.

Insomnia also can cause other serious problems. For example, you may feel drowsy while driving, which could lead to an accident.

Outlook

Secondary insomnia often resolves or improves without treatment if you can stop its cause—especially if you can correct the problem soon after it starts. For example, if caffeine is causing your insomnia, stopping or limiting your intake of the substance may cause your insomnia to go away.

Lifestyle changes, including better sleep habits, often help relieve acute insomnia. For chronic insomnia, your doctor may recommend a type of counseling called cognitive-behavioral therapy or medicines.

What Causes Insomnia?

Secondary Insomnia

Secondary insomnia is the symptom or side effect of another problem. This type of insomnia often is a symptom of an emotional, neurological, or other medical or sleep disorder.

Emotional disorders that can cause insomnia include depression, anxiety, and posttraumatic stress disorder. Alzheimer disease and Parkinson disease are examples of common neurological disorders that can cause insomnia.

A number of other conditions also can cause insomnia, such as the following:

- Conditions that cause chronic pain, such as arthritis and headache disorders
- Conditions that make it hard to breathe, such as asthma and heart failure
- An overactive thyroid
- Gastrointestinal disorders, such as heartburn
- Stroke
- Sleep disorders, such as restless legs syndrome and sleep-related breathing problems
- Menopause and hot flashes

Secondary insomnia also may be a side effect of certain medicines. For example, certain asthma medicines, such as theophylline, and some allergy and cold medicines can cause insomnia. Beta blockers also may cause the condition. These medicines are used to treat heart conditions.

Commonly used substances also may cause insomnia. Examples include caffeine and other stimulants, tobacco or other nicotine products, and alcohol or other sedatives.

Primary Insomnia

Primary insomnia isn't a symptom or side effect of another medical condition. This type of insomnia usually occurs for periods of at least 1 month.

A number of life changes can trigger primary insomnia. It may be due to major or long-lasting stress or emotional upset. Travel or other factors, such as work schedules that disrupt your sleep routine, also may trigger primary insomnia.

Even if these issues are resolved, the insomnia may not go away. Trouble sleeping may persist because of habits formed to deal with the lack of sleep. These habits may include taking naps, worrying about sleep, and going to bed early.

Researchers continue to try to find out whether some people are born with a greater chance of having primary insomnia.

Who Is at Risk for Insomnia?

Insomnia is a common disorder. One in three adults has insomnia sometimes. One in 10 adults has chronic insomnia.

Insomnia affects women more often than men. The condition can occur at any age. However, older adults are more likely to have insomnia than younger people.

People who may be at higher risk for insomnia include those who:

- have a lot of stress;
- are depressed or who have other emotional distress, such as divorce or death of a spouse;
- have lower incomes;
- work at night or have frequent major shifts in their work hours;
- travel long distances with time changes;
- have certain medical conditions or sleep disorders that can disrupt sleep;
- have an inactive lifestyle.

Young and middle-aged African Americans also may be at increased risk for insomnia. Research shows that, compared to Whites, it takes African Americans longer to fall asleep. They also have lighter sleep, don't sleep as well, and take more naps. Sleep-related breathing problems also are more common among African Americans.

What Are the Signs and Symptoms of Insomnia?

The main symptom of insomnia is trouble falling and/or staying asleep, which leads to lack of sleep. If you have insomnia, you may:

- lie awake for a long time before you fall asleep;

- sleep for only short periods;

- be awake for much of the night;

- feel as if you haven't slept at all;

- wake up too early.

The lack of sleep also can cause other symptoms. You may wake up feeling tired or not well rested, and you may feel tired during the day. You also may have trouble focusing on tasks. Insomnia can cause you to feel anxious, depressed, or irritable.

Insomnia may affect your daily activities and cause serious problems. For example, you may feel drowsy while driving. Driving while sleepy leads to more than 100,000 car crashes each year. In older women, research shows that insomnia raises the risk of falling.

If insomnia is affecting your daily activities, see your doctor. Treatment may help you avoid symptoms and problems related to the condition. Also, poor sleep may be a sign of other health problems. Finding and treating those problems could improve both your health and your sleep.

How Is Insomnia Diagnosed?

Usually, your doctor will diagnose insomnia based on your medical and sleep histories and a physical exam. He or she also may recommend a sleep study. For example, you may have a sleep study if the cause of your insomnia is unclear.

Medical History

To find out what's causing your insomnia, your doctor may ask whether you:

- have any new or ongoing health problems;

- have painful injuries or health conditions, such as arthritis;

- take any medicines, either over-the-counter or prescription;

- have symptoms or a history of depression, anxiety, or psychosis;

- are coping with any very stressful life events, such as divorce or death.

Your doctor also may ask questions about your work and leisure habits. For example, he or she may ask about your work and exercise routines; your use of caffeine, tobacco, and alcohol; and your long-distance travel history. Your answers may give clues about what's causing your insomnia.

Your doctor also may ask whether you have any new or ongoing work or personal problems or other stresses in your life. Also, he or she may ask whether you have other family members who have sleep problems.

Sleep History

To get a better sense of your sleep problem, your doctor will ask you details about your sleep habits. Before your visit, think about how to describe your problems, including the following:

- How often you have trouble sleeping and how long you've had the problem

- When you go to bed and get up on workdays and days off

- How long it takes you to fall asleep, how often you wake up at night, and how long it takes to fall back asleep

- Whether you snore loudly and often or wake up gasping or feeling out of breath

- How refreshed you feel when you wake up, and how tired you feel during the day

- How often you doze off or have trouble staying awake during routine tasks, especially driving

To find out what's causing or worsening your insomnia, your doctor also may ask you the following:

- Whether you worry about falling asleep, staying asleep, or getting enough sleep

213

- What you eat or drink, and whether you take medicines before going to bed

- What routine you follow before going to bed

- What the noise level, lighting, and temperature are like where you sleep

- What distractions, such as a TV or computer, are in your bedroom

To help your doctor, consider keeping a sleep diary for 1 or 2 weeks. Write down when you go to sleep, wake up, and take naps. (For example, you might note: Went to bed at 10 a.m.; woke up at 3 a.m. and couldn't fall back asleep; napped after work for 2 hours.)

Also write down how much you sleep each night, as well as how sleepy you feel at various times during the day.

Physical Exam

Your doctor will do a physical exam to rule out other medical problems that might cause insomnia. You also may need blood tests to check for thyroid problems or other conditions that can cause sleep problems.

Sleep Study

Your doctor may recommend a sleep study called a polysomnogram (PSG) if he or she thinks an underlying sleep disorder is causing your insomnia.

A PSG usually is done while you stay overnight at a sleep center. A PSG records brain electrical activity, eye movements, heart rate, breathing, muscle activity, blood pressure, and blood oxygen levels.

How Is Insomnia Treated?

Lifestyle changes often can help relieve acute (short-term) insomnia. These changes may make it easier to fall asleep and stay asleep.

A type of counseling called cognitive-behavioral therapy (CBT) can help relieve the anxiety linked to chronic (ongoing) insomnia. Anxiety tends to prolong insomnia.

Several medicines also can help relieve insomnia and re-establish a regular sleep schedule. However, if your insomnia is the symptom or side effect of another problem, it's important to treat the underlying cause (if possible). Your doctor also may prescribe medicine to help treat your insomnia.

Lifestyle Changes

If you have insomnia, avoid substances that make it worse, such as the following:

- Caffeine, tobacco, and other stimulants taken too close to bedtime: Their effects can last as long as 8 hours.

- Certain over-the-counter and prescription medicines that can disrupt sleep (for example, some cold and allergy medicines): Talk to your doctor about which medicines won't disrupt your sleep.

- Alcohol: An alcoholic drink before bedtime may make it easier for you to fall asleep. However, alcohol triggers sleep that tends to be lighter than normal. This makes it more likely that you will wake up during the night.

Try to adopt good bedtime habits that make it easier to fall asleep and stay asleep. Follow a routine that helps you wind down and relax before bed. For example, read a book, listen to soothing music, or take a hot bath.

Try to schedule your daily exercise at least 5 to 6 hours before going to bed. Don't eat heavy meals or drink a lot before bedtime.

Make your bedroom sleep-friendly. Avoid bright lighting while winding down. Try to limit possible distractions, such as a TV, computer, or pet. Make sure the temperature of your bedroom is cool and comfortable. Your bedroom also should be dark and quiet.

Go to sleep around the same time each night and wake up around the same time each morning, even on weekends. If you can, avoid night shifts, alternating schedules, or other things that may disrupt your sleep schedule.

Cognitive-Behavioral Therapy

CBT for insomnia targets the thoughts and actions that can disrupt sleep. This therapy encourages good sleep habits and uses several methods to relieve sleep anxiety.

For example, relaxation training and biofeedback at bedtime are used to reduce anxiety. These strategies help you better control your breathing, heart rate, muscles, and mood.

CBT also works on replacing sleep anxiety with more positive thinking that links being in bed with being asleep. This method also teaches you what to do if you're unable to fall asleep within a reasonable time.

CBT also may involve talking with a therapist one-on-one or in group sessions to help you consider your thoughts and feelings about sleep. This method may encourage you to describe thoughts racing through your mind in terms of how they look, feel, and sound. The goal is for your mind to settle down and stop racing.

CBT also focuses on limiting the time you spend in bed while awake. This method involves setting a sleep schedule. At first, you will limit your total time in bed to the typical short length of time you're usually asleep.

This schedule may make you even more tired because some of the allotted time in bed will be taken up by problems falling asleep. However, the resulting tiredness is intended to help you get to sleep more quickly. Over time, the length of time spent in bed is increased until you get a full night of sleep.

For success with CBT, you may need to see a therapist who is skilled in this approach weekly over 2 to 3 months. CBT works as well as prescription medicine for many people who have chronic insomnia. It also may provide better long-term relief than medicine alone.

For people who have insomnia and major depressive disorder, CBT combined with antidepressant medicines has shown promise in relieving both conditions.

Medicines

Prescription medicines: Many prescription medicines are used to treat insomnia. Some are meant for short-term use, while others are meant for longer use.

Talk to your doctor about the benefits and side effects of insomnia medicines. For instance, insomnia medicines can help you fall asleep, but some people may feel groggy in the morning after taking them.

Rare side effects may include sleep eating, sleep walking, or driving while asleep. If you have side effects from an insomnia medicine, or if it doesn't work well, tell your doctor. He or she may prescribe a different medicine.

Some insomnia medicines may be habit forming. Talk to your doctor about the benefits and risks of insomnia medicines.

Over-the-counter products: Some over-the-counter (OTC) products claim to treat insomnia. These products include melatonin, L-tryptophan supplements, and valerian teas or extracts.

The Food and Drug Administration doesn't regulate "natural" products and some food supplements. Thus, the dose and purity of these products can vary. How well these products work and how safe they are isn't well understood.

Some OTC products that contain antihistamines are marketed as sleep aids. Although these products may make you sleepy, talk to your doctor before taking them.

Antihistamines pose risks for some people. Also, these products may not offer the best treatment for your insomnia. Your doctor can advise you whether these products can benefit you.

Chapter 23

Teeth Grinding (Bruxism)

Bruxism is when you clench (tightly hold your top and bottom teeth together) or grind (slide your teeth back and forth over each other) your teeth.

Causes

People can clench and grind without being aware of it during both the day and night, although sleep-related bruxism is often the bigger problem because it is harder to control.

The cause of bruxism is not completely agreed upon, but daily stress may be the trigger in many people. Some people probably clench their teeth and never feel symptoms. Whether or not bruxism causes pain and other problems may be a complicated mix of factors:

- How much stress you are under
- How long and tightly you clench and grind
- Whether your teeth are misaligned
- Your posture
- Your ability to relax
- Your diet
- Your sleeping habits

"Bruxism" © 2010 A.D.A.M., Inc. Reprinted with permission.

Each person is probably different.

Symptoms

Clenching the teeth puts pressure on the muscles, tissues, and other structures around your jaw. The symptoms can cause temporomandibular joint problems (TMJ).

Grinding can wear down your teeth. Grinding can be noisy enough at night to bother sleeping partners.

Symptoms include:

- anxiety, stress, and tension;

- depression;

- earache (due in part because the structures of the temporomandibular joint are very close to the ear canal, and because you can feel pain in a different location than its source—this is called referred pain);

- eating disorders;

- headache;

- hot, cold, or sweet sensitivity in the teeth;

- insomnia;

- sore or painful jaw.

Exams and Tests

An examination can rule out other disorders that may cause similar jaw pain or ear pain, including:

- dental disorders;

- ear disorders such as ear infections;

- problems with the temporomandibular joint (TMJ).
  You may have a history of significant stress and tension.

Treatment

The goals of treatment are to reduce pain, prevent permanent damage to the teeth, and reduce clenching as much as possible.

To help relieve pain, there are many self-care steps you can take at home. For example:

- Apply ice or wet heat to sore jaw muscles. Either can have a beneficial effect.

- Avoid eating hard foods like nuts, candies, steak.

- Drink plenty of water every day.

- Get plenty of sleep.

- Learn physical therapy stretching exercises to help restore a normal balance to the action of the muscles and joints on each side of the head.

- Massage the muscles of the neck, shoulders, and face. Search carefully for small, painful nodules called trigger points that can cause pain throughout the head and face.

- Relax your face and jaw muscles throughout the day. The goal is to make facial relaxation a habit.

- Try to reduce your daily stress and learn relaxation techniques.

To prevent damage to the teeth, mouth guards or appliances (splints) have been used since the 1930s to treat teeth grinding, clenching, and TMJ disorders. A splint may help protect the teeth from the pressure of clenching.

A splint may also help reduce clenching, but some people find that it makes their clenching worse. In others, the symptoms go away as long as they use the splint, but pain returns when they stop or the splint loses its effectiveness over time.

There are many different types of splints. Some fit over the top teeth, some on the bottom. They may be designed to keep your jaw in a more relaxed position or provide some other function. If one type doesn't work, another may.

For example, a splint called the NTI-tss [nociceptive trigeminal inhibition-tension suppression system] fits over just the front teeth. The idea is to keep all of your back teeth (molars) completely separated, under the theory that most clenching is done on these back teeth. With the NTI, the only contact is between the splint and a bottom front tooth.

As a next phase after splint therapy, orthodontic adjustment of the bite pattern may help some people. Surgery should be considered a last resort.

Finally, there have been many approaches to try to help people unlearn their clenching behaviors. These are more successful for daytime clenching, since nighttime clenching cannot be consciously stopped.

221

In some people, just relaxing and modifying daytime behavior is enough to reduce nighttime bruxism. Methods to directly modify nighttime clenching have not been well studied. They include biofeedback devices, self-hypnosis, and other alternative therapies.

Outlook (Prognosis)

Bruxism is not a dangerous disorder. However, it can cause permanent damage to the teeth and uncomfortable jaw pain, headaches, or ear pain.

Possible Complications

- Depression
- Eating disorders
- Insomnia
- Increased dental or TMJ problems

Nightly grinding can awaken roommates and sleeping partners.

When to Contact a Medical Professional

There is no recognized TMJ specialty in dentistry. See a dentist immediately if you are having trouble eating or opening your mouth. Keep in mind that a wide variety of possible conditions can cause TMJ symptoms, from arthritis to whiplash injuries. Therefore, see your dentist for a full evaluation if self-care measures do not help within several weeks.

Grinding and clenching does not fall clearly into one medical discipline. For a massage-based approach, look for a massage therapist trained in trigger point therapy, neuromuscular therapy, or clinical massage.

Dentists who have more experience in evaluating and treating TMJ disorders will typically take x-rays and prescribe a mouth guard. Surgery is now considered a last resort for TMJ.

Prevention

Stress reduction and anxiety management may reduce bruxism in people prone to the condition.

Part Three

How Stress Affects Mental Health

Chapter 24

Depression

Chapter Contents

Section 24.1

What Is Depression?

Excerpted from "Depression: When the Blues Don't Go Away," by the
National Institute of Mental Health (NIMH, www.nimh.nih.gov), part
of the National Institutes of Health, 2007.

Everyone occasionally feels blue or sad, but these feelings usually pass within a couple of days. When a person has depression, it interferes with his or her daily life and routine, such as going to work or school, taking care of children, and relationships with family and friends. Depression causes pain for the person who has it and for those who care about him or her.

Depression can be very different in different people or in the same person over time. It is a common but serious illness. Treatment can help those with even the most severe depression get better.

What are the symptoms of depression?

- Ongoing sad, anxious, or empty feelings

- Feelings of hopelessness

- Feelings of guilt, worthlessness, or helplessness

- Feeling irritable or restless

- Loss of interest in activities or hobbies that were once enjoyable, including sex

- Feeling tired all the time

- Difficulty concentrating, remembering details, or difficulty making decisions

- Not able to go to sleep or stay asleep (insomnia); may wake in the middle of the night or sleep all the time

- Overeating or loss of appetite

- Thoughts of suicide or making suicide attempts

- Ongoing aches and pains, headaches, cramps, or digestive problems that do not go away

Not everyone diagnosed with depression will have all of these symptoms. The signs and symptoms may be different in men, women, younger children, and older adults.

Can a person have depression and another illness at the same time?

Often, people have other illnesses along with depression. Sometimes other illnesses come first, but other times the depression comes first. Each person and situation is different, but it is important not to ignore these illnesses and to get treatment for them and the depression. Some illnesses or disorders that may occur along with depression are the following:

- Anxiety disorders, including posttraumatic stress disorder (PTSD), obsessive-compulsive disorder (OCD), panic disorder, social phobia, and generalized anxiety disorder (GAD)

- Alcohol and other substance abuse or dependence

- Heart disease, stroke, cancer, HIV/AIDS [human immunodeficiency virus/acquired immunodeficiency syndrome], diabetes, and Parkinson disease

Studies have found that treating depression can help in treating these other illnesses.

When does depression start?

Young children and teens can get depression but it can occur at other ages also. Depression is more common in women than in men, but men do get depression, too. Loss of a loved one, stress and hormonal changes, or traumatic events may trigger depression at any age.

Why do people get depression?

There is no single cause of depression. Depression happens because of a combination of things including the following:

- **Genes**—Some types of depression tend to run in families. Genes are the blueprints for who we are, and we inherit them from our parents. Scientists are looking for the specific genes that may be involved in depression.

- **Brain chemistry and structure**—When chemicals in the brain are not at the right levels, depression can occur. These chemicals, called neurotransmitters, help cells in the brain communicate with each other. By looking at pictures of the brain, scientists can also see that the structure of the brain in people who have depression looks different than in people who do not have depression.

Scientists are working to figure out why these differences occur. Environmental and psychological factors—trauma, loss of a loved one, a difficult relationship, and other stressors can trigger depression. Scientists are working to figure out why depression occurs in some people but not in others with the same or similar experiences. They are also studying why some people recover quickly from depression and others do not.

What if I or someone I know is in crisis?

If you are thinking about harming yourself, or know someone who is, tell someone who can help immediately.

- Call your doctor.
- Call 911 or go to a hospital emergency room to get immediate help or ask a friend or family member to help you do these things.
- Call the toll-free, 24-hour hotline of the National Suicide Prevention Lifeline at 800-273-TALK (800-273-8255); TTY: 800-799-4TTY (799-4889) to talk to a trained counselor.
- Make sure you or the suicidal person is not left alone.

Section 24.2

Depressed Patients Experience Inflammation under Stress

Individuals with major depression have an exaggerated inflammatory response to psychological stress compared to those who do not suffer from depression, according to a study by researchers at Emory University School of Medicine. Because an overactive inflammatory response may contribute to a number of medical disorders as well as to depression, the findings suggest that increased inflammatory responses to stress in depressed patients may be a link between depression and other diseases, including heart disease, as well as contributing to depression itself.

Results of the study, led by Andrew Miller, MD, and Christine Heim, PhD, of Emory's Department of Psychiatry and Behavioral Sciences, are published in the Sept. 1 [2006] issue of the *American Journal of Psychiatry*. "Several examples of increased resting inflammation in depressed patients already exist in the literature, but this is the first time anyone has shown evidence to suggest that the inflammatory response to stress may be greater in depressed people," says Dr. Miller.

The study included 28 medically healthy male participants, half of whom were diagnosed with major depression and half of whom were not depressed. The participants were exposed to two moderately stressful situations during a 20-minute time period. Blood was collected every 15 minutes starting immediately before and then up to an hour and a half after the test to check for key indicators of inflammation. The researchers measured levels of a pro-inflammatory cytokine (a regulatory protein secreted by the immune system) called interleukin-6, and the activity of a pro-inflammatory signaling molecule in white blood cells called nuclear factor-kB.

While at rest (before the stress challenge), the depressed patients had increased inflammation relative to the control group. Both the depressed and the healthy groups showed an inflammatory response to the stress challenge, but people who were currently depressed exhibited the greatest increases of interleukin-6 and nuclear factor-kB.

"While inflammation is essential for us to fight bacterial and viral infections, too much inflammation can cause harm," says Dr. Miller. "There's always some collateral damage when the immune system gets fired up, and we now believe that too much inflammation, either at rest or during stress, may predispose people to become depressed or stay depressed." In addition, medical research over the last decade has shown that runaway inflammation may play a role in a number of disorders, including heart disease, cancer, and diabetes, all of which have been associated with depression.

People in the study who suffered from depression also had higher rates of early life stressful experiences. "We have found that this kind of personal life history may make people more likely to develop major depression and is actually common in depressed patients," says Dr. Heim.

The study was funded by the National Institute of Mental Health (NIMH) and the National Alliance for Research on Schizophrenia and Depression (NARSAD). It was part of a larger project at the Emory Conte Center for the Neuroscience of Mental Disorders led by Charles B. Nemeroff, MD, PhD, Reunette W. Harris Professor and Chair of Emory's Department of Psychiatry and Behavioral Sciences. The Conte Center is dedicated to understanding the contribution of early life abuse and neglect to the neurobiology of adulthood psychiatric disorders. Ongoing studies by Dr. Miller's team of researchers will attempt to determine how early life experiences contribute to excessive inflammatory stress responses.

"According to the Depression and Bipolar Support Alliance, major depression is the leading cause of disability worldwide and costs the U.S. economy $70 billion annually in medical expenditures, lost productivity, and other expenses," says Thaddeus Pace, PhD, lead author on the paper. "This study is leading us toward finding out what actually causes depression and to identifying what aspects of immune system function are abnormal in depressed people. The goal is to find potential targets within the molecular machinery of the immune system so we can better treat major depression and minimize its consequences on health." Other contributors to the study include Oyetunde Alagbe, MD, Tanja C. Mletzko, MS, and Dominique Musselman, MD, MS.

Section 24.3

Stress Indicators Detected in Depression-Prone Women's Sweat

From "Errant Stress/Immune Indicators Detected in Depression-Prone Women's Sweat," by the National Institute of Mental Health (NIMH, www .nimh.nih.gov), part of the National Institutes of Health, July 29, 2008.

An experimental skin patch test detected abnormal levels of markers for immune function and stress in the sweat of women with histories of depression, researchers say. If confirmed, the non-invasive technique could become an easier alternative to a blood test for predicting risk for inflammatory disorders, such as metabolic syndrome, cardiovascular disease, osteoporosis, and diabetes, which often occur with depression.

"Even though most of them had few symptoms, women with a history of depression showed biomarkers in sweat and blood consistent with a 'fight or flight' stress response," explained Esther Sternberg, MD, chief of NIMH's Section on Neuroendocrine Immunology and Behavior. Inflammation-related immune messenger chemicals soared as much as five-fold and a nerve chemical that normally acts as a brake on the stress response plummeted, while an adrenalin-like nerve chemical was elevated.

Sternberg and her colleagues published their findings online July 29, 2008 in *Biological Psychiatry*.

Although similar abnormalities in stress and immune indicators had previously been linked to depression, the study is the first to demonstrate the feasibility of accurately measuring them in sweat.

In the study, 19 women, most in remission from depression, and 17 healthy controls wore abdominal sweat patches for a day. Variations in marker levels in their sweat correlated strongly with levels in their blood—and also with severity of depression and anxiety symptoms. These changes predispose patients to metabolic syndrome and other inflammatory illnesses, Sternberg said.

In the women with histories of depression, five immune system chemical messengers called cytokines were elevated several-fold, as were three stress-related brain chemicals called neuropeptides.

Cytokines regulate neuropeptides and other brain chemicals that control pain, mood and other behaviors altered in depression. A four-fold drop in levels of a neuropeptide called VIP [vasoactive intestinal peptide] coupled with a rise in an adrenalin-like neuropeptide called NPY [neuropeptide Y] signaled a runaway stress response.

Unlike a blood test, which provides a brief snapshot of marker levels at one point in time, the sweat patch test provides a window into these levels over the course of a day. It may also be a more practical way to monitor the patterns in people on the go. However, larger studies, with patients both on and off antidepressant medications, will be required to confirm the results, and determine whether the method can be applied to other conditions, Sternberg added.

Reference

Cizza G, Marques AH, Eskandari F, Christie IC, Torvik S, Silverman MN, Phillips TM, Sternberg EM. Elevated Neuroimmune Biomarkers in Sweat Patches and Plasma of Premenopausal Women with Major Depressive Disorder in Remission: The P.O.W.E.R. Study. *Biological Psychiatry*

Chapter 25

Anxiety Disorders

Introduction

Anxiety disorders affect about 40 million American adults age 18 years and older (about 18%) in a given year, causing them to be filled with fearfulness and uncertainty. Unlike the relatively mild, brief anxiety caused by a stressful event (such as speaking in public or a first date), anxiety disorders last at least 6 months and can get worse if they are not treated. Anxiety disorders commonly occur along with other mental or physical illnesses, including alcohol or substance abuse, which may mask anxiety symptoms or make them worse. In some cases, these other illnesses need to be treated before a person will respond to treatment for the anxiety disorder. Each anxiety disorder has different symptoms, but all the symptoms cluster around excessive, irrational fear and dread.

Effective therapies for anxiety disorders are available, and research is uncovering new treatments that can help most people with anxiety disorders lead productive, fulfilling lives. If you think you have an anxiety disorder, you should seek information and treatment right away.

Panic Disorder

Panic disorder is a real illness that can be successfully treated. It is characterized by sudden attacks of terror, usually accompanied by a

Excerpted from "Anxiety Disorders," by the National Institute of Mental Health (NIMH, www.nimh.nih.gov), part of the National Institutes of Health, 2009.

pounding heart, sweatiness, weakness, faintness, or dizziness. During these attacks, people with panic disorder may flush or feel chilled; their hands may tingle or feel numb; and they may experience nausea, chest pain, or smothering sensations. Panic attacks usually produce a sense of unreality, a fear of impending doom, or a fear of losing control.

A fear of one's own unexplained physical symptoms is also a symptom of panic disorder. People having panic attacks sometimes believe they are having heart attacks, losing their minds, or on the verge of death. They can't predict when or where an attack will occur, and between episodes many worry intensely and dread the next attack.

Panic attacks can occur at any time, even during sleep. An attack usually peaks within 10 minutes, but some symptoms may last much longer.

Panic disorder affects about 6 million American adults and is twice as common in women as men. Panic attacks often begin in late adolescence or early adulthood, but not everyone who experiences panic attacks will develop panic disorder. Many people have just one attack and never have another. The tendency to develop panic attacks appears to be inherited.

People who have full-blown, repeated panic attacks can become very disabled by their condition and should seek treatment before they start to avoid places or situations where panic attacks have occurred. For example, if a panic attack happened in an elevator, someone with panic disorder may develop a fear of elevators that could affect the choice of a job or an apartment, and restrict where that person can seek medical attention or enjoy entertainment.

Some people's lives become so restricted that they avoid normal activities, such as grocery shopping or driving. About one third become housebound or are able to confront a feared situation only when accompanied by a spouse or other trusted person. When the condition progresses this far, it is called agoraphobia, or fear of open spaces.

Early treatment can often prevent agoraphobia, but people with panic disorder may sometimes go from doctor to doctor for years and visit the emergency room repeatedly before someone correctly diagnoses their condition. This is unfortunate, because panic disorder is one of the most treatable of all the anxiety disorders, responding in most cases to certain kinds of medication or certain kinds of cognitive psychotherapy, which help change thinking patterns that lead to fear and anxiety.

Panic disorder is often accompanied by other serious problems, such as depression, drug abuse, or alcoholism. These conditions need to be treated separately. Symptoms of depression include feelings of sadness or hopelessness, changes in appetite or sleep patterns, low energy, and difficulty concentrating. Most people with depression can be effectively treated with antidepressant medications, certain types of psychotherapy, or a combination of the two.

Obsessive-Compulsive Disorder

People with obsessive-compulsive disorder (OCD) have persistent, upsetting thoughts (obsessions) and use rituals (compulsions) to control the anxiety these thoughts produce. Most of the time, the rituals end up controlling them.

For example, if people are obsessed with germs or dirt, they may develop a compulsion to wash their hands over and over again. If they develop an obsession with intruders, they may lock and relock their doors many times before going to bed. Being afraid of social embarrassment may prompt people with OCD to comb their hair compulsively in front of a mirror—sometimes they get "caught" in the mirror and can't move away from it. Performing such rituals is not pleasurable. At best, it produces temporary relief from the anxiety created by obsessive thoughts.

Other common rituals are a need to repeatedly check things, touch things (especially in a particular sequence), or count things. Some common obsessions include having frequent thoughts of violence and harming loved ones, persistently thinking about performing sexual acts the person dislikes, or having thoughts that are prohibited by religious beliefs. People with OCD may also be preoccupied with order and symmetry, have difficulty throwing things out (so they accumulate), or hoard unneeded items.

Healthy people also have rituals, such as checking to see if the stove is off several times before leaving the house. The difference is that people with OCD perform their rituals even though doing so interferes with daily life and they find the repetition distressing. Although most adults with OCD recognize that what they are doing is senseless, some adults and most children may not realize that their behavior is out of the ordinary.

OCD affects about 2.2 million American adults, and the problem can be accompanied by eating disorders, other anxiety disorders, or depression. It strikes men and women in roughly equal numbers and usually appears in childhood, adolescence, or early adulthood. One third of adults with OCD develop symptoms as children, and research indicates that OCD might run in families.

The course of the disease is quite varied. Symptoms may come and go, ease over time, or get worse. If OCD becomes severe, it can keep a person from working or carrying out normal responsibilities at home. People with OCD may try to help themselves by avoiding situations that trigger their obsessions, or they may use alcohol or drugs to calm themselves.

OCD usually responds well to treatment with certain medications and/or exposure-based psychotherapy, in which people face situations that cause fear or anxiety and become less sensitive (desensitized) to them. NIMH is supporting research into new treatment approaches for people whose OCD does not respond well to the usual therapies. These approaches include combination and augmentation (add-on) treatments, as well as modern techniques such as deep brain stimulation.

Posttraumatic Stress Disorder

Posttraumatic stress disorder (PTSD) develops after a terrifying ordeal that involved physical harm or the threat of physical harm. The person who develops PTSD may have been the one who was harmed, the harm may have happened to a loved one, or the person may have witnessed a harmful event that happened to loved ones or strangers.

PTSD was first brought to public attention in relation to war veterans, but it can result from a variety of traumatic incidents, such as mugging, rape, torture, being kidnapped or held captive, child abuse, car accidents, train wrecks, plane crashes, bombings, or natural disasters such as floods or earthquakes.

People with PTSD may startle easily, become emotionally numb (especially in relation to people with whom they used to be close), lose interest in things they used to enjoy, have trouble feeling affectionate, be irritable, become more aggressive, or even become violent. They avoid situations that remind them of the original incident, and anniversaries of the incident are often very difficult. PTSD symptoms seem to be worse if the event that triggered them was deliberately initiated by another person, as in a mugging or a kidnapping.

Most people with PTSD repeatedly relive the trauma in their thoughts during the day and in nightmares when they sleep. These are called flashbacks. Flashbacks may consist of images, sounds, smells, or feelings, and are often triggered by ordinary occurrences, such as a door slamming or a car backfiring on the street. A person having a flashback may lose touch with reality and believe that the traumatic incident is happening all over again.

Not every traumatized person develops full-blown or even minor PTSD. Symptoms usually begin within 3 months of the incident but occasionally emerge years afterward. They must last more than a month to be considered PTSD. The course of the illness varies. Some people recover within 6 months, while others have symptoms that last much longer. In some people, the condition becomes chronic.

PTSD affects about 7.7 million American adults, but it can occur at any age, including childhood. Women are more likely to develop PTSD than men, and there is some evidence that susceptibility to the disorder may run in families. PTSD is often accompanied by depression, substance abuse, or one or more of the other anxiety disorders.

Certain kinds of medication and certain kinds of psychotherapy usually treat the symptoms of PTSD very effectively.

Social Phobia (Social Anxiety Disorder)

Social phobia, also called social anxiety disorder, is diagnosed when people become overwhelmingly anxious and excessively self-conscious in everyday social situations. People with social phobia have an intense, persistent, and chronic fear of being watched and judged by others and of doing things that will embarrass them. They can worry for days or weeks before a dreaded situation. This fear may become so severe that it interferes with work, school, and other ordinary activities, and can make it hard to make and keep friends.

While many people with social phobia realize that their fears about being with people are excessive or unreasonable, they are unable to overcome them. Even if they manage to confront their fears and be around others, they are usually very anxious beforehand, are intensely uncomfortable throughout the encounter, and worry about how they were judged for hours afterward.

Social phobia can be limited to one situation (such as talking to people, eating or drinking, or writing on a blackboard in front of others) or may be so broad (such as in generalized social phobia) that the person experiences anxiety around almost anyone other than the family.

Physical symptoms that often accompany social phobia include blushing, profuse sweating, trembling, nausea, and difficulty talking. When these symptoms occur, people with social phobia feel as though all eyes are focused on them.

Social phobia affects about 15 million American adults. Women and men are equally likely to develop the disorder, which usually begins in childhood or early adolescence. There is some evidence that genetic factors are involved. Social phobia is often accompanied by other anxiety disorders or depression, and substance abuse may develop if people try to self-medicate their anxiety.

Social phobia can be successfully treated with certain kinds of psychotherapy or medications.

Specific Phobias

A specific phobia is an intense, irrational fear of something that poses little or no actual danger. Some of the more common specific phobias are centered around closed-in places, heights, escalators, tunnels, highway driving, water, flying, dogs, and injuries involving blood. Such phobias aren't just extreme fear; they are irrational fear of a particular thing. You may be able to ski the world's tallest mountains with ease but be unable to go above the 5th floor of an office building. While adults with phobias realize that these fears are irrational, they often find that facing, or even thinking about facing, the feared object or situation brings on a panic attack or severe anxiety.

Specific phobias affect an estimated 19.2 million adult Americans and are twice as common in women as men. They usually appear in childhood or adolescence and tend to persist into adulthood. The causes of specific phobias are not well understood, but there is some evidence that the tendency to develop them may run in families.

If the feared situation or feared object is easy to avoid, people with specific phobias may not seek help; but if avoidance interferes with their careers or their personal lives, it can become disabling and treatment is usually pursued.

Specific phobias respond very well to carefully targeted psychotherapy.

Generalized Anxiety Disorder (GAD)

People with generalized anxiety disorder (GAD) go through the day filled with exaggerated worry and tension, even though there is little or nothing to provoke it. They anticipate disaster and are overly concerned about health issues, money, family problems, or difficulties at work. Sometimes just the thought of getting through the day produces anxiety.

GAD is diagnosed when a person worries excessively about a variety of everyday problems for at least 6 months. People with GAD can't seem to get rid of their concerns, even though they usually realize that their anxiety is more intense than the situation warrants. They can't relax, startle easily, and have difficulty concentrating. Often they have trouble falling asleep or staying asleep. Physical symptoms that often accompany the anxiety include fatigue, headaches, muscle tension, muscle aches, difficulty swallowing, trembling, twitching, irritability, sweating, nausea, lightheadedness, having to go to the bathroom frequently, feeling out of breath, and hot flashes.

When their anxiety level is mild, people with GAD can function socially and hold down a job. Although they don't avoid certain situations as a result of their disorder, people with GAD can have difficulty carrying out the simplest daily activities if their anxiety is severe.

GAD affects about 6.8 million American adults, including twice as many women as men. The disorder develops gradually and can begin at any point in the life cycle, although the years of highest risk are between childhood and middle age.

There is evidence that genes play a modest role in GAD. Other anxiety disorders, depression, or substance abuse often accompany GAD, which rarely occurs alone. GAD is commonly treated with medication or cognitive-behavioral therapy, but co-occurring conditions must also be treated using the appropriate therapies.

Role of Research in Improving the Understanding and Treatment of Anxiety Disorders

NIMH supports research into the causes, diagnosis, prevention, and treatment of anxiety disorders and other mental illnesses. Scientists are looking at what role genes play in the development of these disorders and are also investigating the effects of environmental factors such as pollution, physical and psychological stress, and diet. In addition, studies are being conducted on the "natural history" (what course the illness takes without treatment) of a variety of individual anxiety disorders, combinations of anxiety disorders, and anxiety disorders that are accompanied by other mental illnesses such as depression.

Scientists currently think that, like heart disease and type 1 diabetes, mental illnesses are complex and probably result from a combination of genetic, environmental, psychological, and developmental factors. For instance, although NIMH-sponsored studies of twins and families suggest that genetics play a role in the development of some anxiety disorders, problems such as PTSD are triggered by trauma. Genetic studies may help explain why some people exposed to trauma develop PTSD and others do not.

Several parts of the brain are key actors in the production of fear and anxiety. Using brain imaging technology and neurochemical techniques, scientists have discovered that the amygdala and the hippocampus play significant roles in most anxiety disorders.

The amygdala is an almond-shaped structure deep in the brain that is believed to be a communications hub between the parts of the brain that process incoming sensory signals and the parts that interpret these signals. It can alert the rest of the brain that a threat is present and trigger a fear or anxiety response. It appears that emotional memories are stored in the central part of the amygdala and may play a role in anxiety disorders involving very distinct fears, such as fears of dogs, spiders, or flying.

The hippocampus is the part of the brain that encodes threatening events into memories. Studies have shown that the hippocampus appears to be smaller in some people who were victims of child abuse or who served in military combat. Research will determine what causes this reduction in size and what role it plays in the flashbacks, deficits in explicit memory, and fragmented memories of the traumatic event that are common in PTSD.

By learning more about how the brain creates fear and anxiety, scientists may be able to devise better treatments for anxiety disorders. For example, if specific neurotransmitters are found to play an important role in fear, drugs may be developed that will block them and decrease fear responses; if enough is learned about how the brain generates new cells throughout the lifecycle, it may be possible to stimulate the growth of new neurons in the hippocampus in people with PTSD.

Current research at NIMH on anxiety disorders includes studies that address how well medication and behavioral therapies work in the treatment of OCD, and the safety and effectiveness of medications for children and adolescents who have a combination of anxiety disorders and attention deficit hyperactivity disorder.

Chapter 26

Bipolar Disorder

Bipolar disorder, also known as manic-depressive illness, is a brain disorder that causes unusual shifts in mood, energy, activity levels, and the ability to carry out day-to-day tasks. Symptoms of bipolar disorder are severe. They are different from the normal ups and downs that everyone goes through from time to time. Bipolar disorder symptoms can result in damaged relationships, poor job or school performance, and even suicide. But bipolar disorder can be treated, and people with this illness can lead full and productive lives.

Bipolar disorder often develops in a person's late teens or early adult years. At least half of all cases start before age 25. Some people have their first symptoms during childhood, while others may develop symptoms late in life.

Bipolar disorder is not easy to spot when it starts. The symptoms may seem like separate problems, not recognized as parts of a larger problem. Some people suffer for years before they are properly diagnosed and treated. Like diabetes or heart disease, bipolar disorder is a long-term illness that must be carefully managed throughout a person's life.

Symptoms of Bipolar Disorder

People with bipolar disorder experience unusually intense emotional states that occur in distinct periods called "mood episodes." An overly

Excerpted from "Bipolar Disorder," by the National Institute of Mental Health (NIMH, www.nimh.nih.gov), part of the National Institutes of Health, 2009.

joyful or overexcited state is called a manic episode, and an extremely sad or hopeless state is called a depressive episode. Sometimes, a mood episode includes symptoms of both mania and depression. This is called a mixed state. People with bipolar disorder also may be explosive and irritable during a mood episode.

Extreme changes in energy, activity, sleep, and behavior go along with these changes in mood. It is possible for someone with bipolar disorder to experience a long-lasting period of unstable moods rather than discrete episodes of depression or mania.

A person may be having an episode of bipolar disorder if he or she has a number of manic or depressive symptoms for most of the day, nearly every day, for at least 1 or 2 weeks. Sometimes symptoms are so severe that the person cannot function normally at work, school, or home.

Symptoms of mania or a manic episode are listed in the following text.

Mood Changes

- A long period of feeling "high," or an overly happy or outgoing mood

- Extremely irritable mood, agitation, feeling "jumpy" or "wired"

Behavioral Changes

- Talking very fast, jumping from one idea to another, having racing thoughts

- Being easily distracted

- Increasing goal-directed activities, such as taking on new projects

- Being restless

- Sleeping little

- Having an unrealistic belief in one's abilities

- Behaving impulsively and taking part in a lot of pleasurable, high-risk behaviors, such as spending sprees, impulsive sex, and impulsive business investments

Symptoms of depression or a depressive episode are listed in the following text.

Mood Changes

- A long period of feeling worried or empty
- Loss of interest in activities once enjoyed, including sex

Behavioral Changes

- Feeling tired or "slowed down"
- Having problems concentrating, remembering, and making decisions
- Being restless or irritable
- Changing eating, sleeping, or other habits
- Thinking of death or suicide, or attempting suicide

In addition to mania and depression, bipolar disorder can cause a range of moods.

One side of the scale includes severe depression, moderate depression, and mild low mood. Moderate depression may cause less extreme symptoms, and mild low mood is called dysthymia when it is chronic or long-term. In the middle of the scale is normal or balanced mood.

At the other end of the scale are hypomania and severe mania. Some people with bipolar disorder experience hypomania. During hypomanic episodes, a person may have increased energy and activity levels that are not as severe as typical mania, or he or she may have episodes that last less than a week and do not require emergency care. A person having a hypomanic episode may feel very good, be highly productive, and function well. This person may not feel that anything is wrong even as family and friends recognize the mood swings as possible bipolar disorder. Without proper treatment, however, people with hypomania may develop severe mania or depression.

During a mixed state, symptoms often include agitation, trouble sleeping, major changes in appetite, and suicidal thinking. People in a mixed state may feel very sad or hopeless while feeling extremely energized.

Sometimes, a person with severe episodes of mania or depression has psychotic symptoms too, such as hallucinations or delusions. The psychotic symptoms tend to reflect the person's extreme mood. For example, psychotic symptoms for a person having a manic episode may include believing he or she is famous, has a lot of money, or has special powers. In the same way, a person having a depressive episode may believe he or she is ruined and penniless, or has committed a crime. As a result, people with bipolar disorder who have psychotic symptoms are sometimes wrongly diagnosed as having schizophrenia, another severe mental illness that is linked with hallucinations and delusions.

People with bipolar disorder may also have behavioral problems. They may abuse alcohol or substances, have relationship problems, or perform poorly in school or at work. At first, it's not easy to recognize these problems as signs of a major mental illness.

Bipolar Disorder over Time

Bipolar disorder usually lasts a lifetime. Episodes of mania and depression typically come back over time. Between episodes, many people with bipolar disorder are free of symptoms, but some people may have lingering symptoms.

Doctors usually diagnose mental disorders using guidelines from the *Diagnostic and Statistical Manual of Mental Disorders*, or *DSM*. According to the *DSM*, there are four basic types of bipolar disorder:

1. Bipolar I disorder is mainly defined by manic or mixed episodes that last at least 7 days, or by manic symptoms that are so severe that the person needs immediate hospital care. Usually, the person also has depressive episodes, typically lasting at least 2 weeks. The symptoms of mania or depression must be a major change from the person's normal behavior.

2. Bipolar II disorder is defined by a pattern of depressive episodes shifting back and forth with hypomanic episodes, but no full-blown manic or mixed episodes.

3. Bipolar disorder not otherwise specified (BP-NOS) is diagnosed when a person has symptoms of the illness that do not meet diagnostic criteria for either bipolar I or II. The symptoms may not last long enough, or the person may have too few symptoms, to be diagnosed with bipolar I or II. However, the symptoms are clearly out of the person's normal range of behavior.

4. Cyclothymic disorder, or cyclothymia, is a mild form of bipolar disorder.

People who have cyclothymia have episodes of hypomania that shift back and forth with mild depression for at least 2 years. However, the symptoms do not meet the diagnostic requirements for any other type of bipolar disorder. Some people may be diagnosed with rapid-cycling bipolar disorder. This is when a person has four or more episodes of major depression, mania, hypomania, or mixed symptoms within a year. Some people experience more than one episode in a week, or even within 1 day. Rapid cycling seems to be more common in people who have severe bipolar disorder and may be more common in people who have their first episode at a younger age. One study found that people with rapid cycling had their first episode about 4 years earlier, during mid to late teen years, than people without rapid cycling bipolar disorder. Rapid cycling affects more women than men.

Bipolar disorder tends to worsen if it is not treated. Over time, a person may suffer more frequent and more severe episodes than when the illness first appeared. Also, delays in getting the correct diagnosis and treatment make a person more likely to experience personal, social, and work-related problems.

Proper diagnosis and treatment helps people with bipolar disorder lead healthy and productive lives. In most cases, treatment can help reduce the frequency and severity of episodes.

Illnesses That Often Coexist with Bipolar Disorder

Substance abuse is very common among people with bipolar disorder, but the reasons for this link are unclear. Some people with bipolar disorder may try to treat their symptoms with alcohol or drugs. However, substance abuse may trigger or prolong bipolar symptoms, and the behavioral control problems associated with mania can result in a person drinking too much.

Anxiety disorders, such as post-traumatic stress disorder (PTSD) and social phobia, also co-occur often among people with bipolar disorder. Bipolar disorder also co-occurs with attention deficit hyperactivity disorder (ADHD), which has some symptoms that overlap with bipolar disorder, such as restlessness and being easily distracted.

People with bipolar disorder are also at higher risk for thyroid disease, migraine headaches, heart disease, diabetes, obesity, and other physical illnesses. These illnesses may cause symptoms of mania or depression. They may also result from treatment for bipolar disorder.

Other illnesses can make it hard to diagnose and treat bipolar disorder. People with bipolar disorder should monitor their physical and mental health. If a symptom does not get better with treatment, they should tell their doctor.

Risk Factors for Bipolar Disorder

Scientists are learning about the possible causes of bipolar disorder. Most scientists agree that there is no single cause. Rather, many factors likely act together to produce the illness or increase risk.

Genetics

Bipolar disorder tends to run in families, so researchers are looking for genes that may increase a person's chance of developing the illness. Genes are the "building blocks" of heredity. They help control how the body and brain work and grow. Genes are contained inside a person's cells that are passed down from parents to children.

Children with a parent or sibling who has bipolar disorder are four to six times more likely to develop the illness, compared with children who do not have a family history of bipolar disorder. However, most children with a family history of bipolar disorder will not develop the illness.

Most people with bipolar disorder have:

- missed work because of their illness;
- other illnesses at the same time, especially alcohol and/or substance abuse and panic disorders;
- been treated or hospitalized for bipolar disorder.

Certain traits appear to run in families, including the following:

- History of psychiatric hospitalization
- Co-occurring obsessive-compulsive disorder (OCD)
- Age at first manic episode
- Number and frequency of manic episodes

Scientists continue to study these traits, which may help them find the genes that cause bipolar disorder some day.

But genes are not the only risk factor for bipolar disorder. Studies of identical twins have shown that the twin of a person with bipolar illness does not always develop the disorder. This is important because identical twins share all of the same genes. The study results suggest factors besides genes are also at work. Rather, it is likely that many different genes and a person's environment are involved. However, scientists do not yet fully understand how these factors interact to cause bipolar disorder.

Brain Structure and Functioning

Brain-imaging studies are helping scientists learn what happens in the brain of a person with bipolar disorder. Newer brain-imaging tools, such as functional magnetic resonance imaging (fMRI) and positron emission tomography (PET), allow researchers to take pictures of the living brain at work. These tools help scientists study the brain's structure and activity.

Some imaging studies show how the brains of people with bipolar disorder may differ from the brains of healthy people or people with other mental disorders. For example, one study using MRI found that the pattern of brain development in children with bipolar disorder was similar to that in children with "multidimensional impairment," a disorder that causes symptoms that overlap somewhat with bipolar disorder and schizophrenia. This suggests that the common pattern of brain development may be linked to general risk for unstable moods.

Learning more about these differences, along with information gained from genetic studies, helps scientists better understand bipolar disorder. Someday scientists may be able to predict which types of treatment will work most effectively. They may even find ways to prevent bipolar disorder.

Diagnosing Bipolar Disorder

The first step in getting a proper diagnosis is to talk to a doctor, who may conduct a physical examination, an interview, and lab tests. Bipolar disorder cannot currently be identified through a blood test or a brain scan, but these tests can help rule out other contributing factors, such as a stroke or brain tumor. If the problems are not caused by other illnesses, the doctor may conduct a mental health evaluation. The doctor may also provide a referral to a trained mental health professional, such as a psychiatrist, who is experienced in diagnosing and treating bipolar disorder.

The doctor or mental health professional should conduct a complete diagnostic evaluation. He or she should discuss any family history of bipolar disorder or other mental illnesses and get a complete history of symptoms. The doctor or mental health professionals should also talk to the person's close relatives or spouse and note how they describe the person's symptoms and family medical history.

People with bipolar disorder are more likely to seek help when they are depressed than when experiencing mania or hypomania. Therefore, a careful medical history is needed to assure that bipolar disorder is not mistakenly diagnosed as major depressive disorder, which is also called unipolar depression. Unlike people with bipolar disorder, people who have unipolar depression do not experience mania. Whenever possible, previous records and input from family and friends should also be included in the medical history.

If Someone Is in Crisis

If you are thinking about harming yourself, or know someone who is, tell someone who can help immediately.

- Call your doctor.

- Call 911 or go to a hospital emergency room to get immediate help or ask a friend or family member to help you do these things.

- Call the toll-free, 24-hour hotline of the National Suicide Prevention Lifeline at 800-273-TALK (800-273-8255); TTY: 800-799-4TTY (799-4889) to talk to a trained counselor.

- Make sure you or the suicidal person is not left alone.

Chapter 27

Disordered Eating and Stress

Chapter Contents

Section 27.1

Emotional Eating

Imagine you've had a fight with your best friend. It's a stupid fight, something you'll both get over. But right now you're upset. When you walk in the door, your mom asks what's wrong. How are you most likely to respond?

- Tell your mom what happened and have a long, comforting talk about it.

or

- Tell your mom, "Everything's fine" and head to the freezer for the ice cream.

But can that pint of Rocky Road really help you feel better—or just make you feel sickeningly full?

What Is Emotional Eating?

Emotional eating is when people use food as a way to deal with feelings instead of to satisfy hunger. We've all been there, finishing a whole bag of chips out of boredom or downing cookie after cookie while cramming for a big test. But when done a lot—especially without realizing it—emotional eating can affect weight, health, and overall well-being.

Not many of us make the connection between eating and our feelings. But understanding what drives emotional eating can help people take steps to change it.

One of the biggest myths about emotional eating is that it's prompted by negative feelings. Yes, people often turn to food when they're stressed out, lonely, sad, anxious, or bored. But emotional eating can be linked to positive feelings too, like the romance of sharing dessert on Valentine's Day or the celebration of a holiday feast.

Sometimes emotional eating is tied to major life events, like a death or a divorce. More often, though, it's the countless little daily stresses that cause someone to seek comfort or distraction in food.

Emotional eating patterns can be learned: A child who is given candy after a big achievement may grow up using candy as a reward for a job well done. A kid who is given cookies as a way to stop crying may learn to link cookies with comfort.

It's not easy to "unlearn" patterns of emotional eating. But it is possible. And it starts with an awareness of what's going on.

"Comfort" Foods

We all have our own comfort foods. Interestingly, they may vary according to moods and gender. One study found that happy people seem to want to eat things like pizza, while sad people prefer ice cream and cookies. Bored people crave salty, crunchy things, like chips. Researchers also found that guys seem to prefer hot, homemade comfort meals, like steaks and casseroles. Girls go for chocolate and ice cream.

This brings up a curious question: Does no one take comfort in carrots and celery sticks? Researchers are looking into that, too. What they're finding is that high-fat foods, like ice cream, may activate certain chemicals in the body that create a sense of contentment and fulfillment. This almost addictive quality may actually make you reach for these foods again when feeling upset.

Physical Hunger vs. Emotional Hunger

We're all emotional eaters to some extent (who hasn't suddenly found room for dessert after a filling dinner?). But for some people, emotional eating can be a real problem, causing serious weight gain or cycles of binging and purging.

The trouble with emotional eating (aside from the health issues) is that once the pleasure of eating is gone, the feelings that cause it remain. And you often may feel worse about eating the amount or type of food you did. That's why it helps to know the differences between physical hunger and emotional hunger. Next time you reach for a snack, check in and see which type of hunger is driving it. (See Table 27.1.)

Questions to Ask Yourself

You can also ask yourself these questions about your eating:

Table 27.1. The Difference between Physical Hunger and Emotional Hunger

Physical Hunger	Emotional Hunger
Tends to come on gradually and can be postponed	Feels sudden and urgent
Can be satisfied with any number of foods	Causes very specific cravings (say, for pizza or ice cream)
Once full, you're likely to stop eating	You tend to eat more than you normally would
Doesn't cause feelings of guilt	Can cause guilt afterwards

- Have I been eating larger portions than usual?

- Do I eat at unusual times?

- Do I feel a loss of control around food?

- Am I anxious over something, like school, a social situation, or an event where my abilities might be tested?

- Has there been a big event in my life that I'm having trouble dealing with?

- Am I already overweight or obese, or has there recently been a big jump in my weight or body mass index (BMI)?

- Do other people in my family use food to soothe their feelings too?

If you answered yes to many of these questions, then it's possible that eating has become a coping mechanism instead of a way to fuel your body.

Breaking the Cycle

Managing emotional eating means finding other ways to deal with the situations and feelings that make someone turn to food.

For example, do you come home from school each day and automatically head to the kitchen? Stop and ask yourself, "Am I really hungry?" Is your stomach growling? Are you having difficulty concentrating or feeling irritable? If these signs point to hunger, choose something light and healthy to take the edge off until dinner.

Not really hungry? If the post-school food foraging has just become part of your routine, think about why.

Tips to Try

These three techniques can help:

1. Explore why you're eating and find a replacement activity. For example:

- If you're bored or lonely, call or text a friend or family member.

- If you're stressed out, try a yoga routine. Or listen to some feel-good tunes and let off some steam by jogging in place, doing jumping jacks, or dancing around your room until the urge to eat passes.

- If you're tired, rethink your bedtime routine. Tiredness can feel a lot like hunger, and food won't help if sleepless nights are causing daytime fatigue.

- If you're eating to procrastinate, open those books and get that homework over with. You'll feel better afterwards (honestly!).

2. Write down the emotions that trigger your eating. One of the best ways to keep track is with a mood and food journal. Write down what you ate, how much, and how you felt as you ate (e.g., bored, happy, worried, sad, mad) and whether you were really hungry or just eating for comfort.

Through journaling, you'll start to see patterns emerging between what you feel and what you eat. You'll be able to use this information to make better choices (like choosing to clear your head with a walk around the block instead of a bag of Doritos).

3. Pause and "take 5" before you reach for food. Too often, we rush through the day without really checking in with ourselves. We're so stressed, overscheduled, and plugged-in that we lose out on time to reflect.

Instead of eating when you get in the door, take a few minutes to transition from one part of your day to another. Go over the things that happened that day. Acknowledge how they made you feel: Happy? Grateful? Excited? Angry? Worried? Jealous? Left out?

Getting Help

Even when we understand what's going on, many of us still need help breaking the cycle of emotional eating. It's not easy—especially when emotional eating has already led to weight and self-esteem issues. So don't go it alone when you don't have to.

Take advantage of expert help. Counselors and therapists can help you deal with your feelings. Nutritionists can help you identify your eating patterns and get you on track with a better diet. Fitness experts can get your body's feel-good chemicals firing through exercise instead of food.

If you're worried about your eating, talk to your doctor. He or she can make sure you reach your weight-loss goals safely and put you in touch with professionals who can put you on a path to a new, healthier relationship with food.

Section 27.2

Eating Disorders Linked to Feelings of Extreme Distress

Excerpted from "Eating Disorders," by the National Institute of Mental Health (NIMH, www.nimh.nih.gov), part of the National Institutes of Health, June 12, 2009.

What Are Eating Disorders?

An eating disorder is marked by extremes. It is present when a person experiences severe disturbances in eating behavior, such as extreme reduction of food intake or extreme overeating, or feelings of extreme distress or concern about body weight or shape.

A person with an eating disorder may have started out just eating smaller or larger amounts of food than usual, but at some point, the urge to eat less or more spirals out of control. Eating disorders are very complex, and despite scientific research to understand them, the biological, behavioral, and social underpinnings of these illnesses remain elusive.

The two main types of eating disorders are anorexia nervosa and bulimia nervosa. A third category is eating disorders not otherwise specified (EDNOS), which includes several variations of eating disorders. Most of these disorders are similar to anorexia or bulimia but with slightly different characteristics. Binge-eating disorder, which has received increasing research and media attention in recent years, is one type of EDNOS.

Eating disorders frequently appear during adolescence or young adulthood, but some reports indicate that they can develop during childhood or later in adulthood. Women and girls are much more likely than males to develop an eating disorder. Men and boys account for an estimated 5 to 15 percent of patients with anorexia or bulimia and an estimated 35 percent of those with binge-eating disorder. Eating disorders are real, treatable medical illnesses with complex underlying psychological and biological causes. They frequently co-exist with other psychiatric disorders such as depression, substance abuse, or anxiety disorders. People with eating disorders also can suffer from numerous other physical health complications, such as heart conditions or kidney failure, which can lead to death.

Psychological and medicinal treatments are effective for many eating disorders. However, in more chronic cases, specific treatments have not yet been identified.

In these cases, treatment plans often are tailored to the patient's individual needs that may include medical care and monitoring; medications; nutritional counseling; and individual, group, and/or family psychotherapy. Some patients may also need to be hospitalized to treat malnutrition, to gain weight, or for other reasons.

Anorexia Nervosa

Anorexia nervosa is characterized by emaciation, a relentless pursuit of thinness and unwillingness to maintain a normal or healthy weight, a distortion of body image and intense fear of gaining weight, a lack of menstruation among girls and women, and extremely disturbed eating behavior. Some people with anorexia lose weight by dieting and exercising excessively; others lose weight by self-induced vomiting, or misusing laxatives, diuretics, or enemas.

Many people with anorexia see themselves as overweight, even when they are starved or are clearly malnourished. Eating, food, and weight control become obsessions. A person with anorexia typically weighs herself or himself repeatedly, portions food carefully, and eats only very small quantities of only certain foods. Some who have anorexia recover with treatment after only one episode. Others get well but have relapses. Still others have a more chronic form of anorexia, in which their health deteriorates over many years as they battle the illness.

According to some studies, people with anorexia are up to 10 times more likely to die as a result of their illness compared to those without the disorder. The most common complications that lead to death are cardiac arrest and electrolyte and fluid imbalances. Suicide also can result.

Many people with anorexia also have coexisting psychiatric and physical illnesses, including depression, anxiety, obsessive behavior, substance abuse, cardiovascular and neurological complications, and impaired physical development.

Other symptoms may develop over time, including the following:

- Thinning of the bones (osteopenia or osteoporosis)
- Brittle hair and nails
- Dry and yellowish skin
- Growth of fine hair over body (e.g., lanugo)
- Mild anemia and muscle weakness and loss
- Severe constipation
- Low blood pressure and slowed breathing and pulse
- Drop in internal body temperature, causing a person to feel cold all the time
- Lethargy

Treating anorexia involves three components:

1. Restoring the person to a healthy weight
2. Treating the psychological issues related to the eating disorder
3. Reducing or eliminating behaviors or thoughts that lead to disordered eating and preventing relapse

Some research suggests that the use of medications, such as antidepressants, antipsychotics, or mood stabilizers, may be modestly effective in treating patients with anorexia by helping to resolve mood and anxiety symptoms that often coexist with anorexia. Recent studies, however, have suggested that antidepressants may not be effective in preventing some patients with anorexia from relapsing. In addition, no medication has shown to be effective during the critical first phase of restoring a patient to healthy weight. Overall, it is unclear if and how medications can help patients conquer anorexia, but research is ongoing.

Different forms of psychotherapy, including individual, group, and family-based, can help address the psychological reasons for the illness. Some studies suggest that family-based therapies in which parents assume responsibility for feeding their afflicted adolescent are the most effective in helping a person with anorexia gain weight and improve eating habits and moods.

Shown to be effective in case studies and clinical trials, this particular approach is discussed in some guidelines and studies for treating eating disorders in younger, nonchronic patients.

Others have noted that a combined approach of medical attention and supportive psychotherapy designed specifically for anorexia patients is more effective than just psychotherapy. But the effectiveness of a treatment depends on the person involved and his or her situation. Unfortunately, no specific psychotherapy appears to be consistently effective for treating adults with anorexia. However, research into novel treatment and prevention approaches is showing some promise. One study suggests that an online intervention program may prevent some at-risk women from developing an eating disorder.

Bulimia Nervosa

Bulimia nervosa is characterized by recurrent and frequent episodes of eating unusually large amounts of food (e.g., binge eating), and feeling a lack of control over the eating. This binge eating is followed by a type of behavior that compensates for the binge, such as purging (e.g., vomiting, excessive use of laxatives, or diuretics), fasting, and/or excessive exercise.

Unlike anorexia, people with bulimia can fall within the normal range for their age and weight. But like people with anorexia, they often fear gaining weight, want desperately to lose weight, and are intensely unhappy with their body size and shape. Usually, bulimic behavior is done secretly, because it is often accompanied by feelings of disgust or shame. The binging and purging cycle usually repeats several times a week. Similar to anorexia, people with bulimia often have coexisting psychological illnesses, such as depression, anxiety, and/or substance abuse problems. Many physical conditions result from the purging aspect of the illness, including electrolyte imbalances, gastrointestinal problems, and oral and tooth-related problems.

Other symptoms include the following:

- Chronically inflamed and sore throat
- Swollen glands in the neck and below the jaw
- Worn tooth enamel and increasingly sensitive and decaying teeth as a result of exposure to stomach acids
- Gastroesophageal reflux disorder
- Intestinal distress and irritation from laxative abuse
- Kidney problems from diuretic abuse

• Severe dehydration from purging of fluids

As with anorexia, treatment for bulimia often involves a combination of options and depends on the needs of the individual.

To reduce or eliminate binge and purge behavior, a patient may undergo nutritional counseling and psychotherapy, especially cognitive behavioral therapy (CBT), or be prescribed medication. Some antidepressants, such as fluoxetine (Prozac), which is the only medication approved by the U.S. Food and Drug Administration for treating bulimia, may help patients who also have depression and/or anxiety. It also appears to help reduce binge eating and purging behavior, reduces the chance of relapse, and improves eating attitudes.

CBT that has been tailored to treat bulimia also has shown to be effective in changing binging and purging behavior and eating attitudes. Therapy may be individually oriented or group-based.

Binge-Eating Disorder

Binge-eating disorder is characterized by recurrent binge-eating episodes during which a person feels a loss of control over his or her eating. Unlike bulimia, binge-eating episodes are not followed by purging, excessive exercise, or fasting. As a result, people with binge-eating disorder often are overweight or obese. They also experience guilt, shame, and/or distress about the binge eating, which can lead to more binge eating.

Obese people with binge-eating disorder often have coexisting psychological illnesses including anxiety, depression, and personality disorders. In addition, links between obesity and cardiovascular disease and hypertension are well documented.

Treatment options for binge-eating disorder are similar to those used to treat bulimia. Fluoxetine and other antidepressants may reduce binge-eating episodes and help alleviate depression in some patients.

Patients with binge-eating disorder also may be prescribed appetite suppressants. Psychotherapy, especially CBT, is also used to treat the underlying psychological issues associated with binge eating, in an individual or group environment.

How Are Men And Boys Affected?

Although eating disorders primarily affect women and girls, boys and men are also vulnerable. One in four preadolescent cases of anorexia occurs in boys, and binge-eating disorder affects females and males about equally.

Like females who have eating disorders, males with the illness have a warped sense of body image and often have muscle dysmorphia, a type of disorder that is characterized by an extreme concern with becoming more muscular. Some boys with the disorder want to lose weight, whereas others want to gain weight or "bulk up." Boys who think they are too small are at a greater risk for using steroids or other dangerous drugs to increase muscle mass.

Boys with eating disorders exhibit the same types of emotional, physical, and behavioral signs and symptoms as girls, but for a variety of reasons, boys are less likely to be diagnosed with what is often considered a stereotypically "female" disorder.

Understanding and Treating Eating Disorders

Researchers are unsure of the underlying causes and nature of eating disorders. Unlike a neurological disorder, which generally can be pinpointed to a specific lesion on the brain, an eating disorder likely involves abnormal activity distributed across brain systems. With increased recognition that mental disorders are brain disorders, more researchers are using tools from both modern neuroscience and modern psychology to better understand eating disorders.

One approach involves the study of the human genes. With the publication of the human genome sequence in 2003, mental health researchers are studying the various combinations of genes to determine if any DNA variations are associated with the risk of developing a mental disorder. Neuroimaging, such as the use of magnetic resonance imaging (MRI), may also lead to a better understanding of eating disorders.

Neuroimaging already is used to identify abnormal brain activity in patients with schizophrenia, obsessive-compulsive disorder, and depression. It may also help researchers better understand how people with eating disorders process information, regardless of whether they have recovered or are still in the throes of their illness.

Conducting behavioral or psychological research on eating disorders is even more complex and challenging. As a result, few studies of treatments for eating disorders have been conducted in the past. New studies currently underway, however, are aiming to remedy the lack of information available about treatment.

Researchers also are working to define the basic processes of the disorders, which should help identify better treatments. For example, is anorexia the result of skewed body image, self-esteem problems, obsessive thoughts, compulsive behavior, or a combination of these? Can it be predicted or identified as a risk factor before drastic weight loss occurs, and therefore avoided?

These and other questions may be answered in the future as scientists and doctors think of eating disorders as medical illnesses with certain biological causes. Researchers are studying behavioral questions, along with genetic and brain systems information, to understand risk factors, identify biological markers, and develop medications that can target specific pathways that control eating behavior. Finally, neuroimaging and genetic studies may also provide clues for how each person may respond to specific treatments.

Section 27.3

Binge Eating Disorder

From "Binge Eating Disorder," by the Weight-control Information Network of the National Institute of Diabetes and Digestive and Kidney Diseases (NIDDK, www.niddk.nih.gov), part of the National Institutes of Health, June 2008.

How do I know if I have binge eating disorder?

Most of us overeat from time to time, and some of us often feel we have eaten more than we should have. Eating a lot of food does not necessarily mean that you have binge eating disorder. Experts generally agree that most people with serious binge eating problems often eat an unusually large amount of food and feel their eating is out of control. People with binge eating disorder also may do the following:

- Eat much more quickly than usual during binge episodes

- Eat until they are uncomfortably full

- Eat large amounts of food even when they are not really hungry

- Eat alone because they are embarrassed about the amount of food they eat

- Feel disgusted, depressed, or guilty after overeating

Binge eating also occurs in another eating disorder called bulimia nervosa. Persons with bulimia nervosa, however, usually purge, fast, or do strenuous exercise after they binge eat. Purging means vomiting or using a lot of diuretics (water pills) or laxatives to keep from gaining weight. Fasting is not eating for at least 24 hours. Strenuous exercise, in this case, means exercising for more than an hour just to keep from gaining weight after binge eating. Purging, fasting, and overexercising are dangerous ways to try to control your weight.

How common is binge eating disorder, and who is at risk?

Binge eating disorder is the most common eating disorder. It affects about 3 percent of all adults in the United States. Researchers are looking into how brain chemicals and metabolism (the way the body uses calories) affect binge eating disorder. Binge eating disorder is the most common eating disorder. It affects about 3 percent of all adults in the United States. People of any age can have binge eating disorder, but it is seen more often in adults age 46 to 55. Binge eating disorder is a little more common in women than in men; three women for every two men have it. The disorder affects Blacks as often as Whites, but it is not known how often it affects people in other ethnic groups.

Although most obese people do not have binge eating disorder, people with this problem are usually overweight or obese. Binge eating disorder is more common in people who are severely obese. Normal-weight people can also have the disorder.

People who are obese and have binge eating disorder often became overweight at a younger age than those without the disorder. They might also lose and gain weight more often, a process known as weight cycling or "yo-yo dieting."

What causes binge eating disorder?

No one knows for sure what causes binge eating disorder. As many as half of all people with binge eating disorder are depressed or have been depressed in the past. Whether depression causes binge eating disorder, or whether binge eating disorder causes depression, is not known.

It is also unclear if dieting and binge eating are related, although some people binge eat after dieting. In these cases, dieting means skipping meals, not eating enough food each day, or avoiding certain kinds of food. These are unhealthy ways to try to change your body shape and weight.

Studies suggest that people with binge eating disorder may have trouble handling some of their emotions. Many people who are binge eaters say that being angry, sad, bored, worried, or stressed can cause them to binge eat.

Certain behaviors and emotional problems are more common in people with binge eating disorder. These include abusing alcohol, acting quickly without thinking (impulsive behavior), not feeling in charge of themselves, not feeling a part of their communities, and not noticing and talking about their feelings.

Researchers are looking into how brain chemicals and metabolism (the way the body uses calories) affect binge eating disorder. Other research suggests that genes may be involved in binge eating, since the disorder often occurs in several members of the same family. This research is still in the early stages.

What are the complications of binge eating disorder?

People with binge eating disorder are usually very upset by their binge eating and may become depressed. Research has shown that people with binge eating disorder report more health problems, stress, trouble sleeping, and suicidal thoughts than do people without an eating disorder. Other complications from binge eating disorder could include joint pain, digestive problems, headache, muscle pain, and menstrual problems.

People with binge eating disorder often feel bad about themselves and may miss work, school, or social activities to binge eat.

People with binge eating disorder may gain weight. Weight gain can lead to obesity, and obesity puts people at risk for many health problems, including the following:

- Type 2 diabetes
- High blood pressure
- High blood cholesterol levels
- Gallbladder disease
- Heart disease
- Certain types of cancer

Most people who binge eat, whether they are obese or not, feel ashamed and try to hide their problem. Often they become so good at hiding it that even close friends and family members do not know that their loved one binge eats.

Should people with binge eating disorder try to lose weight?

People with binge eating disorder should get help from a health professional such as a psychiatrist, psychologist, or clinical social worker.

Many people with binge eating disorder are obese and have health problems because of their weight. They should try to lose weight and keep it off; however, research shows that long-term weight loss is more likely when a person has long-term control over his or her binge eating.

People with binge eating disorder who are obese may benefit from a weight-loss program that also offers treatment for eating disorders. However, some people with binge eating disorder may do just as well in a standard weight-loss program as people who do not binge eat. People who are not overweight should avoid trying to lose weight because it may make their binge eating worse.

How can people with binge eating disorder be helped?

People with binge eating disorder should get help from a health care professional such as a psychiatrist, psychologist, or clinical social worker. There are several different ways to treat binge eating disorder.

- Cognitive behavioral therapy teaches people how to keep track of their eating and change their unhealthy eating habits. It teaches them how to change the way they act in tough situations. It also helps them feel better about their body shape and weight.

- Interpersonal psychotherapy helps people look at their relationships with friends and family and make changes in problem areas.

- Drug therapy, such as antidepressants, may be helpful for some people.

The methods mentioned here seem to be equally helpful. Researchers are still trying to find the treatment that is the most helpful in controlling binge eating disorder. Combining drug and behavioral therapy has shown promising results for treating overweight and obese individuals with binge eating disorder. Drug therapy has been shown to benefit weight management and promote weight loss, while behavioral therapy has been shown to improve the psychological components of binge eating.

Other therapies being tried include dialectical behavior therapy, which helps people regulate their emotions; drug therapy with the antiseizure medication topiramate; weight-loss surgery (bariatric surgery); exercise used alone or in combination with cognitive behavioral therapy; and self-help. Self-help books, videos, and groups have helped some people control their binge eating.

If you think you might have binge eating disorder, it is important to know that you are not alone. Most people who have the disorder have tried but failed to control it on their own. You may want to get professional help. Talk to your health care provider about the type of help that may be best for you. The good news is that most people do well in treatment and can overcome binge eating.

Section 27.4

Nocturnal Sleep-Related Eating Disorder

"Sleep Eating," © 2010 Talk About Sleep (www.talkaboutsleep.com).
Reprinted with permission.

Sleep eating is a sleep-related disorder, although some specialists consider it to be a combination of a sleep and an eating disorder. It is a relatively rare and little known condition that is gaining recognition in sleep medicine. Other names for sleep eating are sleep-related eating (disorder), nocturnal sleep-related eating disorder (NS-RED), and sleep-eating syndrome.

Sleep eating is characterized by sleepwalking and excessive nocturnal overeating (compulsive hyperphagia). Sleep eaters are comparable to sleepwalkers in many ways: they are at risk for self-injury during an episode, they may (or may not) experience excessive daytime sleepiness, and they are usually emotionally distressed, tired, angry, or anxious. Sleep eaters are also at risk for the same health complications as compulsive overeaters, with the added dangers of sleepwalking. Common concerns include excessive weight gain, daytime sleepiness, choking while eating, sleep disruption, and injury from cooking or preparing food such as from knives, utensils, or hot cooking surfaces. There is also the potential for starting a fire.

As with sleepwalkers, sleep eaters are unaware and unconscious of their behavior. If there is any memory of the episode, it is usually sketchy. A sleep eater will roam the house, particularly the kitchen, and may eat large quantities of food (as well as non-food items). In the morning, sleep eaters have no recollection of the episode. However, in many cases there are clues to their behavior. One woman woke up with a stomachache and chocolate smeared on her face and hands. Candy wrappers littered the kitchen floor. The next morning her husband informed her that she had been eating during the night. She was shocked and distressed because she had no recollection of the event.

As in the case described above, food consumed by sleep eaters tends to be either high sugar or high fat. Odd combinations of foods, such as potato chips dipped in peanut butter or butter smeared on hot dogs, as well as non-food items, have been reported. Oddly, one person was discovered cutting a bar of soap into slices and then eating it as if it were a slice of cheese!

Sleep eating is classified as a parasomnia. It is a rare version of sleepwalking, which is an arousal disorder. In 1968, Roger Broughton published a paper in *Science* (159: 1070–1078) that outlined the major features of arousal disorders. They are:

- abnormal behavior that occurs during an arousal from slow wave sleep;
- the absence of awareness during the episode;
- automatic and repetitive motor activity;
- slow reaction time and reduced sensitivity to environment;
- difficulty in waking despite vigorous attempts;
- no memory of the episode in the morning (retrograde amnesia); and
- no or little dream recall associated with the event.

How Common Is Sleep Eating?

The actual number of sleep-eating sufferers is unknown; however, it is estimated that 1 to 3 percent of the population is affected by sleep eating. A higher percentage of persons with eating disorders, as many as 10 to 15 percent, are affected. For this reason, sleep eating is more common in younger women. Symptoms typically begin in the late 20s. Episodes may reoccur, in combination with a stressful situation, or an episode may occur only once or twice. Additionally, many parasomnias seem to run in families, which may indicate that sleep eating is genetically linked.

When Should I See a Doctor?

In many cases, sleep eating is the outward sign of an underlying problem. Many sufferers are overweight and dieting. When their control is diminished by sleep, these individuals binge at night to satisfy their hunger. Some sleep eaters have histories of alcoholism, drug abuse, or a primary sleep disorder, such as sleepwalking, restless legs syndrome, or sleep apnea. An article in *Sleep* (October 1991: 14(5): 419–431) suggested that sleep eating is directly linked to the onset of another medical problem.

Because sleep eating occurs in people that are usually dieting and emotionally distressed, attempts at weight loss may be unsuccessful and cause even more stress. Compounded with the dangers of sleepwalking, compulsive eating while asleep is a sleep disorder that results in weight gain, disrupted sleep, and daytime sleepiness. As these consequences of sleep eating impact daily living, the necessity of seeing a healthcare professional becomes more important.

Parasomnias are complex and often serious in nature. If you think you suffer from sleep eating, consult with your physician or a healthcare professional who can refer you to a sleep disorders treatment center. It is strongly recommended that a sleep specialist carry out the diagnosis and treatment. Medical or psychological evaluation should also be investigated.

How Is Sleep Eating Treated?

The first step in treating any sleep disorder is to ascertain any underlying causes. As with most parasomnias, sleep eating is usually the result of an underlying problem, which may include another sleep disorder, prescription drug abuse, nicotine withdrawal, chronic autoimmune hepatitis, encephalitis (or hypothalamic injury), or acute stress (*Sleep* 1991 Oct; 14(5): 419–431).

It is important to keep in mind that throughout life, people experience varying patterns of sleep and nutrition during positive and negative situations. Problems with eating disorders are defined as overeating or not eating enough. Problems with sleeping can be simplified with two symptoms, too much or not enough sleep. Medical attention is required for abnormal behaviors in either or both areas.

For some people who have been diagnosed with sleep eating, interventions without the use of medications have proven helpful. Courses on stress management, group or one-on-one counseling with a therapist, or self-confidence training may alleviate the stress and anxiety that leads to nighttime bingeing. Although considered an alternative treatment, hypnosis may be an option for some sleep eaters. A change in diet that includes avoiding certain foods and eating at specified times of the day, as well as reducing the intake of caffeine or alcohol, may be therapeutic. Professional advice may also suggest avoiding certain medications

If the underlying problem is diagnosed as sleepwalking, medications in the benzodiazepine family have had some success. In sleepwalkers, this class of drugs reduces motor activity during sleep. Another class of drug found to be effective for sleep eaters has been the dopaminergic agents such as Sinemet (carbidopa or levodopa) and Mirapex (pramipexole dihydrochloride).

If the underlying problem is a primary sleep disorder, such as sleep apnea or narcolepsy, check out the sections on http://www.talkabout sleep.com devoted to the treatment of these disorders.

Night Eating: Another Disorder of Sleep and Eating

A similar sleep-related eating disorder has also been clinically described. It is different from sleep eating in that the individual is awake during episodes of nocturnal bingeing. This disorder has many names: nocturnal eating (or drinking) syndrome, nighttime hunger, nocturnal eating, night eating or drinking (syndrome), or the "Dagwood" syndrome. Affected individuals are physically unable to sleep without food intake.

The *Merck Manual* lists night eating under the heading obesity. It states that the disorder "consists of morning anorexia, excessive ingestion of food in the evening, and insomnia." Because night eating is associated with increased weight gain as well as insomnia, this may cause the individual stress, anxiety, or depression.

Night eating or drinking may occur once or many times during the night. It is diagnosed when 50% or more of an individual's diet is consumed between sleeping hours. Unlike sleep eaters, this person will eat foods that are similar to his/her normal diet.

People who are night eaters typically avoid food until noon or later, eat small portions frequently when they do eat, and binge in the evening. They are usually overweight and in adults, overly stressed or anxious. They will also complain of not being able to maintain sleep or not being able to initiate sleep. For night eaters, the urge to eat is an abnormal need, rather than true hunger, according to an article in *Sleep* by Italian researchers (September 1997; 20(9): 734–738).

Night eaters/drinkers are usually children, although the disorder can occur in adults. For children, eating or drinking at night is a conditioned behavior. This is a common occurrence for babies, but most infants can sleep the entire night by the age of 6 months. Sleep disturbance can persist to an older age if the child is allowed a bottle or drinks throughout the night. An older child may consistently wake up during the night and ask for a drink or something to eat and refuse to return to bed until the snack is consumed. In this case, the caregiver should identify actual need versus repeated requests.

According to the International Classification of Sleep Disorders, night eating is characterized as a dyssomnia (as opposed to sleep eating, which is considered a parasomnia). A dyssomnia is a disorder of sleep or wakefulness in which insomnia or excessive daytime sleepiness is a complaint. Within the heading of dyssomnia, night eating is classified as an extrinsic sleep disorder, which means that it originates, develops, or is caused by an external source. Eating or drinking at night is usually a conditioned, conscious behavior; although it is a disorder, in many cases night eating is not caused by a psychological or medical condition.

Night eating may arise because of an ulcer, by dieting during the day, by undue stress, or by a routine expectation (conditioned behavior). Hypoglycemia, or low blood sugar, has also been proposed as a possible cause of nighttime bingeing in some people. This can be determined by a glucose tolerance test.

How Is Night Eating Treated?

For children, treatment of this disorder mainly involves the caregiver. For a young child, weaning from the breast, bottle, or drinks during the night is essential. The adult should evaluate if the request for food or drink is based on real need. If the demand is false, the adult should deny the request.

Eventually, waking up with the urge for food or drink will be eliminated. For an adult, it is important to first recognize that the behavior is not normal. (If the pattern of eating at night has been persistent for a long time, a night eater may only complain of insomnia and weight gain.) Secondly, a night eater should schedule an appointment with a physician. Night eating may be the result of a medical condition or hypoglycemia, both of which can be treated. If not, the habit of eating in the middle of the night can be broken with behavior modification and/or stress reduction. Eating frequent small meals during the day beginning in the morning, reducing carbohydrate intake, and increasing protein intake before bedtime are diet patterns that may help. Protein metabolizes slowly and will stabilize blood sugar levels during sleep. Contrary to protein, sugary snacks raise the blood sugar quickly, then cause it to plunge. So, avoid sweet foods before bedtime.

Night eaters who have conquered their uncontrollable need for nocturnal food or drink often sleep equally as well or better than before they started night eating.

Chapter 28

Obsessive-Compulsive Disorder

People with anxiety disorders feel extremely fearful and unsure. Most people feel anxious about something for a short time now and again, but people with anxiety disorders feel this way most of the time. Their fears and worries make it hard for them to do everyday tasks. About 18% of American adults have anxiety disorders. Children also may have them.

Treatment is available for people with anxiety disorders. Researchers are also looking for new treatments that will help relieve symptoms

This text is about one kind of anxiety disorder called obsessive-compulsive disorder, or OCD.

What Is OCD?

Everyone double-checks things sometimes—for example, checking the stove before leaving the house, to make sure it's turned off. But people with OCD feel the need to check things over and over, or have certain thoughts or perform routines and rituals over and over. The thoughts and rituals of OCD cause distress and get in the way of daily life.

The repeated, upsetting thoughts of OCD are called obsessions. To try to control them, people with OCD repeat rituals or behaviors, which are called compulsions. People with OCD can't control these thoughts and rituals.

From "When Unwanted Thoughts Take Over: Obsessive-Compulsive Disorder," by the National Institute of Mental Health (NIMH, www.nimh.nih.gov), part of the National Institutes of Health, 2009.

Examples of obsessions are fear of germs, of being hurt or of hurting others, and troubling religious or sexual thoughts. Examples of compulsions are repeatedly counting things, cleaning things, washing the body or parts of it, or putting things in a certain order, when these actions are not needed, and checking things over and over.

People with OCD have these thoughts and do these rituals for at least an hour on most days, often longer. The reason OCD gets in the way of their lives is that they can't stop the thoughts or rituals, so they sometimes miss school, work, or meetings with friends, for example.

Symptoms of OCD

People with OCD do or feel the following:

- Have repeated thoughts or images about many different things, such as fear of germs, dirt, or intruders; violence; hurting loved ones; sexual acts; conflicts with religious beliefs; or being overly neat

- Do the same rituals over and over such as washing hands, locking and unlocking doors, counting, keeping unneeded items, or repeating the same steps again and again

- Have unwanted thoughts and behaviors they can't control

- Don't get pleasure from the behaviors or rituals, but get brief relief from the anxiety the thoughts cause

- Spend at least an hour a day on the thoughts and rituals, which cause distress and get in the way of daily life

When OCD Starts

For many people, OCD starts during childhood or the teen years. Most people are diagnosed at about age 19. Symptoms of OCD may come and go and be better or worse at different times.

Help for OCD

There is help for people with OCD. The first step is to go to a doctor or health clinic to talk about symptoms. People who think they have OCD may want to bring this text to the doctor, to help them talk about their symptoms. The doctor will do an exam to make sure that another physical problem isn't causing the symptoms. The doctor may make a referral to a mental health specialist.

There are different kinds of treatment for OCD. Doctors may ask people with OCD to seek psychotherapy with a psychologist, psychiatrist, or licensed social worker. A type of therapy called behavior therapy is especially useful for treating OCD. It teaches a person different ways of thinking, behaving, and reacting to situations that help them feel less anxious and fearful without having obsessive thoughts or acting compulsively.

Doctors also may prescribe medication to help treat OCD. It's important to know that some of these medicines may take several weeks to start working. The kinds of medicines used to treat OCD are antidepressants and anti-anxiety medicines. Some of these medicines are used to treat other problems, such as depression, but also are helpful for OCD. Although these medicines often have mild side effects, they are usually not a problem for most people, especially if the dose starts off low and is increased slowly over time.

Some people do better with therapy, whereas others do better with medicine. Still others do best with a combination of the two. Talk with your doctor about the best treatment for you.

Paying for Treatment

Most insurance plans cover treatment for anxiety disorders. People who are going to have treatment should check with their own insurance companies to find out about coverage. For people who don't have insurance, local city or county governments may offer treatment at a clinic or health center, where the cost is based on income. Medicaid plans also may pay for OCD treatment.

Why Do People Get OCD?

OCD sometimes runs in families, but no one knows for sure why some people have it, whereas others don't. When chemicals in the brain are not at a certain level it may result in OCD. Medications can often help the brain chemicals stay at the correct levels.

To improve treatment, scientists are studying how well different medicines and therapies work. In one kind of research, people with OCD choose to take part in a clinical trial to help physicians find out what treatments work best for most people, or what works best for different symptoms. Usually, the treatment is free. Scientists are learning more about how the brain works, so that they can discover new treatments.

Chapter 29

Substance Abuse, Addiction, and Stress

Chapter Contents

Section 29.1

Stress and Substance Abuse

From "Stress and Substance Abuse," by the National Institute on Drug Abuse (NIDA, www.drugabuse.gov), part of the National Institutes of Health, February 2006.

What Is Stress?

Stress is a term that is hard to define because it means different things to different people. Stress is a normal occurrence in life for people of all ages. The body responds to stress in order to protect itself from emotional or physical distress or, in extreme situations, from danger.

Stressors differ for each of us. What is stressful for one person may or may not be stressful for another, and each of us responds to stress in different ways. How a person copes with stress—by reaching for a beer or cigarette or by heading to the gym—also plays an important role in the impact that stress will have on our bodies.

By using their own support systems, some people are able to cope effectively with the emotional and physical demands brought on by stressful and traumatic experiences. However, individuals who experience prolonged reactions to stress that disrupt their daily functioning may require treatment by a trained and experienced mental health professional.

The Body's Response to Stress

The stress response is mediated by a highly complex, integrated network that involves the central nervous system, the adrenal system, the immune system, and the cardiovascular system.

Stress activates adaptive responses. It releases the neurotransmitter norepinephrine, which is involved in memory. This may be one reason why people remember stressful events more clearly than they do nonstressful situations.

Stress also increases the release of a hormone known as corticotropin-releasing factor (CRF). CRF is found throughout the brain and initiates our biological response to stressors. During all stressful experiences, certain regions of the brain show increased levels of CRF. Interestingly, almost all drugs of abuse have also been found to increase CRF levels, suggesting a neurobiological connection between stress and drug abuse.

Mild or acute stress may cause changes that are useful. For example, stress can actually improve our attention and increase our capacity to store and integrate important and life-protecting information. But if stress is prolonged or chronic, the changes it produces can become harmful.

Stress and Substance Abuse

Stressful events can profoundly influence the abuse of alcohol or other drugs. Stress is a major contributor to the initiation and continuation of alcohol or other drug abuse, as well as to substance abuse relapse after periods of abstinence.

Stress is one of the major factors known to cause relapse to smoking, even after prolonged periods of a smoke-free lifestyle.

Children exposed to severe stress may be more vulnerable to drug abuse. A number of clinical and epidemiological studies show a strong association between psychosocial stressors early in life (e.g., parental loss, child abuse) and an increased risk for depression, anxiety, impulsive behavior, and substance abuse in adulthood.

Stress, Drugs, and Vulnerable Populations

Stressful experiences increase the vulnerability of an individual to relapse to drug use, even after prolonged abstinence.

Individuals who have achieved abstinence from drugs must continue to sustain their abstinence by avoiding environmental triggers, recognizing their psychosocial and emotional triggers, and developing healthy behaviors to handle life's stresses.

A number of relapse prevention approaches have been developed to help clinicians address relapse. Treatment techniques that foster coping skills, problem-solving skills, and social support play a role in successful treatment.

Physicians should be aware of which medications their patients are taking. Some people may need medications for stress-related symptoms or for treatment of depression and anxiety.

What Is PTSD?

Posttraumatic stress disorder (PTSD) is an anxiety disorder that can develop in some people after exposure to a terrifying event or ordeal in which grave physical harm occurred or was threatened.

Generally, PTSD has been associated with the violence of combat. However, PTSD is not limited to battlefield soldiers. PTSD can result from tragic incidents in which people become witnesses, victims, or survivors of violent personal attacks, natural or human-caused disasters, or accidents.

PTSD can develop in people of any age, including children and adolescents.

Symptoms of PTSD can include re-experiencing the trauma; emotional numbness; avoidance of people, places, and thoughts connected to the event; and hyperarousal, which may involve sleeping difficulties, exaggerated startle response, and hypervigilance.

It is not uncommon for people to experience some or all of these symptoms after exposure to a traumatic event; however, if the symptoms persist beyond 1 month and are associated with impaired functioning, then PTSD may be diagnosed.

PTSD and Substance Abuse

Emerging research has documented a strong association between PTSD and substance abuse. In some cases, substance use begins after the exposure to trauma and the development of PTSD, thus making PTSD a risk factor for drug abuse.

Early intervention to help children and adolescents who have suffered trauma from violence or a disaster is critical. Children who witness or are exposed to a traumatic event and are clinically diagnosed with PTSD have a greater likelihood for developing later drug and/or alcohol use disorders.

Among individuals with substance use disorders, 30 to 60 percent meet the criteria for comorbid PTSD.

Patients with substance use disorders tend to suffer from more severe PTSD symptoms than do PTSD patients without substance use disorders.

Helping Those Who Suffer from PTSD and Drug Abuse

Healthcare professionals must be alert to the fact that PTSD frequently co-occurs with depression, other anxiety disorders, and alcohol and other substance abuse. Patients who are experiencing the symptoms of PTSD need support from physicians and healthcare providers to develop coping skills and reduce substance abuse risk.

The likelihood of treatment success increases when these concurrent disorders are appropriately identified and treated.

For substance abuse there are effective medications and behavioral therapies.

For symptoms of PTSD, some antianxiety and antidepressant medications may be useful.

Several behavioral treatments can help individuals who suffer from PTSD. Improvements have been shown with some forms of group therapy and with cognitive-behavioral therapy, especially when it includes an exposure component for trauma victims. Exposure therapy allows patients to gradually and repeatedly re-experience the frightening event(s) under controlled conditions to help them work through the trauma. Exposure therapy is thought to be one of the most effective ways to manage PTSD, when it is conducted by a trained therapist.

Although not widely used for comorbid PTSD and substance abuse, several studies suggest that exposure therapy may be helpful for individuals with PTSD and comorbid cocaine addiction.

Seeking Safety is another example of a cognitive-based behavioral treatment, tested mainly among women with comorbid PTSD and drug abuse. It is currently being evaluated among different populations for its efficacy.

Treatment of patients with comorbid PTSD and addictions will vary, and for some patients, successful treatment may require initial inpatient hospitalization.

Finally, support from family and friends can play an important role in recovery from both disorders.

Section 29.2

Tobacco and Stress

Excerpted and adapted from "Tobacco and Stress—A Bad Combination," by the Center for Health Promotion and Preventive Medicine (CHPPM, www.chppm.com), now part of the United States Army Public Health Command, November 2009.

Many people continue to smoke and use tobacco because they believe it helps them deal with stress. However, research shows that nicotine does not reduce feelings of stress. In fact, nicotine-addicted individuals need nicotine simply to feel normal. Studies show that what appears to be the relaxing effect of smoking is really a reversal of the tension and irritability that develop when nicotine levels in the blood are falling.

Because of the addiction to nicotine, regular tobacco users feel heightened stress between each use of tobacco. This negative mood is repeated throughout the day, making tobacco users feel above-average levels of daily stress. A recent study found that people who use tobacco to specifically reduce stress reported significantly higher stress levels than those who did not use tobacco.

The physical, mental, and emotional changes that result from nicotine addiction make tobacco users even more vulnerable to feelings of stress while under pressure. In fact, just the thought of losing their "fix" can cause tobacco users to feel stressed. This response could reduce a person's ability to focus and adversely impact work performance.

Nicotine withdrawal symptoms such as irritability, anger, frustration, anxiety, depression, impaired concentration, and restlessness are not compatible with duties that depend on concentration, critical thought, or being alert.

Bottom line: Tobacco use increases stress. Studies have found that former tobacco users are less stressed than current tobacco users. So the first step the tobacco user should take when trying to reduce stress is to quit tobacco. Quit tobacco resources can be found at www.UCanQuit2.org.

Section 29.3

Alcohol and Stress

Excerpted from "The Role of Stress in Alcohol Use, Alcoholism Treatment, and Relapse," by Kathleen T. Brady, MD, PhD, and Susan C. Sonne, PharmD, *Alcohol Research and Health,* by the National Institute on Alcohol Abuse and Alcoholism (NIAAA, www.niaaa.nih.gov), part of the National Institutes of Health, 1999. For complete references, visit www.niaaa.nih.gov. Reviewed by David A. Cooke, MD, FACP, November 22, 2010.

Clinicians and researchers consider the addiction to alcohol or other drugs (AODs) a complex problem determined by multiple factors, including psychological and physiological components. Many theories involving numerous variables (e.g., personality and access to AODs) have sought to explain the initiation and maintenance of AOD abuse and dependence. Most of those theoretical models consider stress a major contributor to the initiation and continuation of AOD use as well as to relapse. Accordingly, the relationship between stress and alcohol use has received much attention.

The notion that exposure to stress-inducing factors in everyday life (i.e., life stressors) can cause susceptible people to initiate or relapse to alcohol use has intuitive appeal. Whereas the relationship between stress and AOD use can be studied fairly easily in laboratory animals, a definitive exploration of this connection in humans has been more difficult. Animal studies generally have supported the positive relationship between stress and alcohol use and abuse. Researchers also have begun to focus on an organism's response to stress and the consequences of AOD use and how it affects biological processes in the brain. These studies have identified several neurobiological connections between the changes produced by stress and the changes produced by both short-term (i.e., acute) and long-term (i.e., chronic) AOD use. In the clinical arena, however, the relationship between stress and alcohol use has been more difficult to characterize.

For example, human laboratory studies have not uniformly supported a prominent theory called the tension-reduction hypothesis of alcohol use, which posits that people use alcohol to reduce stress. Furthermore, studies of the relationship between stress and alcohol

279

use are difficult to conduct in alcoholic patients and, as a result, have numerous inherent limitations. Study participants may recall only selective events that have contributed to alcohol use, may be inconsistent about which events to include as stressors, and may have difficulties distinguishing between events that precipitate alcohol use and those that result from alcohol use and relapse.

Because of these difficulties, many studies that have demonstrated an association between AOD use and stress have been unable to establish a causal relationship between the two. For example, heavy alcohol users frequently experience stress related to occupational, social, legal, and financial problems. When interpreting such observations, some investigators have chosen to class stressful events as illness dependent or illness independent, depending on whether they are caused by the AOD use. This classification has not been consistently adopted, however, and many studies fail to determine the degree to which such stressors occur independent of alcohol use, cause alcohol use, or are a consequence of alcohol use.

The type of stressor studied also influences analyses of the relationship between stress and alcohol use. For example, many studies investigating the role of stress in relapse after treatment have limited their focus to stressors that occurred after treatment completion. Some stressful life events that affect the lives of alcoholics after treatment, however, may have occurred before treatment (e.g., a divorce or job loss). Moreover, stressors can range from dramatic and severe events (e.g., a divorce or death of a loved one) to chronic irritants of daily life (e.g., job hassles or financial worries). Both the temporal relationship between stress and alcohol use and the type of stressor studied, however, can profoundly affect study results.

Neurobiological Connections between Stress and Addiction

Animal studies have suggested that exposure to stress facilitates both the initiation and the reinstatement of AOD use after a period of abstinence. To better understand the biological basis of the effects of stress on AOD self-administration in animals, researchers have focused primarily on two neurobiological systems. The first system involves the organism's hormonal and subsequent biological responses to stress and the influence of those responses on the reinforcing effects of AODs. Those studies, which aim mainly to identify specific, stress-induced hormonal changes that mediate the effects of stress on AOD self-administration, primarily have examined the activity of a hormone system called the hypothalamic-pituitary-adrenal (HPA) axis. This hormone system has three components:

- Corticotropin-releasing hormone (CRH), which is produced in a brain region called the hypothalamus

- Adrenocorticotropic hormone (ACTH), which is produced in the pituitary gland located in the brain below the hypothalamus

- Glucocorticoid hormones, such as cortisol in humans and corticosterone in rodents, which are produced in the adrenal glands that are located on top of the kidneys

Glucocorticoid secretion by the adrenal gland is considered one of the central biological responses to stressful events. Studies have shown that both acute stress and alcohol or cocaine administration can activate the HPA axis, probably by acting on CRH. Consistent with this hypothesis, agents that interfere with CRH function also decrease sensitivity to environmental stress in animal models and prevent some of the reinforcing effects of cocaine.

The second neurobiological system investigated in animal studies of stress and AOD use involves the stress-induced changes in the activity of certain brain regions and brain molecules (i.e., neurotransmitters) assumed to play a role in mediating the reinforcing effects of AODs. This approach is based on the hypothesis that stress facilitates AOD self-administration in laboratory animals and humans by enhancing the activity of those neurobiological systems. This research has focused mostly on nerve cells (i.e., neurons) that are located in the midbrain (i.e., mesencephalon) and which use the neurotransmitter dopamine.

Some of these neurons extend to the nucleus accumbens, which is considered one of the primary brain areas involved in mediating the reinforcing effects of various AODs.

One likely explanation for the connection between stress and AOD use is that stress modifies the motivational and/or reinforcing effects of AODs at the neurobiological level. For example, stress increases the activity of the dopaminergic brain systems that are involved in motivation and reward and which also mediate AOD-induced rewarding effects.

Accordingly, stress-induced changes in those systems could enhance the organism's responsiveness to the effects of AODs. Furthermore, when an organism is in a stressful situation, numerous biological systems are activated to help the organism cope with the stress. For example, the adrenal glands release epinephrine to prepare the organism for a "fight or flight" response, and various brain regions secrete pain-relieving chemicals. Similarly, stress possibly results in increased activity in the dopaminergic system in an attempt to counteract the negative emotional state associated with stress.

Animal studies have suggested that another neurotransmitter, serotonin, also may play a role in the relationship between stress and AOD use. For example, alcohol administration increases brain serotonin metabolism in animals. Furthermore, increases in serotonin levels and metabolism have been shown to decrease alcohol consumption in experimental animals.

Studies in nonhuman primates found that animals with low brain serotonin activity are high consumers of alcohol. When these high alcohol-consuming animals were treated with an agent that prevents serotonin breakdown and thus prolongs serotonin's activity in the brain (i.e., a selective serotonin reuptake inhibitor [SSRI]), their alcohol consumption declined substantially. Clinical trials investigating the use of SSRIs in humans, however, have generated mixed results regarding the ability of those agents to decrease alcohol consumption.

In addition, animal studies have indicated that the brain's serotonin systems also affect the brain regions that mediate another stress-related reaction, the fear response. Consistent with this observation, many SSRIs have demonstrated powerful activity in the treatment of anxiety disorders in humans in addition to their antidepressant activity. This association of the serotonin system with both consummatory behaviors and anxiety states further supports the notion that a neurobiological connection exists between stress and AOD use and abuse.

Stress and the Initiation of Alcohol Use

Animal studies have demonstrated that exposure to both acute and repeated stress can increase an animal's potential for initiating AOD self-administration as well as modify the amount and frequency of established AOD self-administration. However, this relationship appears to depend on the timing of the exposure to a stressor and of the AOD exposure. For acute stress to induce AOD administration, the stressful event and the AOD exposure must occur within a short interval. For example, in experiments in which animals were exposed to acute stress by restraining them for a short period of time, AOD self-administration was facilitated only if the stressful situation preceded the AOD exposure by no more than 30 minutes.

When the animals were exposed to stress repeatedly or for prolonged periods, however, the interval between the end of the stressful situation and the AOD exposure did not appear to influence AOD self-administration. Thus, in those instances the animals showed increased AOD self-administration regardless of whether the stressful experiences continued up to the AOD-use assessment or had ended weeks earlier. These observations indicate that repeated stress can induce long-lasting modifications in neural pathways, resulting in a drug-prone state that is independent of the actual presence of the stressor.

Although stressors that have a physical component, such as a mild electric shock to the feet or a pinch in the tail, can lead to increased AOD self-administration, such physical manipulations do not appear to be required for mediating stress effects. In fact, psychological stress alone can also increase drug self-administration. For example, rats that witnessed another animal receiving an electric shock exhibited increased self-administration of cocaine. Similarly, enhanced AOD self-administration occurred in studies in which animals were exposed to stress in the form of social aggression by being placed in an unfamiliar group of animals while being protected from actual physical attacks by a screen grid.

Stress and the Reinstatement of Alcohol Use

Stressful experiences also can contribute to the reinstatement of AOD use after a period of abstinence in animals with a history of AOD self-administration. For example, studies in rats found that a single stressful experience, such as a one-time electrical shock to the feet, induced resumption of drug use in animals that had been previously taught to self-administer cocaine or heroin. This stress-induced reinstatement of AOD use is a well-documented phenomenon. In fact, exposure to stress is the most powerful and reliable experimental manipulation used to induce reinstatement of AOD use.

Animal models of the relationship between stress and alcohol relapse have employed not only animals with a history of alcohol self-administration that had undergone a prolonged period of abstinence but also animals with a history of alcohol dependence that were deprived of alcohol. Studies found that both alcohol-dependent and non-alcohol-dependent animals will increase their response for alcohol (compared to base-like levels) following a period of imposed deprivation.

Researchers have used such an alcohol deprivation model in dependent rats to investigate the effects of two medications used to treat alcoholism in humans, naltrexone and acamprosate. Both of these agents interfere with the actions of the neurotransmitters involved in mediating stress and the reinforcing effects of alcohol. Thus, naltrexone blocks the actions of neurotransmitters called endogenous opioids (i.e., an opioid antagonist), and acamprosate likely interferes with the function of the neurotransmitter glutamate. In alcohol deprivation studies in rats, both agents prevented the increase in alcohol self-administration normally observed in animals that experience stress as a result of a period of forced abstinence. Similarly, opioid antagonists (e.g., naltrexone) prevented the increase in alcohol consumption observed in animals exposed to other types of stress.

Stress in humans often leads to craving, and craving, in turn, frequently results in relapse. Thus, one can reasonably assume that opiate antagonists—which are considered anticraving medications—could reduce stress-induced craving and thereby decrease the risk of a stress-induced relapse. Although human studies have confirmed that naltrexone and another opiate antagonist, nalmefene, are both effective in preventing relapse in abstinent alcoholics, the effects of opiate antagonists on stress-induced relapse have not yet been investigated specifically in humans.

Effects of Alcohol Exposure on the Response to Stress

Not only can exposure to stress induce AOD self-administration in animals, but previous alcohol exposure influences an animal's response to stress. In a study investigating the relationship between alcohol and stress, both alcohol-treated and control rats were repeatedly stressed by restraining their free movement for 2 hours daily for 5 days.

The alcohol-treated rats in that study received alcohol in their drinking water for 2 weeks before being exposed to the restraint stress and continued to receive alcohol during the stress period. A single 2-hour restraining period on the first day of the experiment decreased food intake in both the alcohol-treated and the control rats. On the second and third day of the experiment, however, the control rats showed smaller decreases in food intake, and on the fifth day their food intake had returned to normal levels, suggesting that the animals had adapted to the stress. Among the alcohol-treated rats, however, the decrease in food intake was slightly attenuated after the second-day restraint but did not decrease further on the remaining days of the experiment. These findings suggest that alcohol exposure interfered with the rats' ability to adapt to repeated stress.

In summary, researchers have extensively investigated the effects of stress on AOD self-administration in animals. These studies found that stressful experiences—whether acute or chronic and whether physical or psychological in nature—can contribute significantly to the animals' AOD self-administration.

The Relationship between Stress and Alcohol Use in Humans

Clinical studies indicate that both acute and chronic stress may play a role in the development of AOD use disorders, the initiation of AOD abuse treatment, and the precipitation of relapse in recovering alcoholics.

Stress and the Development of Alcoholism

Clinical and naturalistic studies have assessed the influence of both acute and chronic stress on drinking behavior and the development of alcoholism. Many of those investigations have focused on occupational stress as an example of chronic stress. For example, researchers found in a survey of more than 500 men that drinking problems were closely related to stressful experiences—whether they resulted from acute and severe stressors (e.g., illness or death of a loved one) or from chronic occupational stressors—that were combined with a strong sense of powerlessness. With respect to occupational stress, men in positions combining little freedom in choosing how to fulfill their job obligations (i.e., low job latitude) and high job demands reported the highest drinking levels and most alcohol-related problems.

The extent to which job stress influences drinking behavior also depends on the type of stress experienced. Thus, researchers found that men employed in high-strain jobs (i.e., jobs with high demands and low control) generally had a higher risk of developing alcohol use disorders when compared with men in low-strain occupations (i.e., jobs with low demands and high control). However, this increase was greater for men in positions with high physical demands (three to four times higher risk) than for men in positions with high psychological demands (two to three times higher risk). Other studies noted that chronic, low-level, work-related stressors (e.g., uncooperative coworkers or daily parking problems) also were associated with higher drinking levels.

Several studies have focused specifically on the relationship between stress and alcohol consumption in women. Such analyses are of particular interest, because women may be more susceptible than men are to some of alcohol's harmful health effects. Furthermore, women have been reported to be more likely than men to consider stressful events as being associated with the initiation of problem drinking. The latter association was not confirmed, however, in a critical review of stressful life events and drinking behavior in women. In that review, researchers found no evidence of a gender-specific relationship between stress and alcohol abuse in women, although the researchers noted a high prevalence of stressful life events (e.g., divorce or death of a loved one), particularly among middle-aged women who developed alcohol dependence later in life. Most studies reviewed, however, failed to address the possibility that heavy drinking may be the cause rather than the consequence of life stressors.

Although the general association between stress and drinking behavior in women has remained controversial, some studies have found an important relationship between women's coping styles and stress-related alcohol consumption. In those studies, women who used problem-focused coping strategies (i.e., who took specific measures to eliminate or address the source of the stress) consumed less alcohol during stressful periods in their lives than did women who used coping strategies that focused on emotions or which merely served to relieve the immediate negative emotions (i.e., were palliative) rather than address the problem.

Accordingly, treatment modules teaching problem-focused coping skills may be an important component of effective therapy for some AOD-abusing clients.

Another approach to investigating the role of stress in the development of alcoholism has been to analyze alcohol's stress-response dampening (SRD) effects in different populations. SRD effects are those consequences of alcohol consumption that result in a reduction of both the body's emotional responses (e.g., anxiety, tension, and nervousness) and physiological responses (e.g., changes in heart rate or sweating) to stress. Researchers found that alcohol's SRD effects were more pronounced in nonalcoholic people who demonstrated personality traits that have been associated with a risk for the development of alcoholism (e.g., aggressiveness, impulsivity, and outgoing) than in people without those characteristics. The researchers suggested that because of their enhanced SRD experience, people with those personality traits were likely to find alcohol consumption particularly reinforcing, increasing their risk for alcoholism. More recently, researchers determined that women with a family history of alcoholism or anxiety disorders, who are at increased risk for alcoholism, exhibit a greater SRD effect of alcohol than do women without such a family history.

Again, it is an intriguing notion that this population has an increased risk of alcoholism, because alcohol may be particularly reinforcing as the result of its potent SRD effect. Thus, these studies suggest that an enhanced sensitivity to alcohol's SRD effect may contribute to an increased vulnerability of people with anxiety disorders for initiating and escalating alcohol use.

Stress and Treatment Initiation

Discrete stressful events often provide impetus to an alcoholic person to seek treatment, especially when other resources and responses have failed to alleviate the stressful situation. This correlation between stress and treatment initiation was highlighted in several studies comparing alcoholics who had initiated treatment with alcoholics who received no treatment. In those comparisons, alcoholics entering treatment were more likely to perceive their drinking problems as severe, had more symptoms of alcohol dependence, and experienced more stressors and negative events in various life domains. Of prime importance, these stressors included both chronic hardships (e.g., strains in employment or marriage) and acute stressful events (e.g., accidents, criminal charges, or divorce) that often are associated with drinking.

Alcoholics with greater resources in multiple domains (e.g., those who are employed and have an intact marriage) are likely to seek treatment for alcohol-related problems more quickly than are alcoholics with fewer resources. For example, social resources, such as an extended network of family members and friends, may increase the probability that a drinker's alcohol-related problems are pointed out to him or her by other people, thereby leading to early treatment seeking. This hypothesis contradicts the notion that an alcoholic must lose all his or her resources (i.e., "hit bottom") before seeking treatment; rather, it suggests that resources should be increased ("the bottom should be raised") so that the person seeks treatment before experiencing multiple devastating consequences of alcoholism.

In summary, stress in many cases may play a causal role in the initiation of treatment. This role, however, probably is moderated and mediated by numerous factors, including a drinker's resources, social pressure, problem-solving skills, and coping strategies.

Stress and Relapse

Both discrete, stressful life events and chronic stressors may play a role not only in the development of alcoholism and AOD treatment initiation, but also in the relapse of people recovering from AOD abuse. To explain the association between stress and relapse, as well as the fact that not all AOD abusers relapse when encountering stress, researchers have proposed the stress-vulnerability hypothesis. This hypothesis posits that AOD use in the face of severe stressors is mediated by the presence or absence of both protective factors (e.g., good social support) and risk factors (e.g., homelessness and unemployment). The hypothesis is supported by findings that severe stress (defined as life adversity posing either a high personal threat or chronic coping demands) which occurred prior to and independent of alcohol use was related to relapse after treatment. Thus, during a 3-month followup period after treatment, patients who relapsed had experienced twice as much severe stress before entering treatment compared with patients who remained abstinent. The study also calculated a composite "psychosocial vulnerability score" based on the patient's coping skills, social resources, confidence that he or she would be able to resist an urge to drink, and level of depression.

According to that analysis, people whose scores in these areas improved during treatment had better outcomes (i.e., a lower risk of relapse). These findings emphasize the connection between stress and relapse and suggest that resilience to stress-induced relapse can be improved during treatment.

Another study followed a large group of alcoholics, opiate users, and cigarette smokers in early abstinence to investigate the effects of acute stress and commitment to abstinence on relapse. The commitment to abstinence was measured using a scale that allowed the participants to choose between six different treatment goals, ranging from abstinence to no change in use. The researchers found that commitment to abstinence was the strongest predictor of abstinence during the followup period. Furthermore, an association between elevated stress levels and relapse existed only when the subjects were interviewed after their relapse (i.e., retrospectively) about the factors contributing to their relapse, but not when stress levels were assessed before a relapse occurred (i.e., prospectively). This observation suggests that stress may not actually lead to relapse; instead, the relapse may have resulted in increased stress and the subjects may have used the attribution of stress as causing the relapse as a way to make sense of the relapse. The actual relationship between stress and relapse in this study is difficult to assess, however, because the followup period was rather brief (i.e., 12 weeks) and the study did not assess the effects of chronic stress. Nevertheless, the study results emphasize the need for more careful, prospective studies of the relationship between stress and relapse.

Section 29.4

Drugs, Stress, and Trauma

Excerpted and adapted from "Comorbidity: Addiction and Other
Mental Illnesses," by the National Institute on Drug Abuse (NIDA,
www.drugabuse.gov), part of the National Institutes of Health, 2009.

Definition of Comorbidity

When two disorders or illnesses occur in the same person, simultaneously or sequentially, they are described as comorbid. Comorbidity also implies interactions between the illnesses that affect the course and prognosis of both.

Drug Addiction and Mental Illness

Is drug addiction a mental illness? Yes, because addiction changes the brain in fundamental ways, disturbing a person's normal hierarchy of needs and desires and substituting new priorities connected with procuring and using the drug. The resulting compulsive behaviors that override the ability to control impulses despite the consequences are similar to hallmarks of other mental illnesses.

In fact, the *DSM* [*Diagnostic and Statistical Manual of Mental Disorders*], which is the definitive resource of diagnostic criteria for all mental disorders, includes criteria for drug use disorders, distinguishing between two types: drug abuse and drug dependence. Drug dependence is synonymous with addiction.

By comparison, the criteria for drug abuse hinge on the harmful consequences of repeated use but do not include the compulsive use, tolerance (i.e., needing higher doses to achieve the same effect), or withdrawal (i.e., symptoms that occur when use is stopped) that can be signs of addiction.

Comorbid Drug Use and Other Mental Disorders

Many people who regularly abuse drugs are also diagnosed with mental disorders and vice versa. The high prevalence of this comorbidity has been documented in multiple national population surveys since the 1980s. Data show that persons diagnosed with mood or anxiety disorders are about twice as likely to suffer also from a drug use disorder (abuse or dependence) compared with respondents in general. The same is true for those diagnosed with an antisocial syndrome, such as antisocial personality or conduct disorder. Similarly, persons diagnosed with drug disorders are roughly twice as likely to suffer also from mood and anxiety disorders.

Gender is also a factor in the specific patterns of observed comorbidities. For example, the overall rates of abuse and dependence for most drugs tend to be higher among males than females. Further, males are more likely to suffer from antisocial personality disorder, while women have higher rates of mood and anxiety disorders, all of which are risk factors for substance abuse.

Drug Use Disorders Often Co-Occur with Other Mental Illnesses

The high prevalence of comorbidity between drug use disorders and other mental illnesses does not mean that one caused the other, even if one appeared first. In fact, establishing causality or directionality is difficult for several reasons. Diagnosis of a mental disorder may not occur until symptoms have progressed to a specified level (per *DSM*); however, subclinical symptoms may also prompt drug use, and imperfect recollections of when drug use or abuse started can create confusion as to which came first. Still, three scenarios deserve consideration:

1. Drugs of abuse can cause abusers to experience one or more symptoms of another mental illness. The increased risk of psychosis in some marijuana abusers has been offered as evidence for this possibility.

2. Mental illnesses can lead to drug abuse. Individuals with overt, mild, or even subclinical mental disorders may abuse drugs as a form of self-medication. For example, the use of tobacco products by patients with schizophrenia is believed to lessen the symptoms of the disease and improve cognition.

3. Both drug use disorders and other mental illnesses are caused by overlapping factors such as underlying brain deficits, genetic vulnerabilities, and/or early exposure to stress or trauma.

All three scenarios probably contribute, in varying degrees, to how and whether specific comorbidities manifest themselves.

Common Factors

Overlapping Genetic Vulnerabilities

A particularly active area of comorbidity research involves the search for genes that might predispose individuals to develop both addiction and other mental illnesses, or to have a greater risk of a second disorder occurring after the first appears. It is estimated that 40–60 percent of an individual's vulnerability to addiction is attributable to genetics; most of this vulnerability arises from complex interactions among multiple genes and from genetic interactions with environmental influences. In some instances, a gene product may act directly, as when a protein influences how a person responds to a drug (e.g., whether the drug experience is pleasurable or not) or how long a drug remains in the body. But genes can also act indirectly by altering how an individual responds to stress or by increasing the likelihood of risk-taking and novelty-seeking behaviors, which could influence the development of drug use disorders and other mental illnesses. Several regions of the human genome have been linked to increased risk of both drug use disorders and mental illness, including associations with greater vulnerability to adolescent drug dependence and conduct disorders.

Involvement of Similar Brain Regions

Some areas of the brain are affected by both drug use disorders and other mental illnesses. For example, the circuits in the brain that use the neurotransmitter dopamine—a chemical that carries messages from one neuron to another—are typically affected by addictive substances and may also be involved in depression, schizophrenia, and other psychiatric disorders.

Indeed, some antidepressants and essentially all antipsychotic medications directly target the regulation of dopamine in this system, whereas others may have indirect effects. Importantly, dopamine pathways have also been implicated in the way in which stress can increase vulnerability to drug addiction. Stress is also a known risk factor for a range of mental disorders and therefore provides one likely common neurobiological link between the disease processes of addiction and those of other mental disorders.

The overlap of brain areas involved in both drug use disorders and other mental illnesses suggests that brain changes stemming from one may affect the other. For example, drug abuse that precedes the first symptoms of a mental illness may produce changes in brain structure and function that kindle an underlying propensity to develop that mental illness. If the mental disorder develops first, associated changes in brain activity may increase the vulnerability to abusing substances by enhancing their positive effects, reducing awareness of their negative effects, or alleviating the unpleasant effects associated with the mental disorder or the medication used to treat it.

The Influence of Developmental Stage Adolescence

Although drug abuse and addiction can happen at any time during a person's life, drug use typically starts in adolescence, a period when the first signs of mental illness commonly appear.

It is therefore not surprising that comorbid disorders can already be seen among youth. Significant changes in the brain occur during adolescence, which may enhance vulnerability to drug use and the development of addiction and other mental disorders. Drugs of abuse affect brain circuits involved in learning and memory, reward, decision making, and behavioral control, all of which are still maturing into early adulthood. Thus, understanding the long-term impact of early drug exposure is a critical area of comorbidity research.

Early Occurrence Increases Later Risk

Strong evidence has emerged showing early drug use to be a risk factor for later substance abuse problems; additional findings suggest that it may also be a risk factor for the later occurrence of other mental illnesses. However, this link is not necessarily a simple one and may hinge upon genetic vulnerability, psychosocial experiences, and/or general environmental influences. A 2005 study highlights this complexity, with the finding that frequent marijuana use during adolescence can increase the risk of psychosis in adulthood, but only in individuals who carry a particular gene variant.

It is also true that having a mental disorder in childhood or adolescence can increase the risk of later drug abuse problems, as frequently occurs with conduct disorder and untreated attention deficit hyperactivity disorder (ADHD). This presents a challenge when treating children with ADHD, since effective treatment often involves prescribing stimulant medications with abuse potential. This issue has generated strong interest from the research community, and although the results are not yet conclusive, most studies suggest that ADHD medications do not increase the risk of drug abuse among children with ADHD.

Regardless of how comorbidity develops, it is common in youth as well as adults. Given the high prevalence of comorbid mental disorders and their likely adverse impact on substance abuse treatment outcomes, drug abuse programs for adolescents should include screening and, as needed, treatment for comorbid mental disorders.

Exposure to Traumatic Events Puts People at Higher Risk of Substance Use Disorders

Physically or emotionally traumatized people are at much higher risk of abusing licit, illicit, and prescription drugs. This linkage is of particular concern for returning veterans since nearly one in five military service members back from Iraq and Afghanistan have reported symptoms of post-traumatic stress disorder (PTSD) or major depression.

Recent epidemiological studies suggest that as many as half of all veterans diagnosed with PTSD also have a co-occurring substance use disorder (SUD), which could pose an enormous challenge for our health care system. Many PTSD programs do not accept individuals with active SUDs, and traditional SUD clinics defer treatment of trauma-related issues. Nevertheless, there are treatments at different stages of clinical validation for comorbid PTSD and SUD; these include various combinations of psychosocial (e.g., exposure therapy) and pharmacologic (e.g., mood stabilizers, anxiolytics, and antidepressants) interventions.

However, research is urgently needed to identify the best treatment strategies for addressing PTSD/SUD comorbidities, and to explore whether different treatments might be needed in response to civilian versus combat PTSD.

Diagnosing Comorbidity

The high rate of comorbidity between drug use disorders and other mental illnesses argues for a comprehensive approach to intervention that identifies and evaluates each disorder concurrently, providing treatment as needed. The needed approach calls for broad assessment tools that are less likely to result in a missed diagnosis. Accordingly, patients entering treatment for psychiatric illnesses should also be screened for substance use disorders and vice versa.

Accurate diagnosis is complicated, however, by the similarities between drug-related symptoms such as withdrawal and those of potentially comorbid mental disorders. Thus, when people who abuse drugs enter treatment, it may be necessary to observe them after a period of abstinence in order to distinguish between the effects of substance intoxication or withdrawal and the symptoms of comorbid mental disorders. This practice would allow for a more accurate diagnosis and more targeted treatment.

Treating Comorbid Conditions

A fundamental principle emerging from scientific research is the need to treat comorbid conditions concurrently—which can be a difficult proposition. Patients who have both a drug use disorder and another mental illness often exhibit symptoms that are more persistent, severe, and resistant to treatment compared with patients who have either disorder alone. Nevertheless, steady progress is being made through research on new and existing treatment options for comorbidity and through health services research on implementation of appropriate screening and treatment within a variety of settings, including criminal justice systems.

Medications

Effective medications exist for treating opioid, alcohol, and nicotine addiction and for alleviating the symptoms of many other mental disorders, yet most have not been well studied in comorbid populations. Some medications may benefit multiple problems. For example, evidence suggests that bupropion (trade names: Wellbutrin, Zyban), approved for treating depression and nicotine dependence, might also help reduce craving and use of the drug methamphetamine. Clearly, more research is needed to fully understand and assess the actions of combined or dually effective medications.

Behavioral Therapies

Behavioral treatment (alone or in combination with medications) is the cornerstone to successful outcomes for many individuals with drug use disorders or other mental illnesses. And while behavior therapies continue to be evaluated for use in comorbid populations, several strategies have shown promise for treating specific comorbid conditions.

Most clinicians and researchers agree that broad spectrum diagnosis and concurrent therapy will lead to more positive outcomes for patients with comorbid conditions. Preliminary findings support this notion, but research is needed to identify the most effective therapies (especially studies focused on adolescents).

Barriers to Comprehensive Treatment of Comorbidity

Although research supports the need for comprehensive treatment to address comorbidity, provision of such treatment can be problematic for a number of reasons.

In the United States, different treatment systems address drug use disorders and other mental illnesses separately. Physicians are most often the front line of treatment for mental disorders, whereas drug abuse treatment is provided in assorted venues by a mix of health care professionals with different backgrounds. Thus, neither system may have sufficiently broad expertise to address the full range of problems presented by patients. People also use these health care systems differently, depending on insurance coverage and social factors. For example, when suffering from substance abuse and mental illness comorbidities, women more often seek help from mental health practitioners, whereas men tend to seek help through substance abuse treatment channels.

A lingering bias remains in some substance abuse treatment centers against using any medications, including those necessary to treat serious mental disorders such as depression. Additionally, many substance abuse treatment programs do not employ professionals qualified to prescribe, dispense, and monitor medications.

Many of those needing treatment are in the criminal justice system. It is estimated that about 45 percent of offenders in state and local prisons and jails have a mental health problem comorbid with substance abuse or addiction. However, adequate treatment services for both drug use disorders and other mental illnesses are greatly lacking within these settings. While treatment provision may be burdensome for the criminal justice system, it offers an opportunity to positively affect the public's health and safety. Treatment of comorbid disorders can reduce not only associated medical complications, but also negative social outcomes by mitigating against a return to criminal behavior and reincarceration.

Chapter 30

Bereavement, Mourning, and Grief

Overview

People cope with the loss of a loved one in many ways. For some, the experience may lead to personal growth, even though it is a difficult and trying time. There is no right way of coping with death. The way a person grieves depends on the personality of that person and the relationship with the person who has died. How a person copes with grief is affected by their experience with cancer, the way the disease progressed, the person's cultural and religious background, coping skills, mental history, support systems, and the person's social and financial status.

The terms grief, bereavement, and mourning are often used in place of each other, but they have different meanings.

Grief is the normal process of reacting to the loss. Grief reactions may be felt in response to physical losses (for example, a death) or in response to symbolic or social losses (for example, divorce or loss of a job). Each type of loss means the person has had something taken away. As a family goes through a cancer illness, many losses are experienced, and each triggers its own grief reaction. Grief may be experienced as a mental, physical, social, or emotional reaction. Mental reactions can include anger, guilt, anxiety, sadness, and despair. Physical reactions can include sleeping problems, changes in appetite, physical problems, or illness. Social reactions can include feelings about taking care of

PDQ® Cancer Information Summary. National Cancer Institute; Bethesda, MD. Grief, Bereavement, and Coping with Loss (PDQ®): Patient Version. Updated 08/2010. Available at: http://cancer.gov. Accessed October 14, 2010.

others in the family, seeing family or friends, or returning to work. As with bereavement, grief processes depend on the relationship with the person who died, the situation surrounding the death, and the person's attachment to the person who died. Grief may be described as the presence of physical problems, constant thoughts of the person who died, guilt, hostility, and a change in the way one normally acts.

Bereavement is the period after a loss during which grief is experienced and mourning occurs. The time spent in a period of bereavement depends on how attached the person was to the person who died, and how much time was spent anticipating the loss.

Mourning is the process by which people adapt to a loss. Mourning is also influenced by cultural customs, rituals, and society's rules for coping with loss.

Grief work includes the processes that a mourner needs to complete before resuming daily life. These processes include separating from the person who died, readjusting to a world without him or her, and forming new relationships. To separate from the person who died, a person must find another way to redirect the emotional energy that was given to the loved one. This does not mean the person was not loved or should be forgotten, but that the mourner needs to turn to others for emotional satisfaction. The mourner's roles, identity, and skills may need to change to readjust to living in a world without the person who died. The mourner must give other people or activities the emotional energy that was once given to the person who died in order to redirect emotional energy.

People who are grieving often feel extremely tired because the process of grieving usually requires physical and emotional energy. The grief they are feeling is not just for the person who died, but also for the unfulfilled wishes and plans for the relationship with the person. Death often reminds people of past losses or separations. Mourning may be described as having the following three phases:

- The urge to bring back the person who died

- Disorganization and sadness

- Reorganization

Phases of a Life-Threatening Illness

Understanding how other people cope with a life-threatening illness may help the patient and his or her family prepare to cope with their own illness. A life-threatening illness may be described as having the following four phases:

- Phase before the diagnosis
- The acute phase
- The chronic phase
- Recovery or death

The phase before the diagnosis of a life-threatening illness is the period of time just before the diagnosis when a person realizes that he or she may develop an illness. This phase is not usually a single moment, but extends throughout the period when the person has a physical examination, including various tests, and ends when the person is told of the diagnosis.

The acute phase occurs at the time of the diagnosis when a person is forced to understand the diagnosis and make decisions about his or her medical care.

The chronic phase is the period of time between the diagnosis and the result of treatment. It is the period when a patient tries to cope with the demands of life while also undergoing treatment and coping with the side effects of treatment. In the past, the period between a cancer diagnosis and death usually lasted only a few months, and this time was usually spent in the hospital. Today, people can live for years after being diagnosed with cancer.

In the recovery phase, people cope with the mental, social, physical, religious, and financial effects of cancer.

The final (terminal) phase of a life-threatening illness occurs when death is likely. The focus changes from curing the illness or prolonging life, to providing comfort and relief from pain. Religious concerns are often the focus during this time.

The Pathway to Death

People who are dying may move toward death over longer or shorter periods of time and in different ways. Different causes of death result in different paths toward death.

The pathway to death may be long and slow, sometimes lasting years, or it may be a rapid fall toward death (for example, after a car accident) when the chronic phase of the illness, if it exists at all, is short. The peaks and valleys pathway describes the patient who repeatedly gets better and then worse again (for example, a patient with AIDS [acquired immunodeficiency syndrome] or leukemia). Another pathway to death may be described as a long, slow period of failing health and then a period of stable health (for example, patients whose health gets worse and then stabilizes at a new, more limiting level). Patients on this pathway must readjust to losses in functioning ability.

Deaths from cancer often occur over a long period of time, and may involve long-term pain and suffering, and/or loss of control over one's body or mind. Deaths caused by cancer are likely to drain patients and families physically and emotionally because they occur over a long period of time.

Anticipatory Grief

Anticipatory grief is the normal mourning that occurs when a patient or family is expecting a death. Anticipatory grief has many of the same symptoms as those experienced after a death has occurred. It includes all of the thinking, feeling, cultural, and social reactions to an expected death that are felt by the patient and family.

Anticipatory grief includes depression, extreme concern for the dying person, preparing for the death, and adjusting to changes caused by the death. Anticipatory grief gives the family more time to slowly get used to the reality of the loss. People are able to complete unfinished business with the dying person (for example, saying "good-bye," "I love you," or "I forgive you").

Anticipatory grief may not always occur. Anticipatory grief does not mean that before the death, a person feels the same kind of grief as the grief felt after a death. There is not a set amount of grief that a person will feel. The grief experienced before a death does not make the grief after the death last a shorter amount of time.

Grief that follows an unplanned death is different from anticipatory grief. Unplanned loss may overwhelm the coping abilities of a person, making normal functioning impossible. Mourners may not be able to realize the total impact of their loss. Even though the person recognizes that the loss occurred, he or she may not be able to accept the loss mentally and emotionally. Following an unexpected death, the mourner may feel that the world no longer has order and does not make sense.

Some people believe that anticipatory grief is rare. To accept a loved one's death while he or she is still alive may leave the mourner feeling that the dying patient has been abandoned. Expecting the loss often makes the attachment to the dying person stronger. Although anticipatory grief may help the family, the dying person may experience too much grief, causing the patient to become withdrawn.

Phases of Grief

The process of bereavement may be described as having four phases:

1. **Shock and numbness:** Family members find it difficult to believe the death; they feel stunned and numb.

2. **Yearning and searching:** Survivors experience separation anxiety and cannot accept the reality of the loss. They try to find and bring back the lost person and feel ongoing frustration and disappointment when this is not possible.

3. **Disorganization and despair:** Family members feel depressed and find it difficult to plan for the future. They are easily distracted and have difficulty concentrating and focusing.

4. **Reorganization.**

Treatment

Most of the support that people receive after a loss comes from friends and family. Doctors and nurses may also be a source of support. For people who experience difficulty in coping with their loss, grief counseling or grief therapy may be necessary.

Grief counseling helps mourners with normal grief reactions work through the tasks of grieving. Grief counseling can be provided by professionally trained people, or in self-help groups where bereaved people help other bereaved people. All of these services may be available in individual or group settings.

The goals of grief counseling include the following:

- Helping the bereaved to accept the loss by helping him or her to talk about the loss

- Helping the bereaved to identify and express feelings related to the loss (for example, anger, guilt, anxiety, helplessness, and sadness)

- Helping the bereaved to live without the person who died and to make decisions alone

- Helping the bereaved to separate emotionally from the person who died and to begin new relationships

- Providing support and time to focus on grieving at important times such as birthdays and anniversaries

- Describing normal grieving and the differences in grieving among individuals

- Providing continuous support

- Helping the bereaved to understand his or her methods of coping

- Identifying coping problems the bereaved may have and making recommendations for professional grief therapy

Grief therapy is used with people who have more serious grief reactions. The goal of grief therapy is to identify and solve problems the mourner may have in separating from the person who died. When separation difficulties occur, they may appear as physical or behavior problems, delayed or extreme mourning, conflicted or extended grief, or unexpected mourning (although this is seldom present with cancer deaths).

Grief therapy may be available as individual or group therapy. A contract is set up with the individual that establishes the time limit of the therapy, the fees, the goals, and the focus of the therapy.

In grief therapy, the mourner talks about the deceased and tries to recognize whether he or she is experiencing an expected amount of emotion about the death. Grief therapy may allow the mourner to see that anger, guilt, or other negative or uncomfortable feelings can exist at the same time as more positive feelings about the person who died.

Human beings tend to make strong bonds of affection or attachment with others. When these bonds are broken, as in death, a strong emotional reaction occurs. After a loss occurs, a person must accomplish certain tasks to complete the process of grief. These basic tasks of mourning include accepting that the loss happened, living with and feeling the physical and emotional pain of grief, adjusting to life without the loved one, and emotionally separating from the loved one and going on with life without him or her. It is important that these tasks are completed before mourning can end.

In grief therapy, six tasks may be used to help a mourner work through grief:

1. Develop the ability to experience, express, and adjust to painful grief-related changes

2. Find effective ways to cope with painful changes

3. Establish a continuing relationship with the person who died

4. Stay healthy and keep functioning

5. Re-establish relationships and understand that others may have difficulty empathizing with the grief they experience

6. Develop a healthy image of oneself and the world

Complications in grief may come about due to uncompleted grief from earlier losses. The grief for these earlier losses must be managed in order to handle the current grief. Grief therapy includes dealing with the blockages to the mourning process, identifying unfinished business with the deceased, and identifying other losses that result from the death. The bereaved is helped to see that the loss is final and to picture life after the grief period.

Complicated Grief

Complicated grief reactions require more complex therapies than uncomplicated grief reactions. Adjustment disorders (especially depressed and anxious mood or disturbed emotions and behavior), major depression, substance abuse, and even posttraumatic stress disorder are some of the common problems of complicated bereavement. Complicated grief is identified by the extended length of time of the symptoms, the interference caused by the symptoms, or by the intensity of the symptoms (for example, intense suicidal thoughts or acts).

Complicated or unresolved grief may appear as a complete absence of grief and mourning, an ongoing inability to experience normal grief reactions, delayed grief, conflicted grief, or chronic grief. Factors that contribute to the chance that one may experience complicated grief include the suddenness of the death, the gender of the person in mourning, and the relationship to the deceased (for example, an intense, extremely close, or very contradictory relationship). Grief reactions that turn into major depression should be treated with both drug and psychological therapy. One who avoids any reminders of the person who died, who constantly thinks or dreams about the person who died, and who gets scared and panics easily at any reminders of the person who died may be suffering from posttraumatic stress disorder. Substance abuse may occur, frequently in an attempt to avoid painful feelings about the loss and symptoms (such as sleeplessness), and can also be treated with drugs and psychological therapy.

Children and Grief

In the past, children were thought to be miniature adults and were expected to behave as adults. It is now understood that there are differences in the ways in which children and adults mourn.

Unlike adults, bereaved children do not experience continual and intense emotional and behavioral grief reactions. Children may seem to show grief only occasionally and briefly, but in reality a child's grief usually lasts longer than that of an adult. This may be explained by the fact that a child's ability to experience intense emotions is limited. Mourning in children may need to be addressed again and again as the child gets older. Since bereavement is a process that continues over time, children will think about the loss repeatedly, especially during important times in their life, such as going to camp, graduating from school, getting married, or giving birth to their own children.

A child's grief may be influenced by his or her age, personality, stage of development, earlier experiences with death, and his or her relationship with the deceased. The surroundings, cause of death, and family members' ability to communicate with one another and to continue as a family after the death can also affect grief. The child's ongoing need for care, the child's opportunity to share his or her feelings and memories, the parent's ability to cope with stress, and the child's steady relationships with other adults are also other factors that may influence grief.

Children do not react to loss in the same ways as adults. Grieving children may not show their feelings as openly as adults. Grieving children may not withdraw and dwell on the person who died, but instead may throw themselves into activities (for example, they may be sad one minute and playful the next). Often families think the child doesn't really understand or has gotten over the death. Neither is true; children's minds protect them from what is too powerful for them to handle. Children's grieving periods are shortened because they cannot think through their thoughts and feelings like adults. Also, children have trouble putting their feelings about grief into words. Instead, his or her behavior speaks for the child. Strong feelings of anger and fears of abandonment or death may show up in the behavior of grieving children. Children often play death games as a way of working out their feelings and anxieties. These games are familiar to the children and provide safe opportunities to express their feelings.

Children's Grief and Developmental Stages

Children at different stages of development have different understandings of death and the events near death.

Infants: Infants do not recognize death, but feelings of loss and separation are part of developing an awareness of death. Children who have been separated from their mother may be sluggish, quiet, unresponsive to a smile or a coo, undergo physical changes (for example, weight loss), be less active, and sleep less.

Age 2–3 years: Children at this age often confuse death with sleep and may experience anxiety as early as age 3. They may stop talking and appear to feel overall distress.

Age 3–6 years: At this age children see death as a kind of sleep; the person is alive, but only in a limited way. The child cannot fully separate death from life. Children may think that the person is still living, even though he or she might have been buried, and ask questions about the deceased (for example, how does the deceased eat, go to the toilet, breathe, or play?). Young children know that death occurs physically, but think it is temporary, reversible, and not final. The child's concept of death may involve magical thinking. For example, the child may think that his or her thoughts can cause another person to become sick or die. Grieving children under 5 may have trouble eating, sleeping, and controlling bladder and bowel functions.

Age 6–9 years: Children at this age are commonly very curious about death, and may ask questions about what happens to one's body when it dies. Death is thought of as a person or spirit separate from the person who was alive, such as a skeleton, ghost, angel of death, or bogeyman. They may see death as final and frightening but as something that happens mostly to old people (and not to themselves). Grieving children can become afraid of school, have learning problems, develop antisocial or aggressive behaviors, become overly concerned about their own health (for example, developing symptoms of imaginary illness), or withdraw from others. Or, children this age can become too attached and clinging. Boys usually become more aggressive and destructive (for example, acting out in school), instead of openly showing their sadness. When a parent dies children may feel abandoned by both their deceased parent and their surviving parent because the surviving parent is grieving and is unable to emotionally support the child.

Ages 9 and older: By the time a child is 9 years old, death is known to be unavoidable and is not seen as a punishment. By the time a child is 12 years old, death is seen as final and something that happens to everyone.

In American society, many grieving adults withdraw and do not talk to others. Children, however, often talk to the people around them (even strangers) to see the reactions of others and to get clues for their own responses. Children may ask confusing questions. For example, a child may ask, "I know grandpa died, but when will he come home?" This is a way of testing reality and making sure the story of the death has not changed.

Other Issues for Grieving Children

Children's grief expresses three issues:

- Did I cause the death to happen?
- Is it going to happen to me?
- Who is going to take care of me?

Did I cause the death to happen?

Children often think that they have magical powers. If a mother says in irritation, "You'll be the death of me" and later dies, her child may wonder if he or she actually caused the mother's death. Also, when children argue, one may say (or think), "I wish you were dead." Should that child die, the surviving child may think that his or her thoughts actually caused the death.

Is it going to happen to me?

The death of another child may be especially hard for a child. If the child thinks that the death may have been prevented (by either a parent or a doctor) the child may think that he or she could also die.

Who is going to take care of me?

Since children depend on parents and other adults to take care of them, a grieving child may wonder who will care for him or her after the death of an important person.

Grieving Children: Treatment

A child's grieving process may be made easier by being open and honest with the child about death, using direct language, and incorporating the child into memorial ceremonies for the person who died.

Explanation of death: Not talking about death (which indicates that the subject is off-limits) does not help children learn to cope with loss. When discussing death with children, explanations should be simple and direct. Each child should be told the truth using as much detail as he or she is able to understand. The child's questions should be answered honestly and directly. Children need to be reassured about their own security (they often worry that they will also die, or that their surviving parent will go away). Children's questions should be answered, making sure that the child understands the answers.

Correct language: A discussion about death should include the proper words, such as cancer, died, and death. Substitute words or phrases (for example, "he passed away," "he is sleeping," or "we lost him") should never be used because they can confuse children and lead to misunderstandings.

Planning memorial ceremonies: When a death occurs, children can and should be included in the planning of and participation in memorial ceremonies. These events help children (and adults) remember loved ones. Children should not be forced to be involved in these ceremonies, but they should be encouraged to take part in those portions of the events with which they feel most comfortable. If the child wants to attend the funeral, wake, or memorial service, he or she should be given in advance a full explanation of what to expect. The surviving parent may be too involved in his or her own grief to give their child full attention, therefore, it may be helpful to have a familiar adult or family member care for the grieving child.

Culture and Response to Grief and Mourning

Grief felt for the loss of a loved one, the loss of a treasured possession, or a loss associated with an important life change, occurs across all ages and cultures. However, the role that cultural heritage plays in an individual's experience of grief and mourning is not well understood. Attitudes, beliefs, and practices regarding death must be described according to myths and mysteries surrounding death within different cultures.

Individual, personal experiences of grief are similar in different cultures. This is true even though different cultures have different mourning ceremonies, traditions, and behaviors to express grief.

Helping families cope with the death of a loved one includes showing respect for the family's cultural heritage and encouraging them to decide how to honor the death. Important questions that should be asked of people who are dealing with the loss of a loved one include:

- What are the cultural rituals for coping with dying, the deceased person's body, the final arrangements for the body, and honoring the death?

- What are the family's beliefs about what happens after death?

- What does the family feel is a normal expression of grief and the acceptance of the loss?

- What does the family consider to be the roles of each family member in handling the death?

- Are certain types of death less acceptable (for example, suicide), or are certain types of death especially hard to handle for that culture (for example, the death of a child)?

Death, grief, and mourning spare no one and are normal life events. All cultures have developed ways to cope with death. Interfering with these practices may interfere with the necessary grieving processes. Understanding different cultures' response to death can help physicians recognize the grieving process in patients of other cultures.

Chapter 31

Common Reactions after Trauma

After going through a trauma, survivors often say that their first feeling is relief to be alive. This may be followed by stress, fear, and anger. Trauma survivors may also find they are unable to stop thinking about what happened. Many survivors will show a high level of arousal, which causes them to react strongly to sounds and sights around them.

Most people have some kind of stress reaction after a trauma. Having such a reaction has nothing to do with personal weakness. Stress reactions may last for several days or even a few weeks. For most people, if symptoms occur, they will slowly decrease over time.

All kinds of trauma survivors commonly experience stress reactions. This is true for veterans, children, and disaster rescue or relief workers. If you understand what is happening when you or someone you know reacts to a traumatic event, you may be less fearful and better able to handle things.

Reactions to a trauma may include the following:

- Feeling hopeless about the future

- Feeling detached or unconcerned about others

- Having trouble concentrating or making decisions

- Feeling jumpy and getting startled easily at sudden noises

From the National Center for Posttraumatic Stress Disorder (NCPTSD, www.ptsd.va.gov), part of the Veterans Administration, June 15, 2010.

- Feeling on guard and constantly alert
- Having disturbing dreams and memories or flashbacks
- Having work or school problems

You may also experience more physical reactions such as the following:

- Stomach upset and trouble eating
- Trouble sleeping and feeling very tired
- Pounding heart, rapid breathing, feeling edgy
- Sweating
- Severe headache if thinking of the event
- Failure to engage in exercise, diet, safe sex, regular health care
- Excess smoking, alcohol, drugs, food
- Having your ongoing medical problems get worse

You may have more emotional troubles such as the following:

- Feeling nervous, helpless, fearful, sad
- Feeling shocked, numb, and not able to feel love or joy
- Avoiding people, places, and things related to the event
- Being irritable or having outbursts of anger
- Becoming easily upset or agitated
- Blaming yourself or having negative views of oneself or the world
- Distrust of others, getting into conflicts, being over controlling
- Being withdrawn, feeling rejected or abandoned
- Loss of intimacy or feeling detached

Turn to your family and friends when you are ready to talk. They are your personal support system. Recovery is an ongoing gradual process. It doesn't happen through suddenly being "cured" and it doesn't mean that you will forget what happened. Most people will recover from trauma naturally.

If your stress reactions are getting in the way of your relationships, work, or other important activities, you may want to talk to a counselor or your doctor. Good treatments are available.

Common Problems That Can Occur after a Trauma

Posttraumatic stress disorder (PTSD): PTSD is a condition that can develop after you have gone through a life-threatening event. If you have PTSD, you may have trouble keeping yourself from thinking over and over about what happened to you. You may try to avoid people and places that remind you of the trauma. You may feel numb. Lastly, if you have PTSD, you might find that you have trouble relaxing. You may startle easily and you may feel on guard most of the time.

Depression: Depression involves feeling down or sad more days than not. If you are depressed, you may lose interest in activities that used to be enjoyable or fun. You may feel low in energy and be overly tired. You may feel hopeless or in despair, and you may think that things will never get better. Depression is more likely when you have had losses such as the death of close friends. If you are depressed, at times you might think about hurting or killing yourself. For this reason, getting help for depression is very important.

Self-blame, guilt, and shame: Sometimes in trying to make sense of a traumatic event, you may blame yourself in some way. You may think you are responsible for bad things that happened, or for surviving when others didn't. You may feel guilty for what you did or did not do. Remember, we all tend to be our own worst critics. Most of the time, that guilt, shame, or self-blame is not justified.

Suicidal thoughts: Trauma and personal loss can lead a depressed person to think about hurting or killing themselves. If you think someone you know may be feeling suicidal, you should directly ask them. You will not put the idea in their head. If someone is thinking about killing themselves, call the National Suicide Prevention Lifeline. The phone number is 800-273-TALK (8255). You can also call a counselor, doctor, or 911.

Anger or aggressive behavior: Trauma can be connected with anger in many ways. After a trauma, you might think that what happened to you was unfair or unjust. You might not understand why the event happened and why it happened to you. These thoughts can result in intense anger. Although anger is a natural and healthy emotion, intense feelings of anger and aggressive behavior can cause problems with family, friends, or coworkers. If you become violent when angry, you just make the situation worse. Violence can lead to people being injured, and there may be legal consequences.

Alcohol/drug abuse: Drinking or "self-medicating" with drugs is a common, and unhealthy, way of coping with upsetting events. You may drink too much or use drugs to numb yourself and to try to deal with difficult thoughts, feelings, and memories related to the trauma. While using alcohol or drugs may offer a quick solution, it can actually lead to more problems. If someone close begins to lose control of drinking or drug use, you should try to get them to see a health care provider about managing their drinking or drug use.

Summing It All Up

Right after a trauma, almost every survivor will find him or herself unable to stop thinking about what happened. Stress reactions such as increased fear, nervousness, jumpiness, upsetting memories, and efforts to avoid reminders will gradually decrease over time for most people.

Use your personal support systems, family, and friends when you are ready to talk. Recovery is an ongoing gradual process. It doesn't happen through suddenly being "cured" and it doesn't mean that you will forget what happened. Most people will recover from trauma naturally over time. If your emotional reactions are getting in the way of your relationships, work, or other important activities, you may want to talk to a counselor or your doctor. Good treatments are available.

Chapter 32

Types of Stress-Related Disorders That Develop after Trauma

Chapter Contents

Section 32.1

Dissociative Disorders

Dissociative disorders are so-called because they are marked by a dissociation from or interruption of a person's fundamental aspects of waking consciousness (such as one's personal identity, one's personal history, etc.). Dissociative disorders come in many forms, the most famous of which is dissociative identity disorder (formerly known as multiple personality disorder). All of the dissociative disorders are thought to stem from trauma experienced by the individual with this disorder. The dissociative aspect is thought to be a coping mechanism—the person literally dissociates himself from a situation or experience too traumatic to integrate with his conscious self. Symptoms of these disorders, or even one or more of the disorders themselves, are also seen in a number of other mental illnesses, including post-traumatic stress disorder, panic disorder, and obsessive compulsive disorder.

Dissociative amnesia: This disorder is characterized by a blocking out of critical personal information, usually of a traumatic or stressful nature. Dissociative amnesia, unlike other types of amnesia, does not result from other medical trauma (e.g., a blow to the head). Dissociative amnesia has several subtypes:

- Localized amnesia is present in an individual who has no memory of specific events that took place, usually traumatic. The loss of memory is localized with a specific window of time. For example, a survivor of a car wreck who has no memory of the experience until 2 days later is experiencing localized amnesia.

- Selective amnesia happens when a person can recall only small parts of events that took place in a defined period of time. For example, an abuse victim may recall only some parts of the series of events around the abuse.

- Generalized amnesia is diagnosed when a person's amnesia encompasses his or her entire life.

- Systematized amnesia is characterized by a loss of memory for a specific category of information. A person with this disorder might, for example, be missing all memories about one specific family member.

Dissociative fugue is a rare disorder. An individual with dissociative fugue suddenly and unexpectedly takes physical leave of his or her surroundings and sets off on a journey of some kind. These journeys can last hours, or even several days or months. Individuals experiencing a dissociative fugue have traveled over thousands of miles. An individual in a fugue state is unaware of or confused about his identity, and in some cases will assume a new identity (although this is the exception).

Dissociative identity disorder (DID), which has been known as multiple personality disorder, is the most famous of the dissociative disorders. An individual suffering from DID has more than one distinct identity or personality state that surfaces in the individual on a recurring basis. This disorder is also marked by differences in memory which vary with the individual's "alters," or other personalities. For more information on this, see the NAMI factsheet on dissociative identity disorder [http://www.nami.org/Template.cfm?Section=Helpline&Template=/ContentManagement/ContentDisplay.cfm&ContentID=20562].

Depersonalization disorder is marked by a feeling of detachment or distance from one's own experience, body, or self. These feelings of depersonalization are recurrent. Of the dissociative disorders, depersonalization is the one most easily identified with by the general public; one can easily relate to feeling as they do in a dream, or being "spaced out." Feeling out of control of one's actions and movements is something that people describe when intoxicated. An individual with depersonalization disorder has this experience so frequently and so severely that it interrupts his or her functioning and experience. A person's experience with depersonalization can be so severe that he or she believes the external world is unreal or distorted.

Treatment

Since dissociative disorders seem to be triggered as a response to trauma or abuse, treatment for individuals with such a disorder may stress psychotherapy, although a combination of psychopharmacological and psychosocial treatments is often used. Many of the symptoms of dissociative disorders occur with other disorders, such as anxiety and depression, and can be controlled by the same drugs used to treat those disorders. A person in treatment for a dissociative disorder might benefit from antidepressants or antianxiety medication.

Section 32.2

Acute Stress Disorder

From "Acute Stress Disorder," by the National Center for Posttraumatic Stress Disorder (NCPTSD, www.ptsd.va.gov), part of the Veterans Administration, June 15, 2010.

Acute stress disorder (ASD) is a mental disorder that can occur in the first month following a trauma. The symptoms that define ASD overlap with those for posttraumatic stress disorder (PTSD). One difference, though, is that a PTSD diagnosis cannot be given until symptoms have lasted for 1 month. Also, compared to PTSD, ASD is more likely to involve feelings such as not knowing where you are, or feeling as if you are outside of your body.

How common is ASD?

Studies of ASD vary in terms of the tools used and the rates of ASD found. Overall, within 1 month of a trauma, survivors show rates of ASD ranging from 6% to 33%. Rates differ for different types of trauma. For example, survivors of accidents or disasters such as typhoons show lower rates of ASD. Survivors of violence such as robbery, assaults, and mass shootings show rates at the higher end of that range.

Who is at risk for ASD as a result of trauma?

Several factors can place you at higher risk for developing ASD after a trauma:

- Having gone through other traumatic events
- Having had PTSD in the past
- Having had prior mental health problems

- Tending to have symptoms such as not knowing who or where you are, when confronted with trauma

Does ASD predict PTSD?

If you have ASD, you are very likely to get PTSD. Research has found that over 80% of people with ASD have PTSD 6 months later. Not everyone with ASD will get PTSD, though.

Also, those who do not get ASD can still develop PTSD later on. Studies indicate that a small number (4–13%) of survivors who do not get ASD in the first month after a trauma will get PTSD in later months or years.

Are there effective treatments for ASD?

Yes, a type of treatment called cognitive behavioral therapy (CBT) has been shown to have positive results. Research shows that survivors who get CBT soon after going through a trauma are less likely to get PTSD symptoms later. A mental health care provider trained in treatment for trauma can judge whether CBT may be useful for a trauma survivor.

Another treatment called psychological debriefing (PD) has sometimes been used in the wake of a traumatic event. However, there is little research to back its use for effectively treating ASD or PTSD. It should also be noted that with more severe trauma or reactions such as PTSD, debriefing is not recommended.

Section 32.3

Posttraumatic Stress Disorder (PTSD)

From "Post-Traumatic Stress Disorder," by the National Institute of Mental Health (NIMH, www.nimh.nih.gov), part of the National Institutes of Health, 2008.

What is post-traumatic stress disorder, or PTSD?

PTSD is an anxiety disorder that some people get after seeing or living through a dangerous event. When in danger, it's natural to feel afraid. This fear triggers many split-second changes in the body to prepare to defend against the danger or to avoid it. This "fight-or-flight" response is a healthy reaction meant to protect a person from harm. But in PTSD, this reaction is changed or damaged. People who have PTSD may feel stressed or frightened even when they're no longer in danger.

Who gets PTSD?

Anyone can get PTSD at any age. This includes war veterans and survivors of physical and sexual assault, abuse, accidents, disasters, and many other serious events.

Not everyone with PTSD has been through a dangerous event. Some people get PTSD after a friend or family member experiences danger or is harmed. The sudden, unexpected death of a loved one can also cause PTSD.

What are the symptoms of PTSD?

PTSD can cause many symptoms. These symptoms can be grouped into three categories:

- **Re-experiencing symptoms**
  - Flashbacks—reliving the trauma over and over, including physical symptoms like a racing heart or sweating
  - Bad dreams
  - Frightening thoughts

Re-experiencing symptoms may cause problems in a person's everyday routine. They can start from the person's own thoughts and feelings. Words, objects, or situations that are reminders of the event can also trigger re-experiencing.

- **Avoidance symptoms**

  - Staying away from places, events, or objects that are reminders of the experience

  - Feeling emotionally numb

  - Feeling strong guilt, depression, or worry

  - Losing interest in activities that were enjoyable in the past

  - Having trouble remembering the dangerous event

Things that remind a person of the traumatic event can trigger avoidance symptoms. These symptoms may cause a person to change his or her personal routine. For example, after a bad car accident, a person who usually drives may avoid driving or riding in a car.

- **Hyperarousal symptoms**

  - Being easily startled

  - Feeling tense or "on edge"

  - Having difficulty sleeping and/or having angry outbursts

Hyperarousal symptoms are usually constant, instead of being triggered by things that remind one of the traumatic event. They can make the person feel stressed and angry. These symptoms may make it hard to do daily tasks, such as sleeping, eating, or concentrating.

It's natural to have some of these symptoms after a dangerous event. Sometimes people have very serious symptoms that go away after a few weeks. This is called acute stress disorder, or ASD. When the symptoms last more than a few weeks and become an ongoing problem, they might be PTSD. Some people with PTSD don't show any symptoms for weeks or months.

Do children react differently than adults?

Children and teens can have extreme reactions to trauma, but their symptoms may not be the same as adults. In very young children, these symptoms can include the following:

- Bedwetting, when they'd learned how to use the toilet before
- Forgetting how or being unable to talk
- Acting out the scary event during playtime
- Being unusually clingy with a parent or other adult

Older children and teens usually show symptoms more like those seen in adults. They may also develop disruptive, disrespectful, or destructive behaviors. Older children and teens may feel guilty for not preventing injury or deaths. They may also have thoughts of revenge.

How is PTSD detected?

A doctor who has experience helping people with mental illnesses, such as a psychiatrist or psychologist, can diagnose PTSD. The diagnosis is made after the doctor talks with the person who has symptoms of PTSD.

To be diagnosed with PTSD, a person must have all of the following for at least 1 month:

- At least one re-experiencing symptom
- At least three avoidance symptoms
- At least two hyperarousal symptoms
- Symptoms that make it hard to go about daily life, go to school or work, be with friends, and take care of important tasks

Why do some people get PTSD and other people do not?

It is important to remember that not everyone who lives through a dangerous event gets PTSD. In fact, most will not get the disorder.

Many factors play a part in whether a person will get PTSD. Some of these are risk factors that make a person more likely to get PTSD. Other factors, called resilience factors, can help reduce the risk of the disorder. Some of these risk and resilience factors are present before the trauma and others become important during and after a traumatic event.

Risk factors for PTSD include the following:

- Living through dangerous events and traumas
- Having a history of mental illness
- Getting hurt
- Seeing people hurt or killed

- Feeling horror, helplessness, or extreme fear
- Having little or no social support after the event
- Dealing with extra stress after the event, such as loss of a loved one, pain and injury, or loss of a job or home

Resilience factors that may reduce the risk of PTSD include the following:

- Seeking out support from other people, such as friends and family
- Finding a support group after a traumatic event
- Feeling good about one's own actions in the face of danger
- Having a coping strategy, or a way of getting through the bad event and learning from it
- Being able to act and respond effectively despite feeling fear

Researchers are studying the importance of various risk and resilience factors. With more study, it may be possible someday to predict who is likely to get PTSD and prevent it.

How is PTSD treated?

The main treatments for people with PTSD are psychotherapy ("talk" therapy), medications, or both. Everyone is different, so a treatment that works for one person may not work for another. It is important for anyone with PTSD to be treated by a mental health care provider who is experienced with PTSD. Some people with PTSD need to try different treatments to find what works for their symptoms.

If someone with PTSD is going through an ongoing trauma, such as being in an abusive relationship, both of the problems need to be treated. Other ongoing problems can include panic disorder, depression, substance abuse, and feeling suicidal.

Psychotherapy: Psychotherapy is talk therapy. It involves talking with a mental health professional to treat a mental illness. Psychotherapy can occur one on one or in a group. Talk therapy treatment for PTSD usually lasts 6 to 12 weeks, but can take more time. Research shows that support from family and friends can be an important part of therapy.

Many types of psychotherapy can help people with PTSD. Some types target the symptoms of PTSD directly. Other therapies focus on social, family, or job-related problems. The doctor or therapist may combine different therapies depending on each person's needs.

One helpful therapy is called cognitive behavioral therapy, or CBT. There are several parts to CBT, including the following:

- **Exposure therapy:** This therapy helps people face and control their fear. It exposes them to the trauma they experienced in a safe way. It uses mental imagery, writing, or visits to the place where the event happened. The therapist uses these tools to help people with PTSD cope with their feelings.

- **Cognitive restructuring:** This therapy helps people make sense of the bad memories. Sometimes people remember the event differently than how it happened. They may feel guilt or shame about what is not their fault. The therapist helps people with PTSD look at what happened in a realistic way.

- **Stress inoculation training:** This therapy tries to reduce PTSD symptoms by teaching a person how to reduce anxiety. Like cognitive restructuring, this treatment helps people look at their memories in a healthy way.

Other types of treatment can also help people with PTSD. People with PTSD should talk about all treatment options with their therapist.

Medications: The U.S. Food and Drug Administration (FDA) has approved two medications for treating adults with PTSD: Sertraline (Zoloft) and paroxetine (Paxil).

Both of these medications are antidepressants, which are also used to treat depression. They may help control PTSD symptoms such as sadness, worry, anger, and feeling numb inside. Taking these medications may make it easier to go through psychotherapy.

Sometimes people taking these medications have side effects. The effects can be annoying, but they usually go away. However, medications affect everyone differently. Any side effects or unusual reactions should be reported to a doctor immediately.

The most common side effects of antidepressants like sertraline and paroxetine are the following:

- Headache, which usually goes away within a few days

- Nausea (feeling sick to your stomach), which usually goes away within a few days

- Sleeplessness or drowsiness, which may occur during the first few weeks but then goes away (Sometimes the medication dose needs to be reduced or the time of day it is taken needs to be adjusted to help lessen these side effects.)

- Agitation (feeling jittery)
- Sexual problems, which can affect both men and women, including reduced sex drive and problems having and enjoying sex

Other medications: Doctors may also prescribe other types of medications, such as the ones listed in the following text. There is little information on how well these work for people with PTSD.

- **Benzodiazepines:** These medications may be given to help people relax and sleep. People who take benzodiazepines may have memory problems or become dependent on the medication.

- **Antipsychotics:** These medications are usually given to people with other mental disorders, like schizophrenia. People who take antipsychotics may gain weight and have a higher chance of getting heart disease and diabetes.

- **Other antidepressants:** Like sertraline and paroxetine, the antidepressants fluoxetine (Prozac) and citalopram (Celexa) can help people with PTSD feel less tense or sad. For people with PTSD who also have other anxiety disorders or depression, antidepressants may be useful in reducing symptoms of these co-occurring illnesses.

What about treatment after mass trauma?

Sometimes large numbers of people are affected by the same event. For example, a lot of people needed help after Hurricane Katrina in 2005 and the terrorist attacks of September 11, 2001. Most people will have some PTSD symptoms in the first few weeks after events like these. This is a normal and expected response to serious trauma, and for most people, symptoms generally lessen with time.

Most people can be helped with basic support, such as the following:

- Getting to a safe place
- Seeing a doctor if injured
- Getting food and water
- Contacting loved ones or friends
- Learning what is being done to help

But some people do not get better on their own. A study of Hurricane Katrina survivors found that, over time, more people were having problems with PTSD, depression, and related mental disorders. This pattern is unlike the recovery from other natural disasters, where the number of people who have mental health problems gradually lessens. As communities try to rebuild after a mass trauma, people may experience ongoing stress from loss of jobs and schools, trouble paying bills, finding housing, and getting health care. This delay in community recovery may in turn delay recovery from PTSD.

In the first couple weeks after a mass trauma, brief versions of CBT may be helpful to some people who are having severe distress. Sometimes other treatments are used, but their effectiveness is not known. For example, there is growing interest in an approach called psychological first aid. The goal of this approach is to make people feel safe and secure, connect people to health care and other resources, and reduce stress reactions. There are guides for carrying out the treatment, but experts do not know yet if it helps prevent or treat PTSD.

In single-session psychological debriefing, another type of mass trauma treatment, survivors talk about the event and express their feelings one on one or in a group. Studies show that it is not likely to reduce distress or the risk for PTSD and may actually increase distress and risk.

What efforts are under way to improve the detection and treatment of PTSD?

Researchers have learned a lot in the last decade about fear, stress, and PTSD. Scientists are also learning about how people form memories. This is important because creating very powerful fear-related memories seems to be a major part of PTSD. Researchers are also exploring how people can create "safety" memories to replace the bad memories that form after a trauma.

PTSD research also includes the following examples:

- Researchers are using powerful new research methods, such as brain imaging and the study of genes, to find out more about what leads to PTSD, when it happens, and who is most at risk.

- Researchers are trying to understand why some people get PTSD and others do not. Knowing this can help health care professionals predict who might get PTSD and provide early treatment.

- Scientists are focusing on ways to examine pre-trauma, trauma, and post-trauma risk and resilience factors all at once.

- Researchers are looking for treatments that reduce the impact traumatic memories have on our emotions.

- Clinicians are improving the way people are screened for PTSD, given early treatment, and tracked after a mass trauma.

- Researchers are developing new approaches in self-testing and screening to help people know when it's time to call a doctor.

- Researchers are testing ways to help family doctors detect and treat PTSD or refer people with PTSD to mental health specialists.

How can I help a friend or relative who has PTSD?

If you know someone who has PTSD, it affects you, too. The first and most important thing you can do to help a friend or relative is to help him or her get the right diagnosis and treatment. You may need to make an appointment for your friend or relative and go with him or her to see the doctor. Encourage him or her to stay in treatment or to seek different treatment if his or her symptoms don't get better after 6 to 8 weeks.

To help a friend or relative, you can do the following:

- Offer emotional support, understanding, patience, and encouragement.

- Learn about PTSD so you can understand what your friend or relative is experiencing.

- Talk to your friend or relative, and listen carefully.

- Listen to feelings your friend or relative expresses and be understanding of situations that may trigger PTSD symptoms.

- Invite your friend or relative out for positive distractions such as walks, outings, and other activities.

- Remind your friend or relative that, with time and treatment, he or she can get better.

- Never ignore comments about your friend or relative harming him or herself, and report such comments to your friend's or relative's therapist or doctor.

How can I help myself?

It may be very hard to take that first step to help yourself. It is important to realize that although it may take some time, with treatment, you can get better.

To help yourself, try the following:

- Talk to your doctor about treatment options.

- Engage in mild activity or exercise to help reduce stress.

- Set realistic goals for yourself.

- Break up large tasks into small ones, set some priorities, and do what you can as you can.

- Try to spend time with other people and confide in a trusted friend or relative. Tell others about things that may trigger symptoms.

- Expect your symptoms to improve gradually, not immediately.

- Identify and seek out comforting situations, places, and people.

Where can I go for help?

If you are unsure where to go for help, ask your family doctor. Others who can help are listed in the following text.

- Mental health specialists, such as psychiatrists, psychologists, social workers, or mental health counselors

- Health maintenance organizations

- Community mental health centers

- Hospital psychiatry departments and outpatient clinics

- Mental health programs at universities or medical schools

- State hospital outpatient clinics

- Family services, social agencies, or clergy

- Peer support groups

- Private clinics and facilities

- Employee assistance programs

- Local medical and/or psychiatric societies

You can also check the phone book under "mental health," "health," "social services," "hotlines," or "physicians" for phone numbers and addresses. An emergency room doctor can also provide temporary help and can tell you where and how to get further help.

What if I or someone I know is in crisis?

If you are thinking about harming yourself, or know someone who is, tell someone who can help immediately:

- Call your doctor.

- Call 911 or go to a hospital emergency room to get immediate help or ask a friend or family member to help you do these things.

- Call the toll-free, 24-hour hotline of the National Suicide Prevention Lifeline at 800-273-TALK (800-273-8255); TTY: 800-799-4TTY (4889) to talk to a trained counselor.

- Make sure you or the suicidal person is not left alone.

Chapter 33

Relationships and Traumatic Stress

How does trauma affect relationships?

Trauma survivors with PTSD may have trouble with their close family relationships or friendships. The symptoms of PTSD can cause problems with trust, closeness, communication, and problem solving. These problems may affect the way the survivor acts with others. In turn, the way a loved one responds to him or her affects the trauma survivor. A circular pattern can develop that may sometimes harm relationships.

How might trauma survivors react?

In the first weeks and months following a trauma, survivors may feel angry, detached, tense, or worried in their relationships. In time, most are able to resume their prior level of closeness in relationships. Yet the 5–10% of survivors who develop PTSD may have lasting relationship problems.

Survivors with PTSD may feel distant from others and feel numb. They may have less interest in social or sexual activities. Because survivors feel irritable, on guard, jumpy, worried, or nervous, they may not be able to relax or be intimate. They may also feel an increased need to protect their loved ones. They may come across as tense or demanding.

From "Relationships and PTSD," by the National Center for Posttraumatic Stress Disorder (NCPTSD, www.ptsd.va.gov), part of the Veterans Administration, June 15, 2010.

The trauma survivor may often have trauma memories or flashbacks. He or she might go to great lengths to avoid such memories. Survivors may avoid any activity that could trigger a memory. If the survivor has trouble sleeping or has nightmares, both the survivor and partner may not be able to get enough rest. This may make sleeping together harder.

Survivors often struggle with intense anger and impulses. In order to suppress angry feelings and actions, they may avoid closeness. They may push away or find fault with loved ones and friends. Also, drinking and drug problems, which can be an attempt to cope with PTSD, can destroy intimacy and friendships. Verbal or physical violence can occur.

In other cases, survivors may depend too much on their partners, family members, and friends. This could also include support persons such as health care providers or therapists.

Dealing with these symptoms can take up a lot of the survivor's attention. He or she may not be able to focus on the partner. It may be hard to listen carefully and make decisions together with someone else. Partners may come to feel that talking together and working as a team are not possible.

How might loved ones react?

Partners, friends, or family members may feel hurt, cut off, or down because the survivor has not been able to get over the trauma. Loved ones may become angry or distant toward the survivor. They may feel pressured, tense, and controlled. The survivor's symptoms can make a loved one feel like he or she is living in a war zone or in constant threat of danger. Living with someone who has PTSD can sometimes lead the partner to have some of the same feelings of having been through trauma.

In sum, a person who goes through a trauma may have certain common reactions. These reactions affect the people around the survivor. Family, friends, and others then react to how the survivor is behaving. This in turn comes back to affect the person who went through the trauma.

What are the types of trauma and their effect on relationships?

Certain types of "man-made" traumas can have a more severe effect on relationships. These traumas include the following:

- Childhood sexual and physical abuse

- Rape
- Domestic violence
- Combat
- Terrorism
- Genocide
- Torture
- Kidnapping
- Prisoner of war

Survivors of man-made traumas often feel a lasting sense of terror, horror, endangerment, and betrayal. These feelings affect how they relate to others. They may feel like they are letting down their guard if they get close to someone else and trust them. This is not to say a survivor never feels a strong bond of love or friendship. However, a close relationship can also feel scary or dangerous to a trauma survivor.

Do all trauma survivors have relationship problems?

Many trauma survivors do not develop PTSD. Also, many people with PTSD do not have relationship problems. People with PTSD can create and maintain good relationships by doing the following:

- Building a personal support network to help cope with PTSD while working on family and friend relationships
- Sharing feelings honestly and openly, with respect and compassion
- Building skills at problem solving and connecting with others
- Including ways to play, be creative, relax, and enjoy others

What can be done to help someone who has PTSD?

Relations with others are very important for trauma survivors. Social support is one of the best things to protect against getting PTSD.

Relationships can offset feelings of being alone. Relationships may also help the survivor's self-esteem. This may help reduce depression and guilt. A relationship can also give the survivor a way to help someone else. Helping others can reduce feelings of failure or feeling cut off from others. Lastly, relationships are a source of support when coping with stress.

If you need to seek professional help, try to find a therapist who has skills in treating PTSD as well as working with couples or families.

Many treatment approaches may be helpful for dealing with relationship issues. Options include the following:

- One-to-one and group therapy
- Anger and stress management
- Assertiveness training
- Couples counseling
- Family education classes
- Family therapy

Chapter 34

Traumatic Stress in Children and Teens

What events cause posttraumatic stress disorder (PTSD) in children?

Children and teens could have PTSD if they have lived through an event that could have caused them or someone else to be killed or badly hurt. Such events include sexual or physical abuse or other violent crimes. Disasters such as floods, school shootings, car crashes, or fires might also cause PTSD. Other events that can cause PTSD are war, a friend's suicide, or seeing violence in the area they live.

Child protection services in the United States get around 3 million reports each year. This involves 5.5 million children. Of the reported cases, there is proof of abuse in about 30%. From these cases, we have an idea how often different types of abuse occur:

- Sixty-five percent of cases involve neglect.

- Eighteen percent of cases involve physical abuse.

- Ten percent of cases involve sexual abuse.

- Seven percent of cases involve psychological (mental) abuse.

Also, 3–10 million children witness family violence each year. Around 40–60% of those cases involve child physical abuse. (Note: It is thought that two-thirds of child abuse cases are not reported.)

From "PTSD in Children and Teens," by the National Center for Posttraumatic Stress Disorder (NCPTSD, www.ptsd.va.gov), part of the Veterans Administration, June 15, 2010.

How many children get PTSD?

Studies show that about 15–43% of girls and 14–43% of boys go through at least one trauma. Of those children and teens who have had a trauma, 3–15% of girls and 1–6% of boys develop PTSD.

Rates of PTSD are higher for certain types of trauma survivors. Nearly 100% of children get PTSD if they see a parent being killed or if they see a sexual assault. PTSD develops in 90% of sexually abused children, 77% of children who see a school shooting, and 35% who see violence in the area they live get PTSD.

What are the risk factors for PTSD?

Three factors have been shown to raise the chances that children will get PTSD. These factors are:

- how severe the trauma is;

- how the parents react to the trauma;

- how close or far away the child is from the trauma.

Children and teens that go through the most severe traumas tend to have the highest levels of PTSD symptoms. The PTSD symptoms may be less severe if the child has more family support and if the parents are less upset by the trauma. Lastly, children and teens who are farther away from the event report less distress.

Other factors can also affect PTSD. Events that involve people hurting other people, such as rape and assault, are more likely to result in PTSD than other types of traumas. Also, the more traumas a child goes through, the higher the risk of getting PTSD. Girls are more likely than boys to get PTSD.

It is not clear whether a child's ethnic group may affect PTSD. Some research shows that minorities have higher levels of PTSD symptoms. Other research suggests this may be because minorities may go through more traumas.

Another question is whether a child's age at the time of the trauma has an effect on PTSD. Researchers think it may not be that the effects of trauma differ according to the child's age. Rather, it may be that PTSD looks different in children of different ages.

What does PTSD look like in children?

School-aged children (ages 5–12): These children may not have flashbacks or problems remembering parts of the trauma, the way adults with PTSD often do. Children, though, might put the events of the trauma in the wrong order. They might also think there were signs that the trauma was going to happen. As a result, they think that they will see these signs again before another trauma happens. They think that if they pay attention, they can avoid future traumas.

Children of this age might also show signs of PTSD in their play. They might keep repeating a part of the trauma. These games do not make their worry and distress go away. For example, a child might always want to play shooting games after he sees a school shooting. Children may also fit parts of the trauma into their daily lives. For example, a child might carry a gun to school after seeing a school shooting.

Teens (ages 12–18): Teens are in between children and adults. Some PTSD symptoms in teens begin to look like those of adults. One difference is that teens are more likely than younger children or adults to show impulsive and aggressive behaviors.

What are the other effects of trauma on children?

Besides PTSD, children and teens that have gone through trauma often have other types of problems. Much of what we know about the effects of trauma on children comes from the research on child sexual abuse. This research shows that sexually abused children often have problems with the following:

- Fear, worry, sadness, anger, feeling alone and apart from others

- Feeling as if people are looking down on them, low self-worth, and not being able to trust others

- Behaviors such as aggression, out-of-place sexual behavior, self-harm, and abuse of drugs or alcohol

How is PTSD treated in children and teens?

For many children, PTSD symptoms go away on their own after a few months. Yet some children show symptoms for years if they do not get treatment. There are many treatment options.

Cognitive-behavioral therapy (CBT): CBT is the most effective approach for treating children. One type of CBT is called Trauma-Focused CBT (TF-CBT). In TF-CBT, the child may talk about his or her memory of the trauma. TF-CBT also includes techniques to help lower worry and stress. The child may learn how to assert him or herself.

The therapy may involve learning to change thoughts or beliefs about the trauma that are not correct or true. For example, after a trauma, a child may start thinking, "The world is totally unsafe."

Some may question whether children should be asked to think about and remember events that scared them. However, this type of treatment approach is useful when children are distressed by memories of the trauma. The child can be taught at his or her own pace to relax while they are thinking about the trauma. That way, they learn that they do not have to be afraid of their memories. Research shows that TF-CBT is safe and effective for children with PTSD.

CBT often uses training for parents and caregivers as well. It is important for caregivers to understand the effects of PTSD. Parents need to learn coping skills that will help them help their children.

Psychological first aid/crisis management: Psychological first aid (PFA) has been used with school-aged children and teens that have been through violence where they live. PFA can be used in schools and traditional settings. It involves providing comfort and support, and letting children know their reactions are normal. PFA teaches calming and problem solving skills. PFA also helps caregivers deal with changes in the child's feelings and behavior. Children with more severe symptoms may be referred for added treatment.

Eye movement desensitization and reprocessing (EMDR): EMDR combines cognitive therapy with directed eye movements. EMDR is effective in treating both children and adults with PTSD, yet studies indicate that the eye movements are not needed to make it work.

Play therapy: Play therapy can be used to treat young children with PTSD who are not able to deal with the trauma more directly. The therapist uses games, drawings, and other methods to help children process their traumatic memories.

Other treatments: Special treatments may be needed for children who show out-of-place sexual behaviors, extreme behavior problems, or problems with drugs or alcohol.

What can you do to help?

Reading this information is a first step toward helping your child. Learn about PTSD and pay attention to how your child is doing. Watch for signs such as sleep problems, anger, and avoidance of certain people or places.

Also watch for changes in school performance and problems with friends. You may need to get professional help for your child. Find a mental health provider who has treated PTSD in children. Ask how the therapist treats PTSD, and choose someone who makes you and your child feel at ease. You as a parent might also get help from talking to a therapist on your own.

Chapter 35

Returning from the War Zone: PTSD in Military Personnel

It can be difficult to change to a "civilian" mindset once you are back at home with family, friends, coworkers, and U.S. civilians. However, many people have successfully made this transition—and you can, too. The purpose of this text is to help you shift gears and begin your next phase of life at home with your family.

For those of you who have deployed more than once, you might expect that with each deployment, the emotional cycle will become easier. But things may actually become more difficult. This is especially the case if you have unresolved problems from previous separations and reunions. Each deployment is also different from the last.

Reunion can also be a time of considerable stress for both you and your family. You may find that coming home is, in fact, harder than going to war. In order to get through homecoming as smoothly as possible, you need to know what kinds of issues you might face and make sure you have realistic expectations.

By drawing your attention to potential challenges, we hope to help you and your family experience the smoothest possible readjustment. You are not alone. Many troops wrestle with reintegration issues. Time spent in a war zone changes people. It also changes those back home who welcome them back into family life.

Excerpted and adapted from "Returning from the War Zone: A Guide for Military Personnel," by the National Center for Posttraumatic Stress Disorder (NCPTSD, www.ptsd.va.gov), part of the Veterans Administration, September 2010.

Common Reactions to Trauma

Almost all service members will have reactions after returning from a war zone. These behaviors are normal, especially during the first weeks at home. Most service members will successfully readjust with few major problems. It may take a few months, but you will feel better again.

You, your family, and friends need to be prepared for some common stress reactions. Such predictable reactions do not, by themselves, mean that you have a problem, such as posttraumatic stress disorder (PTSD), which requires professional help. Below are lists of common physical, mental/emotional, and behavioral reactions that you should expect.

Common Physical Reactions

- Trouble sleeping or overly tired
- Stomach upset or trouble eating
- Headaches and sweating when thinking of the war
- Rapid heartbeat or breathing
- Existing health problems become worse
- Experiencing shock, being numb, and unable to feel happy

Common Mental and Emotional Reactions

- Bad dreams or nightmares
- Flashbacks or frequent unwanted memories
- Anger
- Feeling nervous, helpless, or fearful
- Feeling guilty, self-blame, or shame
- Feeling sad, rejected, or abandoned
- Feeling agitated, easily upset, irritated, or annoyed
- Feeling hopeless about the future

Insomnia can occur, and when you do sleep, you may have nightmares. Or you may have no trouble sleeping, but wake up feeling overly tired.

If any of your comrades died during the war, you may be thinking a lot about them. You may feel anger, resentment, or even guilt related to their deaths. Or, you might be in a state of shock, feeling emotionally numb or dazed.

During this time, you may find common family issues more irritating. You may feel anxious or "keyed up." Anger and aggression are common war zone stress reactions, but they may scare your partner, children, and you as well. Minor incidents can lead to severe overreactions, such as yelling at your partner, kids, or others.

Common Behavioral Reactions

- Trouble concentrating

- Edgy, jumpy, and easily startled

- Being on guard, always alert, concerned too much about safety and security

- Avoiding people or places related to the trauma

- Too much drinking, smoking, or drug use

- Lack of exercise, poor diet, or health care

- Problems doing regular tasks at work or school

- Aggressive driving habits

Some avoidance is normal. But if you are constantly avoiding everything that reminds you of your war zone experiences, this can create major difficulties at home. For instance, you may avoid seeing other people for fear that they might ask you about the war. If you are doing this, you can become isolated and withdrawn. Your family and friends will not be able to provide the social support you need, even if you don't know it.

Aggressive driving is also extremely common among service members returning from conflicts in the Middle East. Although you want to drive when you get back, you need to use extra caution. This is particularly true if you're feeling edgy or upset.

Back Home with Family

Common Experiences and Expectations You May Face

There is usually a "honeymoon" phase shortly after demobilization, but honeymoons come to an end. You and members of your family have had unique experiences and have changed. You'll need to get to know each other again and appreciate what each other went through. Very likely, you'll need to renegotiate some of your roles. You will need time to rebuild intimacy and learn how to rely on one another again for support.

In addition, your interests may have changed. You may need to re-examine future plans, dreams, and expectations. You and your family will also need to re-examine common goals.

When you return to life at home, you may experience the following:

- Feel pressured by requests for time and attention from family, friends, and others

- Be expected to perform home, work, and school responsibilities or care for children before you are ready

- Find that your parents are trying to be too involved or treat you like a child again

- Face different relationships with children who now have new needs and behaviors

- Be confronted by the needs of partners who have had their own problems

Financial Concerns

You may have financial issues to handle when you return home. Be careful not to spend impulsively. Seek assistance if making ends meet is hard due to changes in income.

Work Challenges

- Readjusting to work can take time.

- You may feel bored or that you find no meaning in your former work.

- You may have trouble finding a job.

If You Have Children

Children react differently to deployment depending on their age. They can cry, act out, be clingy, withdraw, or rebel. To help you can do the following:

- Provide extra attention, care, and physical closeness.

- Understand that they may be angry and perhaps rightly so.

- Discuss things. Let kids know they can talk about how they feel. Accept how they feel and don't tell them they should not feel that way.

- Tell kids their feelings are normal. Be prepared to tell them many times.

- Maintain routines and plan for upcoming events.

Common Reactions You May Have That Will Affect Family and Friend Relationships

At first, many service members feel disconnected or detached from their partner and/or family. You may be unable to tell your family about what happened. You may not want to scare them by speaking about the war. Or maybe you think that no one will understand. You also may find it's hard to express positive feelings. This can make loved ones feel like they did something wrong or are not wanted anymore. Sexual closeness may also be awkward for a while. Remember, it takes time to feel close again.

When reunited with family, you may also feel the following:

- Mistrusting: During your deployment you trusted only those closest to you, in your unit. It can be difficult to begin to confide in your family and friends again.

- Overcontrolling or overprotective: You might find that you're constantly telling the kids "Don't do that!" or "Be careful, it's not safe!" Rigid discipline may be necessary during wartime, but families need to discuss rules and share in decisions.

- Short tempered: More conflicts with others may be due to poor communication and/or unreasonable expectations.

What Do Families Experience during Deployment?

It's important to remember that those who were at home while you were away faced their own challenges and opportunities. While you were deployed, your family members probably:

- experienced loneliness, concern, and worry;
- learned new skills;
- took on new responsibilities;
- had to deal with problems without your help;
- created new support systems and friendships.

Family Concerns

The separation that occurs while you're deployed to a war zone will affect your family. Most family members are relieved that you've returned home safely, but you all are a little afraid about what to expect. When you're apart, it is harder to share common experiences. You miss one another. Your absence could have created insecurity, misunderstanding, and distance within your family. You may be concerned about the following:

- How much each of you has changed

- Whether you are still needed or loved

- Whether your loved ones understand what you've been through

Your loved ones may think you'll never understand how hard it was to manage things at home without you. Now, they may be having a hard time adjusting back to a two-adult household. For example, they may not want you to take on responsibilities that you had before deployment. They may also be afraid of your reaction to how the family has changed during your absence.

These concerns can be resolved once you return home. If you and family members talk about them, you will all gain an appreciation for what everyone has been through. This deeper understanding can bring you closer as a family.

Healthy Coping for Common Reactions to Trauma

With homecoming, you may need to relearn how to feel safe, comfortable, and trusting with your family. You must get to know one another again. Good communication with your partner, children, parents, siblings, friends, coworkers, and others is the key. Give each other the chance to understand what you have been through. When talking as a family, be careful to listen to one another. Families work best when there is respect for one another, and a willingness to be open and consider alternatives.

Tips for Feeling Better

It's fine for you to spend some time alone. But, if you spend too much time alone or avoid social gatherings, you will be isolated from family and friends. You need the support of these people for a healthy adjustment. You can help yourself to feel better by doing the following:

- Getting back to regular patterns of sleep and exercise

- Pursuing hobbies and creative activities

- Planning sufficient rest, relaxation, and intimate time

- Trying relaxation techniques (meditation, breathing exercises) to reduce stress

- Learning problems to watch out for and how to cope with them

- Striking a balance between staying connected with former war buddies and spending individual time with your partner, kids, other family members, and friends

- Communicating more than the "need-to-know" bare facts

- Talking about your war zone experiences at a time and pace that feels right to you

- Not drinking to excess or when you're feeling depressed or to avoid disturbing memories

- Creating realistic workloads for home, school, and work

Steps to Assuming Normal Routines

Soon after your return, plan to have an open and honest discussion with your family about responsibilities. You all need to decide how they should be split up now that you're home. It's usually best to take on a few tasks at first and then more as you grow accustomed to being home. Be willing to compromise so that both you and your family members feel your needs are understood and respected.

Try to re-establish a normal sleep routine as quickly as possible. Go to bed and get up at the same time every day. Do not drink to help yourself sleep. You might try learning some relaxation techniques, such as deep breathing, yoga, or meditation.

Steps to Controlling Anger

Recognize and try to control your angry feelings. Returning service members don't always realize how angry they are. In fact, you may only recognize your emotion when someone close to you points it out. You can help control your anger by doing the following:

- Counting to 10 or 20 before reacting

- Figuring out the cues or situations that trigger your anger so you can be better prepared

- Learning relaxation techniques (breathing, yoga, meditation)
- Learning ways to deal with irritation and frustration and how not to be provoked into aggressive behavior
- Walking away
- Thinking about the ultimate consequences of your responses
- Writing things down
- Learn tips to controlling anger

Important Points to Remember

- Readjusting to civilian life takes time—don't worry that you're experiencing some challenges. Find solutions to these problems. Don't avoid.
- Take your time adding responsibilities and activities back into your life.
- Reconnect with your social supports. This may be the last thing you feel like doing, but do it anyway. Social support is critical to successful reintegration.
- Remind your loved ones that you love them.
- Realize that you need to talk about the experiences you had during deployment. If you can't talk to family or friends, be sure to talk to a chaplain or counselor.

Red Flags

You now know the reactions that are normal following deployment to war. But sometimes the behaviors that kept you alive in the war zone get on the wrong track. You may not be able to shut them down after you've returned home safely.

Some problems may need outside assistance to solve. Even serious postdeployment psychological problems can be treated successfully and cured.

Being able to admit you have a problem can be tough:

- You might think you should cope on your own.
- You think others can't help you.
- You believe the problem(s) will go away on their own.
- You are embarrassed to talk to someone about it.

Confront Mental Health Stigma

Mental health problems are not a sign of weakness. The reality is that injuries, including psychological injuries, affect the strong and the brave just like everyone else. Some of the most successful officers and enlisted personnel have experienced these problems.

But stigma about mental health issues can be a huge barrier for people who need help. Finding the solution to your problem is a sign of strength and maturity. Getting assistance from others is sometimes the only way to solve something. For example, if you cannot scale a wall on your own and need a comrade to do so, you use them. Knowing when and how to get help is actually part of military training.

Signs to Watch For

If your reactions are causing significant distress or interfering with how you function, you will need outside assistance. Things to watch for include the following:

- Relationship troubles froquent and intense conflicts, poor communication, inability to meet responsibilities

- Work, school, or other community functioning—frequent absences, conflicts, inability to meet deadlines or concentrate, poor performance

- Thoughts of hurting someone or yourself

If you get assistance early, you can prevent more serious problems from developing. If you delay seeking help because of avoidance or stigma, your problems may actually cause you to lose your job, your relationships, and your happiness. Mental and emotional problems can be managed or treated, and early detection is essential.

Many of the common reactions to experience in a war zone are also symptoms of more serious problems such as PTSD. In PTSD, however, they're much more intense and troubling, and they don't go away. If these symptoms don't decrease over a few months, or if they continue to cause significant problems in your daily life, it's time to seek treatment from a professional.

PTSD

PTSD can occur after you have been through a traumatic event. Professionals do not know why it occurs in some and not others. But we do know PTSD is treatable.

Symptoms of PTSD

- **Re-experiencing:** Bad memories of a traumatic event can come back at any time. You may feel the same terror and horror you did when the event took place. Sometimes there's a trigger—a sound, sight, or smell that causes you to relive the event.

- **Avoidance and numbing:** People with PTSD often go to great lengths to avoid things that might remind them of the traumatic event they endured. They also may shut themselves off emotionally in order to protect themselves from feeling pain and fear.

- **Hypervigilance or increased arousal:** Those suffering from PTSD may operate on high alert at all times, often have very short fuses, and startle easily.

How Likely Are You to Get PTSD?

It depends on many factors, such as the following:

- How severe the trauma was
- If you were injured
- The intensity of your reaction to the trauma
- Whether someone you were close to died or was injured
- How much your own life was in danger
- How much you felt you could not control things
- IIow much help and support you got following the event

Steps to Solving the Problem and Getting Help

PTSD is a treatable condition. If you think you have PTSD, or just some of its reactions or symptoms (such as nightmares or racing thoughts), it's important to let your doctor or even a chaplain know. These people can help you set up other appointments as needed.

There are several steps to addressing PTSD:

- Assessment involves having a professional evaluate you with a full interview.

- Educating yourself and your family about PTSD, its symptoms, and how it can affect your life is an important step.

- Some antidepressants can relieve symptoms of PTSD. These medications do not treat the underlying cause, yet do provide some symptom relief.

- Cognitive behavioral therapy (CBT) generally seeks to balance your thinking and help you express and cope with your emotions about the traumatic experience.

There are different types of therapy but in most you will learn the following:

- How the problem affects you and others
- Goal setting about ways to improve your life
- New coping skills
- How to accept your thoughts and feelings and strategies to deal with them

We encourage you to meet with several therapists before choosing one. Finding a therapist involves learning the following:

- What kinds of treatment each therapist offers
- What you can expect from the treatment and the therapist
- What the therapist expects of you

Other Treatable Mental Health Problems

PTSD is not the only serious problem that can occur after deployment. Watch out for signs of these other conditions in yourself and your comrades.

- **Depression:** We all experience sadness or feel down from time to time. That's a normal part of being human. Depression, however, is different. It lasts longer and is more serious than normal sadness or grief. Common symptoms include the following:
    - Feeling down or sad more days than not
    - Losing interest in hobbies or activities that you used to find enjoyable or fun
    - Being excessively low in energy and/or overly tired
    - Feeling that things are never going to get better

- **Suicidal thoughts and suicide:** War experiences and war zone stress reactions, especially those caused by personal loss, can lead a depressed person to think about hurting or killing him- or herself. If you or someone you know is feeling this way, take it seriously, and get help from a suicide hotline: 800-273-TALK (273-8255) and press 1 for veterans.

- **Violence and abuse:** Anger can sometimes turn into violence or physical abuse. It can also result in emotional and/or verbal abuse that can damage relationships. Abuse can take the form of threats, swearing, criticism, throwing things, conflict, pushing, grabbing, and hitting. If you were abused as a child, you are more at risk for abusing your partner or family members. Here are a few warning signs that may lead to domestic violence:

  - Controlling behaviors or jealousy
  - Blaming others for problems or conflict
  - Radical mood changes
  - Verbal abuse such as humiliating, manipulating, and confusing
  - Self-destructive or overly risky actions; heated arguments

- **Substance abuse:** It's common for troops to "self-medicate." They drink or abuse drugs to numb out the difficult thoughts, feelings, and memories related to war zone experiences. While alcohol or drugs may seem to offer a quick solution, they actually lead to more problems. At the same time, a vast majority of people in our society drink. Sometimes it can be difficult to know if your drinking is actually a problem. Warning signs of an alcohol problem include the following:

  - Frequent excessive drinking
  - Having thoughts that you should cut down
  - Feeling guilty or bad about your drinking
  - Others becoming annoyed with you or criticizing how much you drink
  - Drinking in the morning to calm your nerves
  - Problems with work, family, school, or other regular activities caused by drinking

- **Concussions or mild traumatic brain injury (mTBI):** Explosions that produce dangerous blast waves of high pressure rattle your brain inside your skull and can cause mTBI. Helmets cannot protect against this type of impact. In fact, 60 to 80 percent of service members who have injuries from some form of blast may have TBI. Symptoms associated with mild TBI (or concussion) can parallel those of PTSD but also include the following:

- Headaches or dizziness
- Vision problems
- Emotional problems, such as impatience or impulsiveness
- Trouble concentrating, making decisions, or thinking logically
- Trouble remembering things, amnesia
- Lower tolerance for lights and noise

Know that PTSD is often associated with these other conditions. However, there are effective treatments for all of these problems.

Chapter 36

Recent Research on PTSD

Posttraumatic Stress Disorder Research

Posttraumatic stress disorder (PTSD) is an anxiety disorder that some people develop after seeing or living through an event that caused or threatened serious harm or death. Symptoms include flashbacks or bad dreams, emotional numbness, intense guilt or worry, angry outbursts, feeling on edge, or avoiding thoughts and situations that remind them of the trauma. In PTSD, these symptoms last at least 1 month.

To aid those who suffer with PTSD, the National Institute of Mental Health (NIMH) is supporting PTSD-focused research, and related studies on anxiety and fear, to find better ways of helping people cope with trauma, as well as better ways to treat and ultimately prevent the disorder.

Research on Possible Risk Factors for PTSD

Currently, many scientists are focusing on genes that play a role in creating fear memories. Understanding how fear memories are created may help to refine or find new interventions for reducing the

This chapter includes text from "Post-Traumatic Stress Disorder Research," by the National Institute of Mental Health (NIMH, www.nimh.nih.gov), part of the National Institutes of Health, 2007; from "Criminal Behavior and PTSD," by the National Center for Posttraumatic Stress Disorder (NCPTSD, www.ptsd.va.gov), part of the Veterans Administration, August 24, 2010; and from "Study Suggests Some Brain Injuries Reduce the Likelihood of Post-Traumatic Stress Disorder," by the National Institute of Neurological Disorders and Stroke (NINDS, www.ninds.nih.gov), part of the National Institutes of Health, December 23, 2007.

symptoms of PTSD. For example, PTSD researchers have pinpointed genes that make the following:

- **Stathmin, a protein needed to form fear memories:** In one study, mice that did not make stathmin were less likely than normal mice to "freeze," a natural, protective response to danger, after being exposed to a fearful experience. They also showed less innate fear by exploring open spaces more willingly than normal mice.

- **GRP (gastrin-releasing peptide), a signaling chemical in the brain released during emotional events:** In mice, GRP seems to help control the fear response, and lack of GRP may lead to the creation of greater and more lasting memories of fear.

Researchers have also found a version of the 5-HTTLPR [serotonin-transporter-linked polymorphic region] gene, which controls levels of serotonin—a brain chemical related to mood—that appears to fuel the fear response. Like other mental disorders, it is likely that many genes with small effects are at work in PTSD.

Studying parts of the brain involved in dealing with fear and stress also helps researchers to better understand possible causes of PTSD. One such brain structure is the amygdala, known for its role in emotion, learning, and memory. The amygdala appears to be active in fear acquisition, or learning to fear an event (such as touching a hot stove), as well as in the early stages of fear extinction, or learning not to fear.

Storing extinction memories and dampening the original fear response appears to involve the prefrontal cortex (PFC) area of the brain, involved in tasks such as decision-making, problem-solving, and judgment. Certain areas of the PFC play slightly different roles. For example, when it deems a source of stress controllable, the medial PFC suppresses the amygdala, an alarm center deep in the brainstem, and controls the stress response. The ventromedial PFC helps sustain long-term extinction of fearful memories, and the size of this brain area may affect its ability to do so.

Individual differences in these genes or brain areas may only set the stage for PTSD without actually causing symptoms. Environmental factors, such as childhood trauma, head injury, or a history of mental illness, may further increase a person's risk by affecting the early growth of the brain. Also, personality and cognitive factors, such as optimism and the tendency to view challenges in a positive or negative way, as well as social factors, such as the availability and use of social support, appear to influence how people adjust to trauma. More research may show what combinations of these or perhaps other factors could be used someday to predict who will develop PTSD following a traumatic event.

Research on Treating PTSD

Currently, people with PTSD may be treated with psychotherapy (talk therapy), medications, or a combination of the two.

Psychotherapy

Cognitive behavioral therapy (CBT) teaches different ways of thinking and reacting to the frightening events that trigger PTSD symptoms and can help bring those symptoms under control. There are several types of CBT, including the following:

- **Exposure therapy:** This type of therapy uses mental imagery, writing, or visiting the scene of a trauma to help survivors face and gain control of overwhelming fear and distress.

- **Cognitive restructuring:** This type of therapy encourages survivors to talk about upsetting (often incorrect) thoughts about the trauma, question those thoughts, and replace them with more balanced and correct ones.

- **Stress inoculation training:** This type of therapy teaches anxiety reduction techniques and coping skills to reduce PTSD symptoms, and helps correct inaccurate thoughts related to the trauma.

NIMH is currently studying how the brain responds to CBT compared to sertraline (Zoloft), one of the two medications recommended and approved by the U.S. Food and Drug Administration (FDA) for treating PTSD. This research may help clarify why some people respond well to medication and others to psychotherapy.

Medications

In a small study, NIMH researchers recently found that for people already taking a bedtime dose of the medication prazosin (Minipress), adding a daytime dose helped to reduce overall PTSD symptom severity, as well as stressful responses to trauma reminders.

Another medication of interest is D-cycloserine (Seromycin), which boosts the activity of a brain chemical called NMDA [N-methyl-d-aspartate], which is needed for fear extinction. In a study of 28 people with a fear of heights, scientists found that those treated with D-cycloserine before exposure therapy showed reduced fear during the therapy sessions compared to those who did not receive the drug. Researchers are currently studying the effects of using D-cycloserine with therapy to treat PTSD.

Propranolol (Inderal), a type of medicine called a beta-blocker, is also being studied to see if it may help reduce stress following a traumatic event and interrupt the creation of fearful memories. Early studies have successfully reduced or seemingly prevented PTSD in small numbers of trauma victims.

Treatment after Mass Trauma

NIMH researchers are testing creative approaches to making CBT widely available, such as with internet-based self-help therapy and telephone-assisted therapy. Less formal treatments for those experiencing acute stress reactions are also being explored to reduce chances of developing full blown PTSD.

For example, in one preliminary study, researchers created a self-help website using concepts of stress inoculation training. People with PTSD first met face to face with a therapist. After this meeting, participants could log onto the website to find more information about PTSD and ways to cope, and their therapists could also log on to give advice or coaching as needed. Overall, the scientists found delivering therapy this way to be a promising method for reaching a large number of people suffering with PTSD symptoms.

Researchers are also working to improve methods of screening, providing early treatment, and tracking mass trauma survivors; and approaches for guiding survivors through self-evaluation/screening and prompting referral to mental health care providers based on need.

The Next Steps for PTSD Research

In the last decade, rapid progress in research on the mental and biological foundations of PTSD has lead scientists to focus on prevention as a realistic and important goal.

For example, NIMH-funded researchers are exploring new and orphan medications thought to target underlying causes of PTSD in an effort to prevent the disorder. Other research is attempting to enhance cognitive, personality, and social protective factors and to minimize risk factors to ward off full-blown PTSD after trauma. Still other research is attempting to identify what factors determine whether someone with PTSD will respond well to one type of intervention or another, aiming to develop more personalized, effective, and efficient treatments.

The examples described here are only a small sampling of the ongoing work at NIMH. To find more information about ongoing PTSD clinical studies, see NIMH's PTSD clinical trials page [http://www.nimh.nih.gov/trials/post-traumatic-stress-disorder-ptsd.shtml]. As gene research and brain imaging technologies continue to improve, scientists are more likely to be able to pinpoint when and where in the brain PTSD begins. This understanding may then lead to better targeted treatments to suit each person's own needs or even prevent the disorder before it causes harm.

Criminal Behavior and PTSD

At times the symptoms of posttraumatic stress disorder (PTSD) may make it more likely that the sufferer will get in trouble with others or with the law. PTSD affects the way you see, think about, and respond to people and situations. Trauma survivors with PTSD may be more prone to feeling threatened in many situations, even when the feeling of threat is not warranted. Some may act on impulse or go to extremes to protect themselves.

Research shows that aggressive behavior is more common in those with PTSD than those without PTSD. For example, in one study, male Vietnam veterans with PTSD committed more acts of violence against family and others than veterans without PTSD. Also, rates of PTSD in prison inmates are higher than in the general public.

It is also possible that PTSD is not directly related to crime. Rather, a third factor could lead to both PTSD and criminal behavior. Also, keep in mind that the research findings on PTSD and crime vary widely due to different methods used in the studies.

Three areas of functioning may be affected by PTSD: thoughts, level of arousal, and feelings. The following text includes some ways that PTSD symptoms in each of these areas could set the stage for the survivor to act in an aggressive or even criminal way.

Thoughts

Flashbacks: People with this symptom of PTSD believe that they are again going through the trauma. When having a flashback, survivors with PTSD might commit an aggressive or criminal act while thinking that they are in danger again.

Perceived threat: Even without being in an altered state of awareness, those with PTSD are more likely than those without PTSD to see threat around them. Their beliefs and their view of the world are often marked by themes of danger and mistrust. This way of seeing the world makes it more likely that they will be aggressive.

Beliefs about justice: Those with PTSD may hold extreme beliefs about justice based on their having been through trauma. Examples of such beliefs that might lead to crimes include the following:

- Belief in the need for revenge or acting outside the law in order to right the perceived wrongs of others

- Little respect for authority or the law because of perceived and actual abuse by authority figures

Changes in Level of Arousal

Anger and irritability: High levels of arousal are based on the survival instinct to "fight" or "flee" when faced with danger. Triggering of the "fight" instinct may mean that someone with PTSD is more likely to respond aggressively.

Being hyper-alert: Many people with PTSD are always "on guard." This alertness may be extreme. It may lead the person to act out to try to protect him or herself or someone else, even if there is no real danger.

Startle response: Those with PTSD may react on instinct or impulse to any sudden threat. Their responses may be extreme. For example, a person with PTSD may on instinct push back aggressively when accidentally bumped in a crowd.

Changes in Feelings

Distress: When reminded of a trauma, those with PTSD have high levels of distress. This is likely to affect their judgment and make them less able to use reason in their responses.

Negative feelings: Those with PTSD often have high levels of fear, worry, guilt, anger, shame, or depression. These unpleasant feelings may lead them to use drugs and alcohol in an attempt to feel better. Substance use and abuse can in turn cloud judgment and cause them to do things they might not normally do. Also, guilt may lead survivors to commit acts that will likely result in their being punished, injured, or killed.

Feeling numb: At the same time, another class of PTSD symptoms, emotional numbing, may lead to wrongful or criminal behavior because the sufferer experiences the following feelings:

358

- Less empathy, or feeling sorry for, the victim
- Trouble feeling remorse or guilt for their acts
- Trouble sensing how severe and grave their criminal act is, or what the results may be

Numbing could also lead some survivors to engage in thrill-seeking behaviors as they try to feel some type of emotion.

Summing It Up

Symptoms of PTSD can sometimes lead to a lifestyle that makes aggressive or criminal behavior or sudden outbursts of violence more likely to occur. Those with PTSD often suffer from bad memories of the trauma. They may be always tense and fearful. Feeling the need to be always on guard can cause survivors to see threat in normal situations. As a result, they may go to extremes to try to protect themselves. High levels of arousal may result in impulsive, violent behavior that goes beyond what is needed to address the perceived threat.

Further research is needed to make clearer the complex relationship between PTSD and crime. Even with this much-needed research, the role that PTSD may play in criminal behavior should be studied with care on a case-by-case basis.

Study Suggests Some Brain Injuries Reduce the Likelihood of Posttraumatic Stress Disorder

A new study of combat-exposed Vietnam War veterans shows that those with injuries to certain parts of the brain were less likely to develop posttraumatic stress disorder (PTSD). The findings, from the National Institutes of Health (NIH) and the National Naval Medical Center, suggest that drugs or pacemaker-like devices aimed at dampening activity in these brain regions might be effective treatments for PTSD.

PTSD involves the persistent reliving of a traumatic experience through nightmares and flashbacks that may seem real. Twenty percent to 30 percent of Vietnam vets (more than 1 million) have been diagnosed with PTSD, and a similar rate has been reported among Hurricane Katrina survivors in New Orleans. Public health officials are currently tracking the disorder among soldiers returning from Iraq. Yet, while war and natural disasters tend to call the greatest attention to PTSD, it's estimated that millions of Americans suffer from it as a result of assault, rape, child abuse, car accidents, and other traumatic events.

Previous studies have shown that PTSD is associated with changes in brain activity, but those studies couldn't determine whether the changes were contributing to the disorder or merely occurring because of it.

Jordan Grafman, PhD, a senior investigator at the National Institute of Neurological Disorders and Stroke (NINDS), part of NIH, turned to the Vietnam Head Injury Study (VHIS) to make that distinction. The VHIS is a registry of Vietnam veterans who sustained penetrating brain injuries (which are less common in Iraq compared to concussion brain injuries). It has received support from the Department of Defense, the Department of Veterans Affairs and NIH, and is currently supported by NINDS.

"If we could show that lesions in a specific brain region eliminated PTSD, we knew we could say that the region is critical to developing the disorder," says Dr. Grafman. The results of his study appear online in *Nature Neuroscience* [December 23, 2007 issue].

Dr. Grafman and members of his lab, including neuropsychiatrist Vanessa Raymont and postdoctoral fellow Michael Koenigs, studied 193 veterans registered with VHIS and 52 veterans with combat exposure but no head injury. The participants were classified as either having developed PTSD at some point in their lifetime or having never developed PTSD. CT (computerized tomography) scans were used to map their brain injuries.

By comparing the distribution of brain injuries between the PTSD group and the non-PTSD group, the researchers found two regions where damage was rarely associated with PTSD: The amygdala, a structure important in fear and anxiety, and the ventromedial prefrontal cortex (vmPFC), an area involved in higher mental functions and planning.

In another level of analysis, the researchers compared the prevalence of PTSD in subjects who had damage to either the amygdala or vmPFC, subjects who had damage to other parts of the brain and non-head-injured subjects. PTSD occurred in a similar fraction of subjects in the last two groups—40 percent and 48 percent, respectively. In contrast, PTSD occurred in only 18 percent of subjects with damage to the vmPFC and zero (out of 15) subjects with damage to the amygdala. The occurrence of other anxiety disorders was not affected by damage to the amygdala or vmPFC.

"It appears that if you have damage to either of those areas, you're not likely to develop PTSD," says Dr. Grafman. The scientists hypothesize that drugs designed to inhibit the activity of the two structures might provide relief from PTSD. Deep brain stimulation, a technique used to treat Parkinson's disease by modifying the brain's electrical activity, might also prove useful against PTSD if targeted to the amygdala or vmPFC.

Current treatments for PTSD include medications for anxiety and depression, and therapy to help the person confront and deal with traumatic memories. But these treatments vary in effectiveness, a point underscored by the fact that many of the Vietnam veterans in Dr. Grafman's study are still dealing with PTSD some 40 years after the war.

Since the study examined only young men who served in Vietnam, one question is whether the results will extend to women, children, or people exposed to traumatic situations besides wartime combat. Dr. Grafman says similar results probably will be found in those other populations, given that previous studies had connected PTSD to changes in the amygdala and vmPFC, and only some of those studies involved war veterans.

NINDS (www.ninds.nih.gov) is a component of the National Institutes of Health (NIH), and is the nation's primary supporter of biomedical research on the brain and nervous system.

Source: Koenigs M, Huey ED, Raymont V, Cheon B, Solomon J, Wasserman EM, and Grafman J. "Focal Brain Damage Protects Against Post-Traumatic Stress Disorder in Combat Veterans." *Nature Neuroscience,* published online December 23, 2007.

Part Four

Treating
Stress-Related Disorders

Chapter 37

Signs You or a Family Member Need Help for Stress

In spite of your best efforts, your symptoms may progress to the point where they are very uncomfortable, serious, and even dangerous. This is a very important time. It is necessary to take immediate action to prevent a crisis or loss of control. You may be feeling terrible and others may be concerned for your wellness or safety, but you can still do the things that you need to do to help yourself feel better and keep yourself safe.

Signs That Things Are Breaking Down

Get some paper. Write "When Things Are Breaking Down," or something that means that to you. On the first page, make a list of symptoms that indicate to you that things are breaking down or getting much worse. Remember that symptoms and signs vary from person to person. What may mean "things are getting much worse" to one person may mean a "crisis" to another. Your signs or symptoms might include the following:

- Feeling very oversensitive and fragile

- Responding irrationally to events and the actions of others

- Feeling very needy

Excerpted from "Action Planning for Prevention and Recovery," by the Substance Abuse and Mental Health Services Administration (SAMHSA, mentalhealth.samhsa.gov), part of the U.S. Department of Health and Human Services, July 2003. Reviewed by David A. Cooke, MD, FACP, November 8, 2010.

- Being unable to sleep
- Sleeping all the time
- Avoiding eating
- Wanting to be totally alone
- Substance abusing
- Taking out anger on others
- Chain smoking
- Eating too much

On the next page, write an action plan that you think will help reduce your symptoms when they have progressed to this point. The plan now needs to be very direct, with fewer choices and very clear instructions.

Some ideas for an action plan are the following:

- Call my doctor or other health care professional, ask for, and follow his or her instructions.
- Call and talk for as long as necessary to my supporters.
- Arrange for someone to stay with me around the clock until my symptoms subside.
- Make arrangements to get help right away if my symptoms worsen.
- Make sure I am doing everything on my daily checklist.
- Arrange and take at least 3 days off from any responsibilities.
- Have at least two peer counseling sessions.
- Do three deep-breathing relaxation exercises.
- Write in my journal for at least half an hour.
- Schedule a physical examination or doctor appointment or a consultation with another health care provider.
- Ask to have medications checked.

As with the other plans, make note of the parts of your plan that work especially well. If something doesn't work or doesn't work as well as you wish it had, develop a different plan or revise the one you used—when you are feeling better. Always look for new tools that might help you through difficult situations.

Crisis Planning

Identifying and responding to symptoms early reduces the chances that you will find yourself in crisis. It is important to confront the possibility of crisis, because in spite of your best planning and assertive action in your own behalf, you could find yourself in a situation where others will need to take over responsibility for your care. This is a difficult situation—one that no one likes to face. In a crisis, you may feel as if you are totally out of control. Writing a clear crisis plan when you are well, to instruct others about how to care for you when you are not well, helps you maintain responsibility for your own care. It will keep your family members and friends from wasting time trying to figure out what to do for you. It relieves the guilt that may be felt by family members and other caregivers who may have wondered whether they were taking the right action. It also insures that your needs will be met and that you will get better as quickly as possible.

You need to develop your crisis plan when you are feeling well. However, you cannot do it quickly. Decisions like this take time, thought, and often collaboration with health care providers, family members, and other supporters.

The crisis plan differs from the other action plans in that it will be used by others. The other four sections of this planning process are implemented by you alone and need not be shared with anyone else; therefore you can write them using shorthand language that only you need to understand. However, when writing a crisis plan, you need to make it clear, easy to understand, and legible. While you may have developed other plans rather quickly, this plan is likely to take more time. Don't rush the process. Work at it for a while, then leave it for several days and keep coming back to it until you have developed a plan you feel has the best chance of working for you. Once you have completed your crisis plan, give copies of it to the people you name in this plan as your supporters.

This crisis plan sample has nine parts to it, each addressing a particular concern.

Part 1: Feeling Well

Write what you are like when you are feeling well. This can help educate people who might be trying to help you. It might help someone who knows you well to understand you a little better; for someone who doesn't know you well—or at all—it is very important.

Part 2: Symptoms

Describe symptoms that would indicate to others that they need to take over responsibility for your care and make decisions on your behalf. This is hard for everyone. No one likes to think that someone else will have to take over responsibility for his or her care. Yet, through a careful, well-developed description of symptoms that you know would indicate to you that you can't make smart decisions anymore, you can stay in control even when things seem to be out of control. Allow yourself plenty of time to complete this section. Ask your friends, family members, and other supporters for input, but always remember that the final determination is up to you. Be very clear and specific in describing each symptom. Don't just summarize; use as many words as it takes. Your list of symptoms might include the following:

- Being unable to recognize or correctly identify family members and friends

- Uncontrollable pacing; inability to stay still

- Neglecting personal hygiene (for how many days?)

- Not cooking or doing any housework (for how many days?)

- Not understanding what people are saying

- Thinking I am someone I am not

- Thinking I have the ability to do something I don't

- Displaying abusive, destructive, or violent behavior, toward self, others, or property

- Abusing alcohol and/or drugs

- Not getting out of bed (for how long?)

- Refusing to eat or drink

Part 3: Supporters

In this next section of the crisis plan, list these people who you want to take over for you when the symptoms you listed in the previous section arise. Before listing people in this part of your plan though, talk with them about what you'd like from them and make sure they understand and agree to be in the plan. They can be family members, friends, or health care providers. They should be committed to following the plans you have written. When you first develop this plan, your list may be mostly health care providers. But as you work on developing your support system, try to add more family members and friends because they will be more available.

It's best to have at least five people on your list of supporters. If you have only one or two, when they go on vacation or are sick, they might not be available when you really need them. If you don't have that many supporters now, you may need to work on developing new and/or closer relationships with people. Ask yourself how best you can build these kinds of relationships. Seek new friends by doing things such as volunteering and going to support groups and community activities.

In the past, health care providers or family members may have made decisions that were not according to your wishes. You may not want them involved in your care again. If so, write on your plan, "I do not want the following people involved in any way in my care or treatment." Then list those people and why you don't want them involved. They may be people who have treated you badly in the past, have made poor decisions, or who get too upset when you are having a hard time.

Many people like to include a section that describes how they want possible disputes between their supporters settled. For instance, you may want to say that if a disagreement occurs about a course of action, a majority of your supporters can decide or a particular person will make the determination. You also might request that a consumer or advocacy organization become involved in the decision making.

Part 4: Health Care Providers and Medications

Name your physician, pharmacist, and other health care providers, along with their phone numbers. Then list the following:

- The medications you are currently using, the dosage, and why you are using them

- The medications you would prefer to take if medications or additional medications became necessary—like those that have worked well for you in the past—and why you would choose those

- The medications that would be acceptable to you if medications became necessary and why you would choose those

- The medications that must be avoided—like those you are allergic to, that conflict with another medication, or cause undesirable side effects—and give the reasons they should be avoided.

Also list any vitamins, herbs, alternative medications (such as homeopathic remedies), and supplements you are taking. Note which should be increased or decreased if you are in crisis, and which you have discovered are not good for you.

Part 5: Treatments

There may be particular treatments that you like in a crisis situation and others that you would want to avoid. The reason may be as simple as "this treatment has or has not worked in the past," or you may have some concerns about the safety of this treatment. Maybe you just don't like the way a particular treatment makes you feel. Treatments here can mean medical procedures or the many possibilities of alternative therapy (such as injections of B vitamins, massages, or cranial sacral therapy). In this part of your crisis plan, list the following:

- Treatments you are currently undergoing and why

- Treatments you would prefer if treatments or additional treatments became necessary and why you would choose those

- Treatments that would be acceptable to you if treatments were deemed necessary by your support team

- Treatments that must be avoided and why

Part 6: Planning for Your Care

Describe a plan for your care in a crisis that would allow you to stay where you like. Think about your family and friends. Would they be able to take turns providing you with care? Could transportation be arranged to health care appointments? Is there a program in your community that could provide you with care part of the time, with family members and friends taking care of you the rest of the time? Many people who would prefer to stay at home rather than be hospitalized are setting up these kinds of plans. You may need to ask your family members, friends, and health care providers what options are available. If you are having a hard time coming up with a plan, at least write down what you imagine the ideal scenario would be.

Part 7: Treatment Facilities

Describe the treatment facilities you would like to use if family members and friends cannot provide you with care, or if your condition requires hospital care. Your options may be limited by the facilities available in your area and by your insurance coverage. If you are not sure which facilities you would like to use, write down a description of what the ideal facility would be like. Then, talk to family members and friends about the available choices and call the facilities to request information that may help you in making a decision. Also include a list of treatment facilities you would like to avoid—such as places where you received poor care in the past.

Part 8: What You Need from Others

Describe what your supporters can do for you that will help you feel better. This part of the plan is very important and deserves careful attention. Describe everything you can think of that you want your supporters to do (or not do) for you. You may want to get more ideas from your supporters and health care professionals.

Things others could do for you that would help you feel more comfortable might include the following:

- Listen to me without giving me advice, judging me, or criticizing me.
- Hold me (how? how firmly?)
- Let me pace.
- Encourage me to move; help me move.
- Lead me through a relaxation or stress reduction technique.
- Peer counsel with me.
- Provide me with materials so I can draw or paint.
- Give me the space to express my feelings.
- Don't talk to me (or do talk to me).
- Encourage me and reassure me.
- Feed me nutritious food.
- Make sure I take my vitamins and other medications.
- Play me comic videos.
- Play me good music (list the kind).
- Just let me rest.

Include a list of specific tasks you would like others to do for you, who you would like to do which task, and any specific instructions they might need. These tasks might include the following:

371

- Buying groceries
- Watering the plants
- Feeding the pets
- Taking care of the children
- Paying the bills
- Taking out the garbage or trash
- Doing the laundry

You may also want to include a list of things that you do not want others to do for you—things they might otherwise do because they think it would be helpful, but that might even be harmful or worsen the situation. These might include the following:

- Forcing you to do anything, such as walking
- Scolding you
- Becoming impatient with you
- Taking away your cigarettes or coffee
- Talking continuously

Some people also include instructions in this section on how they want to be treated by their caregivers. These instructions might include statements such as "kindly, but firmly, tell me what you are going to do," "don't ask me to make any choices at this point," or "make sure to take my medications out of my top dresser drawer right away."

Part 9: Recognizing Recovery

In the last part of this plan, give your supporters information on how to recognize when you have recovered enough to take care of yourself and they no longer need to use this plan. Some examples are the following:

- When I am eating at least two meals a day
- When I am awake for 6 hours a day
- When I am taking care of my personal hygiene needs daily
- When I can carry on a good conversation
- When I can easily walk around the house

You have now completed your crisis plan. Update it when you learn new information or change your mind about things. Date your crisis plan each time you change it and give revised copies to your supporters.

You can help ensure that your crisis plan will be followed by signing it in the presence of two witnesses. It will further increase potential for use if you appoint and name a durable power of attorney—a person who could legally make decisions for you if you were not able to make them for yourself. Since power of attorney documents vary from state to state, you cannot be absolutely sure the plan will be followed. However, it is your best assurance that your wishes will be honored.

Using Your Action Plans

If you are in a crisis situation, the plans can help you realize it so you can let your supporters know they should take over. However, in certain crisis situations, you may not be aware or willing to admit that you are in crisis. This is why having a strong team of supporters is so important. They will observe the symptoms you have reported and take over responsibility for your care, whether or not you are willing to admit you are in a crisis at that time. Distributing your crisis plan to your supporters and discussing it with them is absolutely essential to your safety and well-being.

You may want to take your plan or parts of your plan to the copy shop to get a reduced-size copy to carry in your pocket, purse, or glove compartment of your car. Then you can refer to the plan if triggers or symptoms come up when you are away from home.

People who are using these plans regularly and updating them as necessary are finding that they have fewer difficult times, and that when they do have a hard time, it is not as bad as it used to be and it doesn't last as long.

Chapter 38

Finding and Choosing a Therapist

The following text contains resources to help you choose and locate a therapist who is right for you. A professional who works well with one person may not be a good choice for another person.

Finding a Therapist

There are many ways to find a therapist. You can start by asking friends and family if they can recommend anyone. Make sure the therapist has skills in treating trauma survivors.

Another way to locate a therapist is to make some phone calls.

- Contact your local mental health agency or family doctor.

- Call your state psychological association.

- Call the psychology department at a local college.

- Call the National Center for Victims of Crime's toll-free information and referral service at 800-FYI-CALL (394-2255). This service uses agencies from across the country that support crime victims.

- If you work for a large company, call the human resources office to see if they make referrals.

From "Finding and Choosing a Therapist," by the National Center for Post-traumatic Stress Disorder (NCPTSD, www.ptsd.va.gov), part of the Veterans Administration, June 15, 2010.

- If you are a member of a health maintenance organization (HMO), call to find out about mental health services.

Some mental health services are listed in the phone book. In the blue government pages, look in the "County Government Offices" section. In that section, look for "Health Services (Dept. of)" or "Department of Health Services." Then in that section, look under "Mental Health."

In the yellow pages, therapists are listed under "counseling," "psychologists," "social workers," "psychotherapists," "social and human services," or "mental health."

Information can also be found using the internet. You may find a list of therapists in your area. Some lists include the therapists' areas of practice. The following text contains some suggested websites:

- Center for Mental Health Services Locator [http://store.samhsa.gov/mhlocator]: This services locator is on the Substance Abuse and Mental Health Services Administration (SAMHSA) website.

- Anxiety Disorders Association of America [http://www.adaa.org/findatherapist]: This organization offers a referral network.

- ABCT Find a Therapist Service [http://www.abct.org/Members/?m=FindTherapist&fa=FT_Form&nolm=1]: The Association for Advancement of Behavioral and Cognitive Therapies (ABCT, formerly AABT) maintains a database of therapists.

- Sidran [http://www.sidran.org/sub.cfm?sectionID=5]: This organization offers a referral list of therapists, as well as a fact sheet on how to choose a therapist for PTSD and dissociative disorders.

Your health insurance may pay for mental health services. Also, some services are available at low cost according to your ability to pay.

Help for Veterans

VA Medical Centers and Vet Centers provide veterans with mental health services. These services may cost little or nothing, according to a Veteran's benefits and ability to pay. Following discharge after deployment to a combat zone, you should enroll for VA services. You are then qualified for care for conditions that may be related to your service.

VHA Facilities Locator [http://www2.va.gov/directory/guide/home.asp?isFlash=1]. Use this online tool to find a VA Medical Center or Vet Center near you. You can also go online to read more about services at Vet Centers.

Other resources include the following:

- The VA Health Benefits Service Center (877-222-8387)
- The Vet Centers' national number (800-905-4675)
- VA Office of Mental Health OEF/OIF Veterans Page [http://www .mentalhealth.va.gov/returningservicevets.asp]
- VA Returning Service Members (OEF/OIF) Page [http://www .oefoif.va.gov]
- My HealtheVet [http://www.myhealth.va.gov]

VA Medical Centers and Vet Centers are listed in the phone book. In the blue government pages, look under "United States Government Offices." Then look for "Veterans Affairs, Dept. of." In that section, look under "Medical Care" and "Vet Centers—Counseling and Guidance."

Finding a Support Group

The National Center for PTSD does not provide PTSD support groups. Many local VA Medical Centers have various types of groups. To find support groups online or in your area, try the following resources:

- Anxiety Disorders Association of America [http://www.adaa.org/ finding-help/getting-support/support-groups] offers a self-help group network.
- National Alliance for Mental Illness (NAMI) [http://www.nami .org] has a website with information for those with mental illness. You may also find family support groups in different states.
- About.com's trauma resource page [http://ptsd.about.com/ ?once=true&] offers information, resources, links, and support groups (see Forums). These resources cover many trauma topics including incest and child abuse.

Choosing a Therapist

There are many things to consider in choosing a therapist. Some practical issues are location, cost, and what insurance the therapist accepts. Other issues include the therapist's background, training, and the way he or she works with people.

Some people meet with a few therapists before deciding which one to work with. Most, however, try to see someone known in their area.

Then they go with that person unless a problem occurs. Either way, here is a list of questions you may want to ask a possible therapist.

- What is your education? Are you licensed? How many years have you been practicing?

- What are your special areas of practice?

- Have you ever worked with people who have been through trauma? Do you have any special training in PTSD treatment?

- What kinds of PTSD treatments do you use? Have they been proven effective for dealing with my kind of problem or issue?

- What are your fees? (Fees are usually based on a 45-minute to 50-minute session.) Do you have any discounted fees? How much therapy would you recommend?

- What types of insurance do you accept? Do you file insurance claims? Do you contract with any managed care organizations? Do you accept Medicare or Medicaid insurance?

Types of Mental Health Professionals

There are many types of professionals who can provide therapy for trauma issues. The following text describes some of the most common of these professionals.

Clinical Psychologists

Psychologists are trained in the area of human behavior. Clinical psychologists focus on mental health assessment and treatment.

Psychologists use scientifically proven methods to help people change their thoughts, feelings, and behaviors.

Licensed psychologists have doctoral degrees (PhD, PsyD, EdD). Their graduate training is in clinical, counseling, or school psychology. In addition to their graduate study, licensed psychologists must have another 1 to 2 years of supervised clinical experience. A license is granted after passing an exam given by the American Board of Professional Psychology. Psychologists have the title of "doctor," but they cannot prescribe medicine.

Clinical Social Workers

The purpose of social work is to enhance human well-being. Social workers help meet the basic human needs of all people. They help people manage the forces around them that contribute to problems in living.

Certified social workers have a master's degree or doctoral degree in social work (MSW, DSW, or PhD). To be licensed, clinical social workers must pass an exam given by the Academy of Certified Social Workers (ACSW).

Master's Level Clinicians

Master's Level Clinicians have a master's degree in counseling, psychology, or marriage and family therapy (MA, MFT). They have at least 2 years of training beyond the 4-year college degree. To be licensed, master's level clinicians must meet requirements that vary by state.

Psychiatrists

Psychiatrists have a Doctor of Medicine degree (MD). After they complete 4 years of medical school, they must have 3 to 4 years of residency training. Board certified psychiatrists have also passed written and oral exams given by the American Board of Psychiatry and Neurology. Since they are medical doctors, psychiatrists can prescribe medicine. Some also provide psychotherapy.

Chapter 39

Psychotherapies for Stress-Related Disorders

What Is Psychotherapy?

Psychotherapy, or "talk therapy," is a way to treat people with a mental disorder by helping them understand their illness. It teaches people strategies and gives them tools to deal with stress and unhealthy thoughts and behaviors. Psychotherapy helps patients manage their symptoms better and function at their best in everyday life

Sometimes psychotherapy alone may be the best treatment for a person, depending on the illness and its severity. Other times, psychotherapy is combined with medications. Therapists work with an individual or families to devise an appropriate treatment plan.

What Are the Different Types of Psychotherapy?

Many kinds of psychotherapy exist. There is no "one-size-fits-all" approach. In addition, some therapies have been scientifically tested more than others. Some people may have a treatment plan that includes only one type of psychotherapy. Others receive treatment that includes elements of several different types. The kind of psychotherapy a person receives depends on his or her needs.

Excerpted from "Psychotherapies," by the National Institute of Mental Health (NIMH, www.nimh.nih.gov), part of the National Institutes of Health, May 13, 2010.

This text explains several of the most commonly used psychothera-pies. However, it does not cover every detail about psychotherapy. Pa-tients should talk to their doctor or a psychotherapist about planning treatment that meets their needs.

Cognitive Behavioral Therapy

Cognitive behavioral therapy (CBT) is a blend of two therapies: cognitive therapy (CT) and behavioral therapy. CT was developed by psychotherapist Aaron Beck, MD, in the 1960s. CT focuses on a person's thoughts and beliefs, and how they influence a person's mood and ac-tions, and aims to change a person's thinking to be more adaptive and healthy. Behavioral therapy focuses on a person's actions and aims to change unhealthy behavior patterns.

CBT helps a person focus on his or her current problems and how to solve them. Both patient and therapist need to be actively involved in this process. The therapist helps the patient learn how to identify distorted or unhelpful thinking patterns, recognize and change in-accurate beliefs, relate to others in more positive ways, and change behaviors accordingly.

CBT can be applied and adapted to treat many specific mental disorders.

CBT for depression: Many studies have shown that CBT is a par-ticularly effective treatment for depression, especially minor or moderate depression. Some people with depression may be successfully treated with CBT only. Others may need both CBT and medication. CBT helps people with depression restructure negative thought patterns. Doing so helps people interpret their environment and interactions with others in a positive and realistic way. It may also help a person recognize things that may be contributing to the depression and help him or her change behaviors that may be making the depression worse.

CBT for anxiety disorders: CBT for anxiety disorders aims to help a person develop a more adaptive response to a fear. A CBT thera-pist may use "exposure" therapy to treat certain anxiety disorders, such as a specific phobia, posttraumatic stress disorder, or obsessive compulsive disorder. Exposure therapy has been found to be effective in treating anxiety-related disorders. It works by helping a person confront a specific fear or memory while in a safe and supportive en-vironment. The main goals of exposure therapy are to help the patient learn that anxiety can lessen over time and give him or her the tools to cope with fear or traumatic memories. A recent study sponsored by the Centers for Disease Control and Prevention concluded that CBT is effective in treating trauma-related disorders in children and teens.

CBT for bipolar disorder: People with bipolar disorder usually need to take medication, such as a mood stabilizer. But CBT is often used as an added treatment. The medication can help stabilize a person's mood so that he or she is receptive to psychotherapy and can get the most out of it. CBT can help a person cope with bipolar symptoms and learn to recognize when a mood shift is about to occur. CBT also helps a person with bipolar disorder stick with a treatment plan to reduce the chances of relapse (e.g., when symptoms return).

CBT for eating disorders: Eating disorders can be very difficult to treat. However, some small studies have found that CBT can help reduce the risk of relapse in adults with anorexia who have restored their weight. CBT may also reduce some symptoms of bulimia, and it may also help some people reduce binge-eating behavior.

CBT for schizophrenia: Treating schizophrenia with CBT is challenging. The disorder usually requires medication first. But research has shown that CBT, as an add-on to medication, can help a patient cope with schizophrenia. CBT helps patients learn more adaptive and realistic interpretations of events. Patients are also taught various coping techniques for dealing with "voices" or other hallucinations. They learn how to identify what triggers episodes of the illness, which can prevent or reduce the chances of relapse.

CBT for schizophrenia also stresses skill-oriented therapies. Patients learn skills to cope with life's challenges. The therapist teaches social, daily functioning, and problem-solving skills. This can help patients with schizophrenia minimize the types of stress that can lead to outbursts and hospitalizations.

Dialectical Behavior Therapy

Dialectical behavior therapy (DBT), a form of CBT, was developed by Marsha Linehan, PhD. At first, it was developed to treat people with suicidal thoughts and actions. It is now also used to treat people with borderline personality disorder (BPD). BPD is an illness in which suicidal thinking and actions are more common.

The term "dialectical" refers to a philosophic exercise in which two opposing views are discussed until a logical blending or balance of the two extremes—the middle way—is found. In keeping with that philosophy, the therapist assures the patient that the patient's behavior and feelings are valid and understandable. At the same time, the therapist coaches the patient to understand that it is his or her personal responsibility to change unhealthy or disruptive behavior.

DBT emphasizes the value of a strong and equal relationship between patient and therapist. The therapist consistently reminds the patient when his or her behavior is unhealthy or disruptive—when boundaries are overstepped—and then teaches the skills needed to better deal with future similar situations. DBT involves both individual and group therapy. Individual sessions are used to teach new skills, while group sessions provide the opportunity to practice these skills.

Research suggests that DBT is an effective treatment for people with BPD. A recent NIMH-funded study found that DBT reduced suicide attempts by half compared to other types of treatment for patients with BPD.

Interpersonal Therapy

Interpersonal therapy (IPT) is most often used on a one-on-one basis to treat depression or dysthymia (a more persistent but less severe form of depression). The current manual-based form of IPT used today was developed in the 1980s by Gerald Klerman, MD, and Myrna Weissman, MD.

IPT is based on the idea that improving communication patterns and the ways people relate to others will effectively treat depression. IPT helps identify how a person interacts with other people. When a behavior is causing problems, IPT guides the person to change the behavior. IPT explores major issues that may add to a person's depression, such as grief, or times of upheaval or transition. Sometimes IPT is used along with antidepressant medications.

IPT varies depending on the needs of the patient and the relationship between the therapist and patient. Basically, a therapist using IPT helps the patient identify troubling emotions and their triggers. The therapist helps the patient learn to express appropriate emotions in a healthy way. The patient may also examine relationships in his or her past that may have been affected by distorted mood and behavior. Doing so can help the patient learn to be more objective about current relationships. Studies vary as to the effectiveness of IPT. It may depend on the patient, the disorder, the severity of the disorder, and other variables. In general, however, IPT is found to be effective in treating depression.

A variation of IPT called interpersonal and social rhythm therapy (IPSRT) was developed to treat bipolar disorder. IPSRT combines the basic principles of IPT with behavioral psychoeducation designed to help patients adopt regular daily routines and sleep/wake cycles, stick with medication treatment, and improve relationships. Research has found that when IPSRT is combined with medication, it is an effective treatment for bipolar disorder. IPSRT is as effective as other types of psychotherapy combined with medication in helping to prevent a relapse of bipolar symptoms.

Family-Focused Therapy

Family-focused therapy (FFT) was developed by David Miklowitz, PhD, and Michael Goldstein, PhD, for treating bipolar disorder. It was designed with the assumption that a patient's relationship with his or her family is vital to the success of managing the illness. FFT includes family members in therapy sessions to improve family relationships, which may support better treatment results.

Therapists trained in FFT work to identify difficulties and conflicts among family members that may be worsening the patient's illness. Therapy is meant to help members find more effective ways to resolve those difficulties. The therapist educates family members about their loved one's disorder, its symptoms and course, and how to help their relative manage it more effectively. When families learn about the disorder, they may be able to spot early signs of a relapse and create an action plan that involves all family members. During therapy, the therapist will help family members recognize when they express unhelpful criticism or hostility toward their relative with bipolar disorder. The therapist will teach family members how to communicate negative emotions in a better way. Several studies have found FFT to be effective in helping a patient become stabilized and preventing relapses.

FFT also focuses on the stress family members feel when they care for a relative with bipolar disorder. The therapy aims to prevent family members from "burning out" or disengaging from the effort. The therapist helps the family accept how bipolar disorder can limit their relative. At the same time, the therapist holds the patient responsible for his or her own well-being and actions to a level that is appropriate for the person's age.

Generally, the family and patient attend sessions together. The needs of each patient and family are different, and those needs determine the exact course of treatment. However, the main components of a structured FFT usually include the following:

- Family education on bipolar disorder
- Building communication skills to better deal with stress
- Solving problems together as a family

It is important to acknowledge and address the needs of family members. Research has shown that primary caregivers of people with bipolar disorder are at increased risk for illness themselves. For example, a 2007 study based on results from the NIMH-funded Systematic Treatment Enhancement Program for Bipolar Disorder (STEP-BD) trial found that primary caregivers of participants were at high risk for developing sleep problems and chronic conditions, such as high blood pressure. However, the caregivers were less likely to see a doctor for their own health issues. In addition, a 2005 study found that 33 percent of caregivers of bipolar patients had clinically significant levels of depression.

Are Psychotherapies Different for Children and Adolescents?

Psychotherapies can be adapted to the needs of children and adolescents, depending on the mental disorder. For example, the NIMH-funded Treatment of Adolescents with Depression Study (TADS) found that CBT, when combined with antidepressant medication, was the most effective treatment over the short term for teens with major depression. CBT by itself was also an effective treatment, especially over the long term. Studies have found that individual and group-based CBT are effective treatments for child and adolescent anxiety disorders. Other studies have found that IPT is an effective treatment for child and adolescent depression.

Psychosocial treatments that involve a child's parents and family also have been shown to be effective, especially for disruptive disorders such as conduct disorder or oppositional defiant disorder. Some effective treatments are designed to reduce the child's problem behaviors and improve parent-child interactions. Focusing on behavioral parent management training, parents are taught the skills they need to encourage and reward positive behaviors in their children. Similar training helps parents manage their child's attention deficit/hyperactivity disorder (ADHD). This approach, which has been shown to be effective, can be combined with approaches directed at children to help them learn problem-solving, anger management, and social interaction skills.

Family-based therapy may also be used to treat adolescents with eating disorders. One type is called the Maudsley approach, named after the Maudsley Hospital in London, where the approach was developed. This type of outpatient family therapy is used to treat anorexia nervosa in adolescents. It considers the active participation of parents to be essential in the recovery of their teen. The Maudsley approach proceeds through three phases:

- **Weight restoration:** Parents become fully responsible for ensuring that their teen eats. A therapist helps parents better understand their teen's disease. Parents learn how to avoid criticizing their teen, but they also learn to make sure that their teen eats.

- **Returning control over eating to the teen:** Once the teen accepts the control parents have over his or her eating habits, parents may begin giving up that control. Parents are encouraged to help their teen take more control over eating again.

- **Establishing healthy adolescent identity:** When the teen has reached and maintained a healthy weight, the therapist helps him or her begin developing a healthy sense of identity and autonomy.

Several studies have found the Maudsley approach to be successful in treating teens with anorexia. Currently a large-scale, NIMH-funded study on the approach is under way.

What Other Types of Therapies Are Used?

In addition to the therapies listed in the preceding text, many more approaches exist. Some types have been scientifically tested more than others. Also, some of these therapies are constantly evolving. They are often combined with more established psychotherapies. A few examples of other therapies are described here.

Psychodynamic therapy: Historically, psychodynamic therapy was tied to the principles of psychoanalytic theory, which asserts that a person's behavior is affected by his or her unconscious mind and past experiences. Now therapists who use psychodynamic therapy rarely include psychoanalytic methods. Rather, psychodynamic therapy helps people gain greater self-awareness and understanding about their own actions. It helps patients identify and explore how their nonconscious emotions and motivations can influence their behavior. Sometimes ideas from psychodynamic therapy are interwoven with other types of therapy, like CBT or IPT, to treat various types of mental disorders. Research on psychodynamic therapy is mixed. However, a review of 23 clinical trials involving psychodynamic therapy found it to be as effective as other established psychotherapies.

Light therapy: Light therapy is used to treat seasonal affective disorder (SAD), a form of depression that usually occurs during the autumn and winter months, when the amount of natural sunlight decreases. Scientists think SAD occurs in some people when their bodies' daily rhythms are upset by short days and long nights. Research has found that the hormone melatonin is affected by this seasonal change. Melatonin normally works to regulate the body's rhythms and responses to light and dark. During light therapy, a person sits in front of a "light box" for periods of time, usually in the morning. The box emits a full spectrum light, and sitting in front of it appears to help reset the body's daily rhythms. Also, some research indicates that a low dose of melatonin, taken at specific times of the day, can also help treat SAD.

Other types of therapies are sometimes used in conjunction with the more established therapies.

Expressive or creative arts therapy: Expressive or creative arts therapy is based on the idea that people can help heal themselves through art, music, dance, writing, or other expressive acts. One study has found that expressive writing can reduce depression symptoms among women who were victims of domestic violence. It also helps college students at risk for depression.

Animal-assisted therapy: Working with animals, such as horses, dogs, or cats, may help some people cope with trauma, develop empathy, and encourage better communication. Companion animals are sometimes introduced in hospitals, psychiatric wards, nursing homes, and other places where they may bring comfort and have a mild therapeutic effect. Animal-assisted therapy has also been used as an added therapy for children with mental disorders. Research on the approach is limited, but a recent study found it to be moderately effective in easing behavioral problems and promoting emotional well-being.

Play therapy: This therapy is used with children. It involves the use of toys and games to help a child identify and talk about his or her feelings, as well as establish communication with a therapist. A therapist can sometimes better understand a child's problems by watching how he or she plays. Research in play therapy is minimal.

Chapter 40

Medications for Stress-Related Disorders

Mental Health Medications

Medications are used to treat the symptoms of mental disorders such as schizophrenia, depression, bipolar disorder (sometimes called manic-depressive illness), anxiety disorders, and attention deficit-hyperactivity disorder (ADHD). Sometimes medications are used with other treatments such as psychotherapy. This text describes the following:

- Types of medications used to treat mental disorders
- Side effects of medications
- Directions for taking medications
- Warnings about medications from the U.S. Food and Drug Administration (FDA)

This text does not provide information about diagnosing mental disorders. Choosing the right medication, medication dose, and treatment plan should be based on a person's individual needs and medical situation, and under a doctor's care.

This chapter contains text excerpted from "Mental Health Medications," by the National Institute of Mental Health (NIMH, www.nimh.nih.gov), part of the National Institutes of Health, February 24, 2010, and from "Side Effects of Sleep Drugs," by the U.S. Food and Drug Administration (FDA, www.fda.gov), June 16, 2010.

What are psychiatric medications?

Psychiatric medications treat mental disorders. Sometimes called psychotropic or psychotherapeutic medications, they have changed the lives of people with mental disorders for the better. Many people with mental disorders live fulfilling lives with the help of these medications. Without them, people with mental disorders might suffer serious and disabling symptoms.

How are medications used to treat mental disorders?

Medications treat the symptoms of mental disorders. They cannot cure the disorder, but they make people feel better so they can function.

Medications work differently for different people. Some people get great results from medications and only need them for a short time. For example, a person with depression may feel much better after taking a medication for a few months, and may never need it again. People with disorders like schizophrenia or bipolar disorder or people who have long-term or severe depression or anxiety may need to take medication for a much longer time.

Some people get side effects from medications and other people don't. Doses can be small or large, depending on the medication and the person. Factors that can affect how medications work in people include the following:

- Type of mental disorder, such as depression, anxiety, bipolar disorder, and schizophrenia

- Age, sex, and body size

- Physical illnesses

- Habits like smoking and drinking

- Liver and kidney function

- Genetics

- Other medications and herbal/vitamin supplements

- Diet

- Whether medications are taken as prescribed

What medications are used to treat schizophrenia?

Antipsychotic medications are used to treat schizophrenia and schizophrenia-related disorders. Some of these medications have been available since the mid-1950s. They are also called conventional "typical" antipsychotics. Some of the more commonly used medications include the following:

- Chlorpromazine (Thorazine)
- Haloperidol (Haldol)
- Perphenazine (generic only)
- Fluphenazine (generic only)

In the 1990s, new antipsychotic medications were developed. These new medications are called second generation, or "atypical" antipsychotics.

One of these medications was clozapine (Clozaril). It is a very effective medication that treats psychotic symptoms, hallucinations, and breaks with reality, such as when a person believes he or she is the president. But clozapine can sometimes cause a serious problem called agranulocytosis, which is a loss of the white blood cells that help a person fight infection. Therefore, people who take clozapine must get their white blood cell counts checked every week or two. This problem and the cost of blood tests make treatment with clozapine difficult for many people. Still, clozapine is potentially helpful for people who do not respond to other antipsychotic medications.

Other atypical antipsychotics were developed. All of them are effective, and none cause agranulocytosis. These include the following:

- Risperidone (Risperdal)
- Olanzapine (Zyprexa)
- Quetiapine (Seroquel)
- Ziprasidone (Geodon)
- Aripiprazole (Abilify)
- Paliperidone (Invega)

The antipsychotics listed are some of the medications used to treat symptoms of schizophrenia.

Note: The FDA issued a Public Health Advisory for atypical antipsychotic medications. The FDA determined that death rates are higher for elderly people with dementia when taking this medication. A review of data has found a risk with conventional antipsychotics as well. Antipsychotic medications are not FDA-approved for the treatment of behavioral disorders in patients with dementia.

Some people have side effects when they start taking these medications. Most side effects go away after a few days and often can be managed successfully.

People who are taking antipsychotics should not drive until they adjust to their new medication. Side effects of many antipsychotics include the following:

- Drowsiness

- Dizziness when changing positions

- Blurred vision

- Rapid heartbeat

- Sensitivity to the sun

- Skin rashes

- Menstrual problems for women

Atypical antipsychotic medications can cause major weight gain and changes in a person's metabolism. This may increase a person's risk of getting diabetes and high cholesterol. A person's weight, glucose levels, and lipid levels should be monitored regularly by a doctor while taking an atypical antipsychotic medication.

Typical antipsychotic medications can cause side effects related to physical movement, such as the following:

- Rigidity

- Persistent muscle spasms

- Tremors

- Restlessness

Long-term use of typical antipsychotic medications may lead to a condition called tardive dyskinesia (TD). TD causes muscle movements a person can't control. The movements commonly happen around the mouth. TD can range from mild to severe, and in some people the problem cannot be cured. Sometimes people with TD recover partially or fully after they stop taking the medication.

Every year, an estimated 5 percent of people taking typical antipsychotics get TD. The condition happens to fewer people who take the new, atypical antipsychotics, but some people may still get TD. People who think that they might have TD should check with their doctor before stopping their medication.

Antipsychotics are usually pills that people swallow or liquid they can drink. Some antipsychotics are shots that are given once or twice a month.

Symptoms of schizophrenia, such as feeling agitated and having hallucinations, usually go away within days. Symptoms like delusions usually go away within a few weeks. After about 6 weeks, many people will see a lot of improvement.

However, people respond in different ways to antipsychotic medications, and no one can tell beforehand how a person will respond. Sometimes a person needs to try several medications before finding the right one. Doctors and patients can work together to find the best medication or medication combination and dose.

Some people may have a relapse—their symptoms come back or get worse. Usually, relapses happen when people stop taking their medication, or when they only take it sometimes. Some people stop taking the medication because they feel better or they may feel they don't need it anymore. But no one should stop taking an antipsychotic medication without talking to his or her doctor. When a doctor says it is okay to stop taking a medication, it should be gradually tapered off, never stopped suddenly.

Antipsychotics can produce unpleasant or dangerous side effects when taken with certain medications. For this reason, all doctors treating a patient need to be aware of all the medications that person is taking. Doctors need to know about prescription and over-the-counter medicine, vitamins, minerals, and herbal supplements. People also need to discuss any alcohol or other drug use with their doctor.

To find out more about how antipsychotics work, the National Institute of Mental Health (NIMH) funded a study called CATIE (Clinical Antipsychotic Trials of Intervention Effectiveness). This study compared the effectiveness and side effects of five antipsychotics used to treat people with schizophrenia. In general, the study found that the older medication perphenazine worked as well as the newer, atypical medications. But because people respond differently to different medications, it is important that treatments be designed carefully for each person.

What medications are used to treat depression?

Depression is commonly treated with antidepressant medications. Antidepressants work to balance some of the natural chemicals in our brains. These chemicals are called neurotransmitters, and they affect our mood and emotional responses.

Antidepressants work on neurotransmitters such as serotonin, nor-epinephrine, and dopamine.

The most popular types of antidepressants are called selective serotonin reuptake inhibitors (SSRIs). These include the following:

- Fluoxetine (Prozac)

- Citalopram (Celexa)

- Sertraline (Zoloft)

- Paroxetine (Paxil)

- Escitalopram (Lexapro)

Other types of antidepressants are serotonin and norepinephrine reuptake inhibitors (SNRIs). SNRIs are similar to SSRIs and include venlafaxine (Effexor) and duloxetine (Cymbalta). Another antidepressant that is commonly used is bupropion (Wellbutrin). Bupropion, which works on the neurotransmitter dopamine, is unique in that it does not fit into any specific drug type. SSRIs and SNRIs are popular because they do not cause as many side effects as older classes of antidepressants. Older antidepressant medications include tricyclics, tetracyclics, and monoamine oxidase inhibitors (MAOIs). For some people, tricyclics, tetracyclics, or MAOIs may be the best medications.

Antidepressants may cause mild side effects that usually do not last long. Any unusual reactions or side effects should be reported to a doctor immediately.

The most common side effects associated with SSRIs and SNRIs include the following:

- Headache, which usually goes away within a few days

- Nausea (feeling sick to your stomach), which usually goes away within a few days

- Sleeplessness or drowsiness, which may happen during the first few weeks but then goes away (Sometimes the medication dose needs to be reduced or the time of day it is taken needs to be adjusted to help lessen these side effects.)

- Agitation (feeling jittery)

- Sexual problems, which can affect both men and women and may include reduced sex drive and problems having and enjoying sex

Tricyclic antidepressants can cause side effects, including the following:

- Dry mouth

- Constipation

- Bladder problems (It may be hard to empty the bladder or the urine stream may not be as strong as usual. Older men with enlarged prostate conditions may be more affected.)

- Sexual problems, which can affect both men and women and may include reduced sex drive and problems having and enjoying sex

- Blurred vision, which usually goes away quickly

- Drowsiness (Usually, antidepressants that make you drowsy are taken at bedtime.)

People taking MAOIs need to be careful about the foods they eat and the medicines they take. Foods and medicines that contain high levels of a chemical called tyramine are dangerous for people taking MAOIs. Tyramine is found in some cheeses, wines, and pickles. The chemical is also in some medications, including decongestants and over-the-counter cold medicine.

Mixing MAOIs and tyramine can cause a sharp increase in blood pressure, which can lead to stroke. People taking MAOIs should ask their doctors for a complete list of foods, medicines, and other substances to avoid. An MAOI skin patch has recently been developed and may help reduce some of these risks. A doctor can help a person figure out if a patch or a pill will work for him or her.

People taking antidepressants need to follow their doctors' directions. The medication should be taken in the right dose for the right amount of time. It can take 3 or 4 weeks until the medicine takes effect. Some people take the medications for a short time, and some people take them for much longer periods. People with long-term or severe depression may need to take medication for a long time.

Once a person is taking antidepressants, it is important not to stop taking them without the help of a doctor. Sometimes people taking antidepressants feel better and stop taking the medication too soon, and the depression may return.

When it is time to stop the medication, the doctor will help the person slowly and safely decrease the dose. It's important to give the body time to adjust to the change. People don't get addicted, or "hooked," on the medications, but stopping them abruptly can cause withdrawal symptoms.

If a medication does not work, it is helpful to be open to trying another one. A study funded by NIMH found that if a person with difficult-to-treat depression did not get better with a first medication, chances of getting better increased when the person tried a new one or added a second medication to his or her treatment. The study was called STAR*D (Sequenced Treatment Alternatives to Relieve Depression).

The herbal medicine St. John's wort has been used for centuries in many folk and herbal remedies. Today in Europe, it is used widely to treat mild-to-moderate depression. In the United States, it is one of the top-selling botanical products.

The National Institutes of Health conducted a clinical trial to determine the effectiveness of treating adults who have major depression with St. Johns wort.

The study included 340 people diagnosed with major depression. One third of the people took the herbal medicine, one third took an SSRI, and one third took a placebo, or sugar pill. The people did not know what they were taking. The study found that St. John's wort was no more effective than the placebo in treating major depression. A study currently in progress is looking at the effectiveness of St. John's wort for treating mild or minor depression.

Other research has shown that St. John's wort can dangerously interact with other medications, including those used to control HIV [human immunodeficiency virus]. On February 10, 2000, the FDA issued a Public Health Advisory letter stating that the herb appears to interfere with certain medications used to treat heart disease, depression, seizures, certain cancers, and organ transplant rejection. Also, St. John's wort may interfere with oral contraceptives.

Because St. John's wort may not mix well with other medications, people should always talk with their doctors before taking it or any herbal supplement.

FDA warning on antidepressants: Antidepressants are safe and popular, but some studies have suggested that they may have unintentional effects, especially in young people. In 2004, the FDA looked at published and unpublished data on trials of antidepressants that involved nearly 4,400 children and adolescents. They found that 4 percent of those taking antidepressants thought about or tried suicide (although no suicides occurred), compared to 2 percent of those receiving placebos (sugar pill).

In 2005, the FDA decided to adopt a "black box" warning label—the most serious type of warning—on all antidepressant medications. The warning says there is an increased risk of suicidal thinking or attempts in children and adolescents taking antidepressants. In 2007, the FDA proposed that makers of all antidepressant medications extend the warning to include young adults up through age 24.

The warning also says that patients of all ages taking antidepressants should be watched closely, especially during the first few weeks of treatment. Possible side effects to look for are depression that gets worse, suicidal thinking or behavior, or any unusual changes in behavior such as trouble sleeping, agitation, or withdrawal from normal social situations. Families and caregivers should report any changes to the doctor.

Results of a comprehensive review of pediatric trials conducted between 1988 and 2006 suggested that the benefits of antidepressant medications likely outweigh their risks to children and adolescents with major depression and anxiety disorders. The study was funded in part by NIMH.

Finally, the FDA has warned that combining the newer SSRI or SNRI antidepressants with one of the commonly-used "triptan" medications used to treat migraine headaches could cause a life-threatening illness called "serotonin syndrome." A person with serotonin syndrome may be agitated, have hallucinations (see or hear things that are not real), have a high temperature, or have unusual blood pressure changes. Serotonin syndrome is usually associated with the older antidepressants called MAOIs, but it can happen with the newer antidepressants as well, if they are mixed with the wrong medications.

What medications are used to treat bipolar disorder?

Bipolar disorder, also called manic-depressive illness, is commonly treated with mood stabilizers. Sometimes, antipsychotics and antidepressants are used along with a mood stabilizer.

Mood stabilizers: People with bipolar disorder usually try mood stabilizers first. In general, people continue treatment with mood stabilizers for years. Lithium is a very effective mood stabilizer. It was the first mood stabilizer approved by the FDA in the 1970s for treating both manic and depressive episodes.

Anticonvulsant medications also are used as mood stabilizers. They were originally developed to treat seizures, but they were found to help control moods as well. One anticonvulsant commonly used as a mood stabilizer is valproic acid, also called divalproex sodium (Depakote). For some people, it may work better than lithium. Other anticonvulsants used as mood stabilizers are carbamazepine (Tegretol), lamotrigine (Lamictal), and oxcarbazepine (Trileptal).

397

Atypical antipsychotics: Atypical antipsychotic medications are sometimes used to treat symptoms of bipolar disorder. Often, antipsychotics are used along with other medications. Antipsychotics used to treat people with bipolar disorder include the following:

- Olanzapine (Zyprexa), which helps people with severe or psychotic depression, which often is accompanied by a break with reality, hallucinations, or delusions

- Aripiprazole (Abilify), which can be taken as a pill or as a shot

- Risperidone (Risperdal)

- Ziprasidone (Geodon)

- Clozapine (Clozaril), which is often used for people who do not respond to lithium or anticonvulsants.

Antidepressants: Antidepressants are sometimes used to treat symptoms of depression in bipolar disorder. Fluoxetine (Prozac), paroxetine (Paxil), or sertraline (Zoloft) are a few that are used. However, people with bipolar disorder should not take an antidepressant on its own. Doing so can cause the person to rapidly switch from depression to mania, which can be dangerous. To prevent this problem, doctors give patients a mood stabilizer or an antipsychotic along with an antidepressant.

Research on whether antidepressants help people with bipolar depression is mixed. An NIMH-funded study found that antidepressants were no more effective than a placebo to help treat depression in people with bipolar disorder. The people were taking mood stabilizers along with the antidepressants.

Treatments for bipolar disorder have improved over the last 10 years. But everyone responds differently to medications. If you have any side effects, tell your doctor right away. He or she may change the dose or prescribe a different medication.

Different medications for treating bipolar disorder may cause different side effects. Some medications used for treating bipolar disorder have been linked to unique and serious symptoms, which are described in the following text.

Lithium can cause several side effects, and some of them may become serious. They include the following:

- Loss of coordination

- Excessive thirst

- Frequent urination

- Blackouts
- Seizures
- Slurred speech
- Fast, slow, irregular, or pounding heartbeat
- Hallucinations (seeing things or hearing voices that do not exist)
- Changes in vision
- Itching, rash
- Swelling of the eyes, face, lips, tongue, throat, hands, feet, ankles, or lower legs

If a person with bipolar disorder is being treated with lithium, he or she should visit the doctor regularly to check the levels of lithium in the blood, and make sure the kidneys and the thyroid are working normally.

Some possible side effects linked with valproic acid/divalproex sodium include the following:

- Changes in weight
- Nausea
- Stomach pain
- Vomiting
- Anorexia
- Loss of appetite

Valproic acid may cause damage to the liver or pancreas, so people taking it should see their doctors regularly.

Valproic acid may affect young girls and women in unique ways. Sometimes, valproic acid may increase testosterone (a male hormone) levels in teenage girls and lead to a condition called polycystic ovarian syndrome (PCOS). PCOS is a disease that can affect fertility and make the menstrual cycle become irregular, but symptoms tend to go away after valproic acid is stopped. It also may cause birth defects in women who are pregnant.

Lamotrigine can cause a rare but serious skin rash that needs to be treated in a hospital. In some cases, this rash can cause permanent disability or be life-threatening.

In addition, valproic acid, lamotrigine, carbamazepine, oxcarbazepine, and other anticonvulsant medications have an FDA warning.

The warning states that their use may increase the risk of suicidal thoughts and behaviors. People taking anticonvulsant medications for bipolar or other illnesses should be closely monitored for new or worsening symptoms of depression, suicidal thoughts or behavior, or any unusual changes in mood or behavior. People taking these medications should not make any changes without talking to their health care professional.

Other medications for bipolar disorder may also be linked with rare but serious side effects. Always talk with the doctor or pharmacist about any potential side effects before taking the medication.

Medications should be taken as directed by a doctor. Sometimes a person's treatment plan needs to be changed. When changes in medicine are needed, the doctor will guide the change. A person should never stop taking a medication without asking a doctor for help.

There is no cure for bipolar disorder, but treatment works for many people. Treatment works best when it is continuous, rather than on and off. However, mood changes can happen even when there are no breaks in treatment. Patients should be open with their doctors about treatment. Talking about how treatment is working can help it be more effective.

It may be helpful for people or their family members to keep a daily chart of mood symptoms, treatments, sleep patterns, and life events. This chart can help patients and doctors track the illness. Doctors can use the chart to treat the illness most effectively.

Because medications for bipolar disorder can have serious side effects, it is important for anyone taking them to see the doctor regularly to check for possibly dangerous changes in the body.

What medications are used to treat anxiety disorders?

Antidepressants, antianxiety medications, and beta-blockers are the most common medications used for anxiety disorders.

Anxiety disorders include the following:

- Obsessive-compulsive disorder (OCD)
- Post-traumatic stress disorder (PTSD)
- Generalized anxiety disorder (GAD)
- Panic disorder
- Social phobia

Antidepressants: Antidepressants were developed to treat depression, but they also help people with anxiety disorders. SSRIs such as fluoxetine (Prozac), sertraline (Zoloft), escitalopram (Lexapro), paroxetine (Paxil), and citalopram (Celexa) are commonly prescribed for panic disorder, OCD, PTSD, and social phobia. The SNRI venlafaxine (Effexor) is commonly used to treat GAD. The antidepressant bupropion (Wellbutrin) is also sometimes used. When treating anxiety disorders, antidepressants generally are started at low doses and increased over time.

Some tricyclic antidepressants work well for anxiety. For example, imipramine (Tofranil) is prescribed for panic disorder and GAD. Clomipramine (Anafranil) is used to treat OCD. Tricyclics are also started at low doses and increased over time.

MAOIs are also used for anxiety disorders. Doctors sometimes prescribe phenelzine (Nardil), tranylcypromine (Parnate), and isocarboxazid (Marplan).

People who take MAOIs must avoid certain food and medicines that can interact with their medicine and cause dangerous increases in blood pressure.

Benzodiazepines (antianxiety medications): The antianxiety medications called benzodiazepines can start working more quickly than antidepressants. The ones used to treat anxiety disorders include the following:

- Clonazepam (Klonopin), which is used for social phobia and GAD

- Lorazepam (Ativan), which is used for panic disorder

- Alprazolam (Xanax), which is used for panic disorder and GAD

- Buspirone (BuSpar), an antianxiety medication used to treat GAD, which unlike benzodiazepines, takes at least 2 weeks for buspirone to begin working

Beta-blockers: Beta-blockers control some of the physical symptoms of anxiety, such as trembling and sweating. Propranolol (Inderal) is a beta-blocker usually used to treat heart conditions and high blood pressure. The medicine also helps people who have physical problems related to anxiety. For example, when a person with social phobia must face a stressful situation, such as giving a speech, or attending an important meeting, a doctor may prescribe a beta-blocker. Taking the medicine for a short period of time can help the person keep physical symptoms under control.

The most common side effects for benzodiazepines are drowsiness and dizziness. Other possible side effects include the following:

- Upset stomach
- Blurred vision
- Headache
- Confusion
- Grogginess
- Nightmares

Possible side effects from buspirone (BuSpar) include the following:

- Dizziness
- Headaches
- Nausea
- Nervousness
- Lightheadedness
- Excitement
- Trouble sleeping

Common side effects from beta-blockers include the following:

- Fatigue
- Cold hands
- Dizziness
- Weakness

In addition, beta-blockers generally are not recommended for people with asthma or diabetes because they may worsen symptoms.

People can build a tolerance to benzodiazepines if they are taken over a long period of time and may need higher and higher doses to get the same effect. Some people may become dependent on them. To avoid these problems, doctors usually prescribe the medication for short periods, a practice that is especially helpful for people who have substance abuse problems or who become dependent on medication easily. If people suddenly stop taking benzodiazepines, they may get withdrawal symptoms, or their anxiety may return. Therefore, they should be tapered off slowly.

Buspirone and beta-blockers are similar. They are usually taken on a short-term basis for anxiety. Both should be tapered off slowly. Talk to the doctor before stopping any antianxiety medication.

Which groups have special needs when taking psychiatric medications?

Psychiatric medications are taken by all types of people, but some groups have special needs, including the following:

- Children and adolescents
- Older adults
- Women who are pregnant or may become pregnant

Children and adolescents: Most medications used to treat young people with mental illness are safe and effective. However, many medications have not been studied or approved for use with children. Researchers are not sure how these medications affect a child's growing body. Still, a doctor can give a young person an FDA-approved medication on an "off-label" basis. This means that the doctor prescribes the medication to help the patient even though the medicine is not approved for the specific mental disorder or age.

For these reasons, it is important to watch young people who take these medications. Young people may have different reactions and side effects than adults. Also, some medications, including antidepressants and ADHD medications, carry FDA warnings about potentially dangerous side effects for young people.

More research is needed on how these medications affect children and adolescents. NIMH has funded studies on this topic. For example, NIMH funded the Preschoolers with ADHD Treatment Study (PATS), which involved 300 preschoolers (3 to 5 years old) diagnosed with ADHD. The study found that low doses of the stimulant methylphenidate are safe and effective for preschoolers. However, children of this age are more sensitive to the side effects of the medication, including slower growth rates. Children taking methylphenidate should be watched closely.

In addition to medications, other treatments for young people with mental disorders should be considered. Psychotherapy, family therapy, educational courses, and behavior management techniques can help everyone involved cope with the disorder.

Older adults: Because older people often have more medical problems than other groups, they tend to take more medications than younger people, including prescribed, over-the-counter, and herbal medications. As a result, older people have a higher risk for experiencing bad drug interactions, missing doses, or overdosing.

Older people also tend to be more sensitive to medications. Even healthy older people react to medications differently than younger people because their bodies process it more slowly. Therefore, lower or less frequent doses may be needed.

Sometimes memory problems affect older people who take medications for mental disorders. An older adult may forget his or her regular dose and take too much or not enough. A good way to keep track of medicine is to use a 7-day pill box, which can be bought at any pharmacy. At the beginning of each week, older adults and their caregivers fill the box so that it is easy to remember what medicine to take. Many pharmacies also have pillboxes with sections for medications that must be taken more than once a day.

Women who are pregnant or may become pregnant: The research on the use of psychiatric medications during pregnancy is limited. The risks are different depending on what medication is taken, and at what point during the pregnancy the medication is taken. Research has shown that antidepressants, especially SSRIs, are safe during pregnancy. Birth defects or other problems are possible, but they are very rare.

However, antidepressant medications do cross the placental barrier and may reach the fetus. Some research suggests the use of SSRIs during pregnancy is associated with miscarriage or birth defects, but other studies do not support this. Studies have also found that fetuses exposed to SSRIs during the third trimester may be born with "withdrawal" symptoms such as breathing problems, jitteriness, irritability, trouble feeding, or hypoglycemia (low blood sugar).

Most studies have found that these symptoms in babies are generally mild and short-lived, and no deaths have been reported. On the flip side, women who stop taking their antidepressant medication during pregnancy may get depression again and may put both themselves and their infant at risk.

In 2004, the FDA issued a warning against the use of certain antidepressants in the late third trimester. The warning said that doctors may want to gradually taper pregnant women off antidepressants in the third trimester so that the baby is not affected. After a woman delivers, she should consult with her doctor to decide whether to return to a full dose during the period when she is most vulnerable to postpartum depression.

Some medications should not be taken during pregnancy. Benzodiazepines may cause birth defects or other infant problems, especially if taken during the first trimester. Mood stabilizers are known to cause birth defects. Benzodiazepines and lithium have been shown to cause "floppy baby syndrome," which is when a baby is drowsy and limp, and cannot breathe or feed well.

Research suggests that taking antipsychotic medications during pregnancy can lead to birth defects, especially if they are taken during the first trimester. But results vary widely depending on the type of antipsychotic. The conventional antipsychotic haloperidol has been studied more than others, and has been found not to cause birth defects.

After the baby is born, women and their doctors should watch for postpartum depression, especially if they stopped taking their medication during pregnancy.

In addition, women who nurse while taking psychiatric medications should know that a small amount of the medication passes into the breast milk. However, the medication may or may not affect the baby. It depends on the medication and when it is taken. Women taking psychiatric medications and who intend to breastfeed should discuss the potential risks and benefits with their doctors.

Decisions on medication should be based on each woman's needs and circumstances. Medications should be selected based on available scientific research, and they should be taken at the lowest possible dose. Pregnant women should be watched closely throughout their pregnancy and after delivery.

What should I ask my doctor if I am prescribed a psychiatric medication?

You and your family can help your doctor find the right medications for you. The doctor needs to know your medical history; family history; information about allergies; other medications, supplements, or herbal remedies you take; and other details about your overall health. You or a family member should ask the following questions when a medication is prescribed:

- What is the name of the medication?
- What is the medication supposed to do?
- How and when should I take it?
- How much should I take?
- What should I do if I miss a dose?
- When and how should I stop taking it?
- Will it interact with other medications I take?

- Do I need to avoid any types of food or drink while taking the medication?

- What should I avoid?

- Should it be taken with or without food?

- Is it safe to drink alcohol while taking this medication?

- What are the side effects? What should I do if I experience them?

- Is the Patient Package Insert for the medication available?

After taking the medication for a short time, tell your doctor how you feel, if you are having side effects, and any concerns you have about the medicine.

Side Effects of Sleep Drugs

Eating a little bit of chocolate was a treat that Teresa Wood looked forward to after work. The Fairfax Station, Virginia, resident allowed herself two small pieces of chocolate candy a day.

But after taking a drug to help her sleep at night, Wood awoke in the morning to find an empty box on the table in place of a pound of chocolates that had been there the night before.

"I couldn't believe it," says Wood. "I started looking all around the house—I even looked under the bed. I thought for sure someone came into the house during the night and ate them." But she was alone.

A few weeks later, Wood awoke to find a near-full box of chocolates gone again. "I just don't remember eating all that candy," she says.

Do sleep drugs cause complex sleep-related behaviors?

Wood and her doctor determined that she had been getting up during the night and "sleep eating," an occurrence known as a complex sleep-related behavior. Other behaviors include making phone calls, having sex, and getting into the car and driving while not fully awake. Most people do not remember these events later.

Complex behaviors are a potential side effect of sedative-hypnotic products—a class of drugs used to help a person fall asleep and stay asleep.

"Complex behaviors, such as sleep-driving, could be potentially dangerous to both the patients and to others," says Russell Katz, MD, Director of the Food and Drug Administration's Division of Neurology Products.

Do sleep drugs cause allergic reactions?

Other rare but potential side effects of sedative-hypnotic drugs are a severe allergic reaction (anaphylaxis) and severe facial swelling (angioedema), which can occur as early as the first time the product is taken.

"Severe allergic reactions can affect a patient's ability to breathe and can affect other body systems as well, and can even be fatal at times," says Katz. "Although these allergic reactions are probably very rare, people should be aware that they can occur, because these reactions may be difficult to notice as people are falling asleep."

Are stronger warnings needed?

To make known the risks of these products, FDA requested in early 2007 that all manufacturers of sedative-hypnotic drug products strengthen their product labeling to include warnings about complex sleep-related behaviors and anaphylaxis and angioedema.

"There are a number of prescription sleep aids available that are well-tolerated and effective for many people," says Steven Galson, MD, MPH, Director of FDA's Center for Drug Evaluation and Research However, after reviewing the available information on adverse events that occurred after the sedative-hypnotic drugs were on the market, FDA concluded that labeling changes were necessary to inform health care providers and consumers about risks, says Galson.

In addition to the labeling changes, FDA has requested that manufacturers of sedative-hypnotic products do the following:

- They should send letters to health care providers to notify them about the new warnings (Manufacturers sent these letters beginning in March 2007.)

- They should develop Patient Medication Guides for the products to inform consumers about risks and advise them of precautions that can be taken. (Patient Medication Guides are handouts given to patients, families, and caregivers when a medicine is dispensed. The guides will contain FDA-approved information, such as proper use and the recommendation to avoid ingesting alcohol or other central nervous system depressants.)

- They should conduct clinical studies to investigate the frequency with which sleep-driving and other complex behaviors occur in association with individual drug products.

The revised labeling and other actions to make risks known affect these sedative-hypnotic products:

- Ambien and Ambien CR (zolpidem tartrate)
- Butisol sodium
- Carbitol (pentobarbital and carbromal)
- Dalmane (flurazepam hydrochloride)
- Doral (quazepam)
- Halcion (triazolam)
- Lunesta (eszopiclone)
- Placidyl (ethchlorvynol)
- ProSom (estazolam)
- Restoril (temazepam)
- Rozerem (ramelteon)
- Seconal (secobarbital sodium)
- Sonata (zaleplon)

What precautions should I take?

FDA advises people who are treated with any of these products to take the following precautions:

- Talk to your health care provider before you start these medications and if you have any questions or concerns.
- Read the Medication Guide, when available, before taking the product.
- Do not increase the dose prescribed by your health care provider. Complex sleep-related behaviors are more likely to occur with higher than appropriate doses.
- Do not drink alcohol or take other drugs that depress the nervous system.
- Do not discontinue the use of these medications without first talking to your health care provider.

What about over-the-counter sleep aids?

Not all sleep medications are prescription. FDA has approved over-the-counter (OTC) medications for use up to 2 weeks to help relieve occasional sleepiness in people ages 12 and older. "If you continue to have sleeping problems beyond 2 weeks, you should see a doctor," says Marina Chang, RPh, pharmacist, and team leader in FDA's Division of Nonprescription Regulation Development.

OTC sleep aids are non-habit-forming and do not present the risk of allergic reactions and complex sleep-related behaviors that are known to occur with sedative-hypnotic drugs.

But just because they're available over-the-counter doesn't mean they don't have side effects, says Chang. "They don't have the same level of precision as the prescription drugs. They don't completely stop working after 8 hours—many people feel drowsy for longer than 8 hours after taking them."

Chang advises reading the product label and exercising caution when taking OTC sleep aids until you learn how they will affect you. "They affect people differently," she says. "They are not for everybody."

What are some tips for better sleep?

- Go to bed and get up at the same time each day.

- Avoid caffeine, nicotine, beer, wine, and liquor in the 4 to 6 hours before bedtime.

- Don't exercise within 2 hours of bedtime.

- Don't eat large meals within 2 hours of bedtime.

- Don't nap later than 3 p.m.

- Sleep in a dark, quiet room that isn't too hot or cold for you.

- If you can't fall asleep within 20 minutes, get up and do something quiet until you feel sleepy.

- Wind down in the 30 minutes before bedtime by doing something relaxing, such as reading or listening to music.

Chapter 41

Complementary and Alternative Medicine Therapies

Chapter Contents

Section 41.1

Overview of Stress Management Strategies

From "Alternative Approaches to Mental Health Care," by the Substance Abuse and Mental Health Services Administration (SAMHSA, mentalhealth. samhsa.gov), part of the U.S. Department of Health and Human Services, April 2003. Reviewed by David A. Cooke, MD, FACP, November 22, 2010.

An alternative approach to mental health care is one that emphasizes the interrelationship between mind, body, and spirit. Although some alternative approaches have a long history, many remain controversial. It is crucial to consult with your health care providers about the approaches you are using to achieve mental wellness.

Self-Help

Many people with mental illnesses find that self-help groups are an invaluable resource for recovery and for empowerment. Self-help generally refers to groups or meetings that do the following:

- Involve people who have similar needs

- Are facilitated by a consumer, survivor, or other layperson

- Assist people to deal with a life-disrupting event, such as a death, abuse, serious accident, addiction, or diagnosis of a physical, emotional, or mental disability, for oneself or a relative

- Are operated on an informal, free-of-charge, and nonprofit basis

- Provide support and education

- Are voluntary, anonymous, and confidential

Diet and Nutrition

Adjusting both diet and nutrition may help some people with mental illnesses manage their symptoms and promote recovery. For example, research suggests that eliminating milk and wheat products can reduce the severity of symptoms for some people who have schizophrenia and some children with autism. Similarly, some holistic/natural physicians use herbal treatments, B-complex vitamins, riboflavin, magnesium, and thiamine to treat anxiety, autism, depression, drug-induced psychoses, and hyperactivity.

Pastoral Counseling

Some people prefer to seek help for mental health problems from their pastor, rabbi, or priest, rather than from therapists who are not affiliated with a religious community. Counselors working within traditional faith communities increasingly are recognizing the need to incorporate psychotherapy and/or medication, along with prayer and spirituality, to effectively help some people with mental disorders.

Animal-Assisted Therapies

Working with an animal (or animals) under the guidance of a health care professional may benefit some people with mental illness by facilitating positive changes, such as increased empathy and enhanced socialization skills. Animals can be used as part of group therapy programs to encourage communication and increase the ability to focus. Developing self-esteem and reducing loneliness and anxiety are just some potential benefits of individual-animal therapy.

Expressive Therapies

Art therapy: Drawing, painting, and sculpting help many people to reconcile inner conflicts, release deeply repressed emotions, and foster self-awareness, as well as personal growth. Some mental health providers use art therapy as both a diagnostic tool and as a way to help treat disorders such as depression, abuse-related trauma, and schizophrenia. You may be able to find a therapist in your area who has received special training and certification in art therapy.

Dance/movement therapy: Some people find that their spirits soar when they let their feet fly. Others—particularly those who prefer more structure or who feel they have "two left feet"—gain the same sense of release and inner peace from the Eastern martial arts, such as Aikido and Tai Chi. Those who are recovering from physical, sexual, or emotional abuse may find these techniques especially helpful for gaining a sense of ease with their own bodies. The underlying premise to dance/movement therapy is that it can help a person integrate the emotional, physical, and cognitive facets of self.

Music/sound therapy: It is no coincidence that many people turn on soothing music to relax or fast tunes to help feel upbeat. Research suggests that music stimulates the body's natural feel-good chemicals (opiates and endorphins). This stimulation results in improved blood flow, blood pressure, pulse rate, breathing, and posture changes. Music or sound therapy has been used to treat disorders such as stress, grief, depression, schizophrenia, and autism in children, and to diagnose mental health needs.

Culturally Based Healing Arts

Traditional Oriental medicine (such as acupuncture, shiatsu, and Reiki), Indian systems of health care (such as Ayurveda and yoga), and Native American healing practices (such as the Sweat Lodge and Talking Circles) all incorporate the following beliefs:

* Wellness is a state of balance between the spiritual, physical, and mental/emotional "selves."

* An imbalance of forces within the body is the cause of illness.

* Herbal/natural remedies, combined with sound nutrition, exercise, and meditation/prayer, will correct this imbalance.

Acupuncture: The Chinese practice of inserting needles into the body at specific points manipulates the body's flow of energy to balance the endocrine system. This manipulation regulates functions such as heart rate, body temperature, and respiration, as well as sleep patterns and emotional changes. Acupuncture has been used in clinics to assist people with substance abuse disorders through detoxification; to relieve stress and anxiety; to treat attention deficit and hyperactivity disorder in children; to reduce symptoms of depression; and to help people with physical ailments.

Ayurveda: Ayurvedic medicine is described as "knowledge of how to live." It incorporates an individualized regimen—such as diet, meditation, herbal preparations, or other techniques—to treat a variety of conditions, including depression, to facilitate lifestyle changes, and to teach people how to release stress and tension through yoga or transcendental meditation.

Yoga/meditation: Practitioners of this ancient Indian system of health care use breathing exercises, posture, stretches, and meditation to balance the body's energy centers. Yoga is used in combination with other treatment for depression, anxiety, and stress-related disorders.

Native American traditional practices: Ceremonial dances, chants, and cleansing rituals are part of Indian Health Service programs to heal depression, stress, trauma (including those related to physical and sexual abuse), and substance abuse.

Cuentos: Based on folktales, this form of therapy originated in Puerto Rico. The stories used contain healing themes and models of behavior such as self-transformation and endurance through adversity. Cuentos is used primarily to help Hispanic children recover from depression and other mental health problems related to leaving one's homeland and living in a foreign culture.

Relaxation and Stress Reduction Techniques

Biofeedback: Learning to control muscle tension and involuntary body functioning, such as heart rate and skin temperature, can be a path to mastering one's fears. It is used in combination with, or as an alternative to, medication to treat disorders such as anxiety, panic, and phobias. For example, a person can learn to retrain his or her breathing habits in stressful situations to induce relaxation and decrease hyperventilation. Some preliminary research indicates it may offer an additional tool for treating schizophrenia and depression.

Guided imagery or visualization: This process involves going into a state of deep relaxation and creating a mental image of recovery and wellness. Physicians, nurses, and mental health providers occasionally use this approach to treat alcohol and drug addictions, depression, panic disorders, phobias, and stress.

Massage therapy: The underlying principle of this approach is that rubbing, kneading, brushing, and tapping a person's muscles can help release tension and pent emotions. It has been used to treat trauma-related depression and stress. A highly unregulated industry, certification for massage therapy varies widely from state to state. Some states have strict guidelines, while others have none.

Technology-Based Applications

The boom in electronic tools at home and in the office makes access to mental health information just a telephone call or a mouse click away. Technology is also making treatment more widely available in once-isolated areas.

Telemedicine: Plugging into video and computer technology is a relatively new innovation in health care. It allows both consumers and providers in remote or rural areas to gain access to mental health or specialty expertise. Telemedicine can enable consulting providers to speak to and observe patients directly. It also can be used in education and training programs for generalist clinicians.

Telephone counseling: Active listening skills are a hallmark of telephone counselors. These also provide information and referral to interested callers. For many people telephone counseling often is a first step to receiving in-depth mental health care. Research shows that such counseling from specially trained mental health providers reaches many people who otherwise might not get the help they need. Before calling, be sure to check the telephone number for service fees; a 900 area code means you will be billed for the call, an 800 or 888 area code means the call is toll-free.

Electronic communications: Technologies such as the internet, bulletin boards, and electronic mail lists provide access directly to consumers and the public on a wide range of information. Online consumer groups can exchange information, experiences, and views on mental health, treatment systems, alternative medicine, and other related topics.

Radio psychiatry: Another relative newcomer to therapy, radio psychiatry was first introduced in the United States in 1976. Radio psychiatrists and psychologists provide advice, information, and referrals in response to a variety of mental health questions from callers. The American Psychiatric Association and the American Psychological Association have issued ethical guidelines for the role of psychiatrists and psychologists on radio shows.

Section 41.2

Acupuncture

From "Acupuncture May Help Symptoms of Posttraumatic Stress Disorder," by the National Center for Complementary and Alternative Medicine (NCCAM, nccam.nih.gov), part of the National Institutes of Health, 2010.

A pilot study shows that acupuncture may help people with posttraumatic stress disorder. Posttraumatic stress disorder (PTSD) is an anxiety disorder that can develop after exposure to a terrifying event or ordeal in which grave physical harm occurred or was threatened. Traumatic events that may trigger PTSD include violent personal assaults, natural or human-caused disasters, accidents, or military combat.

Michael Hollifield, MD, and colleagues conducted a clinical trial examining the effect of acupuncture on the symptoms of PTSD. The researchers analyzed depression, anxiety, and impairment in 73 people with a diagnosis of PTSD. The participants were assigned to receive either acupuncture or group cognitive-behavioral therapy over 12 weeks, or were assigned to a wait-list as part of the control group. The people in the control group were offered treatment or referral for treatment at the end of their participation.

The researchers found that acupuncture provided treatment effects similar to group cognitive-behavioral therapy; both interventions were superior to the control group. Additionally, treatment effects of both the acupuncture and the group therapy were maintained for 3 months after the end of treatment.

The limitations of the study are consistent with preliminary research. For example, this study had a small group of participants that lacked diversity, and the results do not account for outside factors that may have affected the treatments' results.

Reference

Michael Hollifield, Nityamo Sinclair-Lian, Teddy D. Warner, and Richard Hammerschlag, "Acupuncture for Posttraumatic Stress Disorder: A Randomized Controlled Pilot Trial." *The Journal of Nervous and Mental Disease,* June 2007.

Section 41.3

Herbal Supplements May Improve Stress Symptoms

This section contains text from "Kava," and "Valerian," documents produced by the National Center for Complementary and Alternative Medicine (NCCAM, nccam.nih.gov), part of the National Institutes of Health, July 2010.

Kava

Kava is native to the islands of the South Pacific and is a member of the pepper family. Kava has been used as a ceremonial beverage in the South Pacific for centuries.

Common names for kava include kava kava, awa, and kava pepper; the Latin name is *Piper methysticum*.

What Kava Is Used For

Kava has been used to help people fall asleep and fight fatigue, as well as to treat asthma and urinary tract infections.

Topically, kava has been used as a numbing agent.

Today, kava is used primarily for anxiety, insomnia, and menopausal symptoms.

How Kava Is Used

The root and rhizome (underground stem) of kava are used to prepare beverages, extracts, capsules, tablets, and topical solutions.

What the Science Says

Although scientific studies provide some evidence that kava may be beneficial for the management of anxiety, the U.S. Food and Drug Administration (FDA) has issued a warning that using kava supplements has been linked to a risk of liver damage.

Kava is not a proven therapy for other uses. NCCAM-funded studies on kava were suspended after the FDA issued its warning.

Side Effects and Cautions

Kava has been reported to cause liver damage, including hepatitis and liver failure (which can cause death).

Kava has been associated with several cases of dystonia (abnormal muscle spasm or involuntary muscle movements). Kava may interact with several drugs, including drugs used for Parkinson disease.

Long-term and/or heavy use of kava may result in scaly, yellowed skin. Avoid driving and operating heavy machinery while taking kava because the herb has been reported to cause drowsiness.

Tell all your health care providers about any complementary and alternative practices you use. Give them a full picture of what you do to manage your health. This will help ensure coordinated and safe care.

Valerian

Valerian is a plant native to Europe and Asia; it is also found in North America. Valerian has been used as a medicinal herb since at least the time of ancient Greece and Rome. Its therapeutic uses were described by Hippocrates, and in the 2nd century, Galen prescribed valerian for insomnia.

Common names for valerian include all-heal and garden heliotrope; the Latin name is *Valeriana officinalis*.

What Valerian Is Used For

Valerian has long been used for sleep disorders and anxiety.

Valerian has also been used for other conditions, such as headaches, depression, irregular heartbeat, and trembling.

How Valerian Is Used

The roots and rhizomes (underground stems) of valerian are typically used to make supplements, including capsules, tablets, and liquid extracts, as well as teas.

What the Science Says

Research suggests that valerian may be helpful for insomnia, but there is not enough evidence from well-designed studies to confirm this.

There is not enough scientific evidence to determine whether valerian works for other conditions, such as anxiety or depression.

NCCAM-funded research on valerian includes studies on the herb's effects on sleep in healthy older adults and in people with Parkinson disease.

NCCAM-funded researchers are also studying the potential of valerian and other herbal products to relieve menopausal symptoms.

Side Effects and Cautions

Studies suggest that valerian is generally safe to use for short periods of time (for example, 4 to 6 weeks).

No information is available about the long-term safety of valerian.

Valerian can cause mild side effects, such as headaches, dizziness, upset stomach, and tiredness the morning after its use.

Tell all your health care providers about any complementary and alternative practices you use. Give them a full picture of what you do to manage your health. This will help ensure coordinated and safe care.

Section 41.4

Massage Therapy

From "Massage Therapy: An Introduction," by the National Center for
Complementary and Alternative Medicine (NCCAM, nccam.nih.gov),
part of the National Institutes of Health, August 2010.

Massage therapy has a long history in cultures around the world.
Today, people use many different types of massage therapy for a variety of health-related purposes. In the United States, massage therapy
is often considered part of complementary and alternative medicine
(CAM), although it does have some conventional uses.

History of Massage

Massage therapy dates back thousands of years. References to
massage appear in writings from ancient China, Japan, India, Arabic
nations, Egypt, Greece (Hippocrates defined medicine as "the art of
rubbing"), and Rome.

Massage became widely used in Europe during the Renaissance. In
the 1850s, two American physicians who had studied in Sweden introduced massage therapy in the United States, where it became popular
and was promoted for a variety of health purposes. With scientific and
technological advances in medical treatment during the 1930s and
1940s, massage fell out of favor in the United States. Interest in massage revived in the 1970s, especially among athletes.

Use of Massage Therapy in the United States

According to the 2007 National Health Interview Survey, which
included a comprehensive survey of CAM use by Americans, an estimated 18 million U.S. adults and 700,000 children had received massage therapy in the previous year.

People use massage for a variety of health-related purposes, including to relieve pain, rehabilitate sports injuries, reduce stress, increase relaxation, address anxiety and depression, and aid general
wellness.

421

Defining Massage Therapy

The term "massage therapy" encompasses many different techniques. In general, therapists press, rub, and otherwise manipulate the muscles and other soft tissues of the body. They most often use their hands and fingers, but may use their forearms, elbows, or feet.

There are many types of massage therapy. In Swedish massage, the therapist uses long strokes, kneading, deep circular movements, vibration, and tapping. Sports massage is similar to Swedish massage, adapted specifically to the needs of athletes. Among the many other examples are deep tissue massage and trigger point massage, which focuses on myofascial trigger points—muscle "knots" that are painful when pressed and can cause symptoms elsewhere in the body.

The Practice of Massage Therapy

Massage therapists work in a variety of settings, including private offices, hospitals, nursing homes, studios, and sport and fitness facilities. Some also travel to patients' homes or workplaces. They usually try to provide a calm, soothing environment.

Therapists usually ask new patients about symptoms, medical history, and desired results. They may also perform an evaluation through touch, to locate painful or tense areas and determine how much pressure to apply.

Typically, the patient lies on a table, either in loose-fitting clothing or undressed (covered with a sheet, except for the area being massaged). The therapist may use oil or lotion to reduce friction on the skin. Sometimes, people receive massage therapy while sitting in a chair. A massage session may be fairly brief, but may also last an hour or even longer.

Research Status

Although scientific research on massage therapy—whether it works and, if so, how—is limited, there is evidence that massage may benefit some patients. Conclusions generally cannot yet be drawn about its effectiveness for specific health conditions.

According to one analysis, however, research supports the general conclusion that massage therapy is effective. The studies included in the analysis suggest that a single session of massage therapy can reduce "state anxiety" (a reaction to a particular situation), blood pressure, and heart rate, and multiple sessions can reduce "trait anxiety" (general anxiety-proneness), depression, and pain. In addition, recent studies suggest that massage may benefit certain conditions, for example:

- A 2008 review of 13 clinical trials found evidence that massage might be useful for chronic low-back pain. Clinical practice guidelines issued in 2007 by the American Pain Society and the American College of Physicians recommend that physicians consider using certain CAM therapies, including massage (as well as acupuncture), when patients with chronic low-back pain do not respond to conventional treatment.

- A multisite study of more than 300 hospice patients with advanced cancer concluded that massage may help to relieve pain and improve mood for these patients.

- A study of 64 patients with chronic neck pain found that therapeutic massage was more beneficial than a self-care book, in terms of improving function and relieving symptoms.

There are numerous theories about how massage therapy may affect the body. For example, the "gate control theory" suggests that massage may provide stimulation that helps to block pain signals sent to the brain. Other theories suggest that massage might stimulate the release of certain chemicals in the body, such as serotonin or endorphins, or cause beneficial mechanical changes in the body. However, additional studies are needed to test the various theories.

Safety

Massage therapy appears to have few serious risks—if it is performed by a properly trained therapist and if appropriate cautions are followed. The number of serious injuries reported is very small. Side effects of massage therapy may include temporary pain or discomfort, bruising, swelling, and a sensitivity or allergy to massage oils.

Cautions about massage therapy include the following:

- Vigorous massage should be avoided by people with bleeding disorders or low blood platelet counts, and by people taking blood-thinning medications such as warfarin.

- Massage should not be done in any area of the body with blood clots, fractures, open or healing wounds, skin infections, or weakened bones (such as from osteoporosis or cancer), or where there has been a recent surgery.

- Although massage therapy appears to be generally safe for cancer patients, they should consult their oncologist before having a massage that involves deep or intense pressure. Any direct pressure over a tumor usually is discouraged. Cancer patients should discuss any concerns about massage therapy with their oncologist.

- Pregnant women should consult their health care provider before using massage therapy.

Training, Licensing, and Certification

There are approximately 1,500 massage therapy schools and training programs in the United States. In addition to hands-on practice of massage techniques, students generally learn about the body and how it works, business practices, and ethics. Massage training programs generally are approved by a state board. Some may also be accredited by an independent agency, such as the Commission on Massage Therapy Accreditation (COMTA).

As of 2010, 43 states and the District of Columbia had laws regulating massage therapy. In some states, regulation is by town ordinance.

The National Certification Board for Therapeutic Massage and Bodywork certifies practitioners who pass a national examination. Increasingly, states that license massage therapists require them to have a minimum of 500 hours of training at an accredited institution, pass a national exam, meet specific continuing education requirements, and carry malpractice insurance.

In addition to massage therapists, health care providers such as chiropractors and physical therapists may have training in massage.

If You Are Thinking about Using Massage Therapy

- Do not use massage therapy to replace your regular medical care or as a reason to postpone seeing a health care provider about a medical problem.

- If you have a medical condition and are unsure whether massage therapy would be appropriate for you, discuss your concerns with your health care provider. Your health care provider may also be able to help you select a massage therapist. You might also look for published research articles on massage therapy for your condition.

- Before deciding to begin massage therapy, ask about the therapist's training, experience, and credentials. Also ask about the number of treatments that might be needed, the cost, and insurance coverage.

- If a massage therapist suggests using other CAM practices (for example, herbs or other supplements, or a special diet), discuss it first with your regular health care provider.

- Tell all your health care providers about any complementary and alternative practices you use. Give them a full picture of what you do to manage your health. This will ensure coordinated and safe care.

NCCAM-Funded Research on Massage Therapy

Recent NCCAM-sponsored studies have been investigating the following:

- The effects of massage on chronic neck pain and low-back pain

- Massage to treat anxiety disorder, alleviate depression in patients with advanced AIDS [acquired immunodeficiency syndrome], and promote recovery in women who were victims of sexual abuse as children

- Massage to relieve fatigue in cancer patients undergoing chemotherapy, reduce treatment-related swelling of the arms in breast cancer patients, and alleviate pain and distress in cancer patients at the end of life

- Whether massage improves weight gain and immune system function in preterm infants

- Whether massage given at home by a trained family member helps reduce pain from sickle cell anemia

Section 41.5

Meditation

This section contains text from "Meditation: An Introduction," by the National Center for Complementary and Alternative Medicine (NCCAM, www.nccam.nih.gov), part of the National Institutes of Health, June 2010, and from "Transcendental Meditation Helps Young Adults Cope with Stress," by the NCCAM, December 2009.

Meditation: An Introduction

Meditation is a mind-body practice in complementary and alternative medicine (CAM). There are many types of meditation, most of which originated in ancient religious and spiritual traditions. Generally, a person who is meditating uses certain techniques, such as a specific posture, focused attention, and an open attitude toward distractions. Meditation may be practiced for many reasons, such as to increase calmness and physical relaxation, to improve psychological balance, to cope with illness, or to enhance overall health and well-being.

Overview

The term meditation refers to a group of techniques, such as mantra meditation, relaxation response, mindfulness meditation, and Zen Buddhist meditation. Most meditative techniques started in Eastern religious or spiritual traditions. These techniques have been used by many different cultures throughout the world for thousands of years. Today, many people use meditation outside of its traditional religious or cultural settings, for health and well-being.

In meditation, a person learns to focus attention. Some forms of meditation instruct the practitioner to become mindful of thoughts, feelings, and sensations and to observe them in a nonjudgmental way. This practice is believed to result in a state of greater calmness and physical relaxation, and psychological balance. Practicing meditation can change how a person relates to the flow of emotions and thoughts.

Most types of meditation have four elements in common:

- **A quiet location:** Meditation is usually practiced in a quiet place with as few distractions as possible. This can be particularly helpful for beginners.

- **A specific, comfortable posture:** Depending on the type being practiced, meditation can be done while sitting, lying down, standing, walking, or in other positions.

- **A focus of attention:** Focusing one's attention is usually a part of meditation. For example, the meditator may focus on a mantra (a specially chosen word or set of words), an object, or the sensations of the breath. Some forms of meditation involve paying attention to whatever is the dominant content of consciousness.

- **An open attitude:** Having an open attitude during meditation means letting distractions come and go naturally without judging them. When the attention goes to distracting or wandering thoughts, they are not suppressed; instead, the meditator gently brings attention back to the focus. In some types of meditation, the meditator learns to "observe" thoughts and emotions while meditating.

Meditation used as CAM is a type of mind-body medicine. Generally, mind-body medicine focuses on the interactions among the brain/mind, the rest of the body, and behavior and the ways in which emotional, mental, social, spiritual, and behavioral factors can directly affect health.

Uses of Meditation for Health in the United States

A 2007 national government survey that asked about CAM use in a sample of 23,393 U.S. adults found that 9.4 percent of respondents (representing more than 20 million people) had used meditation in the past 12 months—compared with 7.6 percent of respondents (representing more than 15 million people) in a similar survey conducted in 2002. The 2007 survey also asked about CAM use in a sample of 9,417 children; 1 percent (representing 725,000 children) had used meditation in the past 12 months.

People use meditation for various health problems, such as the following:

- Anxiety

- Pain

- Depression

- Stress

- Insomnia

- Physical or emotional symptoms that may be associated with
  chronic illnesses (such as heart disease, HIV/AIDS [human immunodeficiency virus/acquired immunodeficiency syndrome],
  and cancer) and their treatment

Meditation is also used for overall wellness.

Examples of Meditation Practices

Mindfulness meditation and Transcendental Meditation (also known
as TM) are two common forms of meditation. NCCAM-sponsored research projects are studying both types of meditation.

Mindfulness meditation is an essential component of Buddhism. In
one common form of mindfulness meditation, the meditator is taught
to bring attention to the sensation of the flow of the breath in and out
of the body. The meditator learns to focus attention on what is being
experienced, without reacting to or judging it. This is seen as helping
the meditator learn to experience thoughts and emotions in normal
daily life with greater balance and acceptance.

The TM technique is derived from Hindu traditions. It uses a mantra (a word, sound, or phrase repeated silently) to prevent distracting
thoughts from entering the mind. The goal of TM is to achieve a state
of relaxed awareness.

How Meditation Might Work

Practicing meditation has been shown to induce some changes in
the body. By learning more about what goes on in the body during
meditation, researchers hope to be able to identify diseases or conditions for which meditation might be useful.

Some types of meditation might work by affecting the autonomic
(involuntary) nervous system. This system regulates many organs and
muscles, controlling functions such as heartbeat, sweating, breathing,
and digestion. It has two major parts:

- The sympathetic nervous system helps mobilize the body for
  action. When a person is under stress, it produces the "fight-or-
  flight response": The heart rate and breathing rate go up and
  blood vessels narrow (restricting the flow of blood).

- The parasympathetic nervous system causes the heart rate and
  breathing rate to slow down, the blood vessels to dilate (improving blood flow), and the flow of digestive juices increases.

It is thought that some types of meditation might work by reducing activity in the sympathetic nervous system and increasing activity in the parasympathetic nervous system.

In one area of research, scientists are using sophisticated tools to determine whether meditation is associated with significant changes in brain function. A number of researchers believe that these changes account for many of meditation's effects.

It is also possible that practicing meditation may work by improving the mind's ability to pay attention. Since attention is involved in performing everyday tasks and regulating mood, meditation might lead to other benefits.

A 2007 NCCAM-funded review of the scientific literature found some evidence suggesting that meditation is associated with potentially beneficial health effects. However, the overall evidence was inconclusive. The reviewers concluded that future research needs to be more rigorous before firm conclusions can be drawn.

Side Effects and Risks

Meditation is considered to be safe for healthy people. There have been rare reports that meditation could cause or worsen symptoms in people who have certain psychiatric problems, but this question has not been fully researched.

People with physical limitations may not be able to participate in certain meditative practices involving physical movement. Individuals with existing mental or physical health conditions should speak with their health care providers prior to starting a meditative practice and make their meditation instructor aware of their condition.

If You Are Thinking about Using Meditation Practices

- Do not use meditation as a replacement for conventional care or as a reason to postpone seeing a doctor about a medical problem.

- Ask about the training and experience of the meditation instructor you are considering.

- Look for published research studies on meditation for the health condition in which you are interested.

Tell all your health care providers about any complementary and alternative practices you use. Give them a full picture of what you do to manage your health. This will help ensure coordinated and safe care.

Transcendental Meditation Helps Young Adults Cope with Stress

A recent study found that transcendental meditation (TM) helped college students decrease psychological distress and increase coping ability. For a group of students at high risk for developing hypertension, these changes also were associated with decreases in blood pressure. This could be good news for the many students experiencing academic, financial, and social pressures that can lead to psychological distress—especially in light of evidence that college-age people with even slightly elevated blood pressure are three times more likely to develop hypertension within 30 years.

Funded in part by NCCAM, researchers from Maharishi University of Management and American University studied 298 students from American University and other schools in the Washington, DC, area. The researchers randomly assigned students to a TM group or a control (wait-list) group. They also created a high-risk subgroup, based on blood pressure readings, family history, and weight. The TM group received a seven-step course in TM techniques, with invitations to attend refresher meetings, and kept track of how often they practiced TM. At the beginning of the study and after 3 months, researchers tested all participants for blood pressure and psychological measures. The researchers noted that 30 percent of the participants dropped out before the end of the study.

Blood pressure decreased in the TM group and increased in the control group, but the differences were not significant overall (TM-control blood pressure differences were significant within the high-risk subgroup). However, compared with controls, the TM group had significant improvement in total psychological distress, anxiety, depression, anger/hostility, and coping ability. Changes in psychological distress and coping paralleled changes in blood pressure.

According to the researchers, these findings suggest that young adults at risk of developing hypertension may be able to reduce that risk by practicing TM. The researchers recommend that future studies of TM in college students evaluate long-term effects on blood pressure and psychological distress.

Source: Nidich SI, Rainforth MV, Haaga DAF, et al. A randomized controlled trial on effects of the Transcendental Meditation program on blood pressure, psychological distress, and coping in young adults. *American Journal of Hypertension;* Dec 2009; 22(12):1326–1331.

Section 41.6

Spirituality May Alleviate Distress

Excerpted and adapted from PDQ® Cancer Information Summary. National Cancer Institute; Bethesda, MD. Spirituality in Cancer Care (PDQ®): Patient Version. Updated 12/2010. Available at: http://cancer.gov. Accessed December 22, 2010.

Religious and spiritual values are important to patients coping with physical and mental health issues, such as stress-related disorders.

Studies have shown that religious and spiritual values are important to Americans. Most American adults say that they believe in God and that their religious beliefs affect how they live their lives. However, people have different ideas about life after death, belief in miracles, and other religious beliefs. Such beliefs may be based on gender, education, and ethnic background.

Many patients with health conditions rely on spiritual or religious beliefs and practices to help them cope with their disease. This is called spiritual coping. Many caregivers also rely on spiritual coping. Each person may have different spiritual needs, depending on cultural and religious traditions. For some seriously ill patients, spiritual well-being may affect how much anxiety they feel about death. For others, it may affect what they decide about treatments. Some patients and their family caregivers may want doctors to talk about spiritual concerns, but may feel unsure about how to bring up the subject.

There is a growing understanding that doctors' support of spiritual well-being in very ill patients helps improve their quality of life. Health care providers are looking at new ways to help them with religious and spiritual concerns. Doctors may ask patients which spiritual issues are important to them.

Spirituality and Religion May Have Different Meanings

The terms spirituality and religion are often used in place of each other, but for many people they have different meanings. Religion may be defined as a specific set of beliefs and practices, usually within an organized group. Spirituality may be defined as an individual's sense of peace, purpose, and connection to others, and beliefs about the meaning of life. Spirituality may be found and expressed through an organized religion or in other ways. Patients may think of themselves as spiritual or religious or both.

Serious illness may cause spiritual distress. Serious illnesses like cancer may cause patients or family caregivers to have doubts about their beliefs or religious values and cause much spiritual distress. Some studies show that patients may feel that they are being punished by God or may have a loss of faith after being diagnosed. Other patients may have mild feelings of spiritual distress when coping with illness.

Spiritual and Religious Well-Being May Help Improve Quality of Life

It is not known for sure how spirituality and religion are related to health. Some studies show that spiritual or religious beliefs and practices create a positive mental attitude that may help a patient feel better and improve the well-being of family caregivers.

Spiritual and religious well-being may help improve health and quality of life in the following ways:

- Decrease anxiety, depression, anger, and discomfort

- Decrease the sense of isolation (feeling alone) and the risk of suicide

- Decrease alcohol and drug abuse

- Lower blood pressure and the risk of heart disease

- Help the patient adjust to the effects of disease, mental illness, and its treatment

- Increase the ability to enjoy life during treatment

- Give a feeling of personal growth as a result of living with health concerns

- Increase positive feelings, including the following:
  - Hope and optimism
  - Freedom from regret
  - Satisfaction with life
  - A sense of inner peace

Spiritual and Religious Well-Being May Also Help a Patient Live Longer

Spiritual distress may also affect health. Spiritual distress may make it harder for patients to cope. Health care providers may encourage patients to meet with experienced spiritual or religious leaders to help deal with their spiritual issues. This may improve their health, quality of life, and ability to cope.

Spiritual Assessment

A spiritual assessment may help the doctor understand how religious or spiritual beliefs will affect the way a patient copes with his or her health concern.

A spiritual assessment is a method or tool used by doctors to understand the role that religious and spiritual beliefs have in the patient's life. This may help the doctor understand how these beliefs affect the way the patient responds to the diagnosis and decisions about treatment. Some doctors or caregivers may wait for the patient to bring up spiritual concerns. Others may use an interview or a questionnaire.

A spiritual assessment explores religious beliefs and spiritual practices and may include questions about the following:

- Religious denomination, if any
- Beliefs or philosophy of life
- Important spiritual practices or rituals
- Using spirituality or religion as a source of strength
- Being part of a community of support
- Using prayer or meditation
- Loss of faith
- Conflicts between spiritual or religious beliefs and treatments
- Ways that health care providers and caregivers may help with the patient's spiritual needs
- Concerns about death and afterlife

The health care team may not ask about every issue the patient feels is important. Patients should bring up other spiritual or religious issues that they think may affect their care.

433

Meeting the Patient's Spiritual and Religious Needs

To help patients with spiritual needs, medical staff will listen to the wishes of the patient.

Spirituality and religion are very personal issues. Patients should expect doctors and caregivers to respect their religious and spiritual beliefs and concerns. Patients who rely on spirituality to cope should be able to count on the health care team to give them support. This may include giving patients information about people or groups that can help with spiritual or religious needs. Most hospitals have chaplains, but not all outpatient settings do. Patients who do not want to discuss spirituality during care should also be able to count on the health care team to respect their wishes.

Doctors and caregivers will try to respond to their patients' concerns, but may not take part in patients' religious practices or discuss specific religious beliefs.

The health care team will help with a patient's spiritual needs when setting goals and planning treatment. The health care team may help with a patient's spiritual needs in the following ways:

- Suggest goals and options for care that honor the patient's spiritual and/or religious views

- Support the patient's use of spiritual coping during the illness

- Encourage the patient to speak with his/her religious or spiritual leader

- Refer the patient to a hospital chaplain or support group that can help with spiritual issues during illness

- Refer the patient to other therapies that have been shown to increase spiritual well-being

Other therapies may include mindfulness relaxation, such as yoga or meditation, or creative arts programs, such as writing, drawing, or music therapy.

Section 41.7

Yoga

This section includes text excerpted from "Yoga for Health: An Introduction," by the National Center for Complementary and Alternative Medicine (NCCAM, www.nccam.nih.gov), part of the National Institutes of Health, May 2008; and from "Long-Term Yoga Practice May Decrease Women's Stress," by the NCCAM, February 2010.

Yoga

Yoga is a mind-body practice in complementary and alternative medicine (CAM) with origins in ancient Indian philosophy.

The various styles of yoga that people use for health purposes typically combine physical postures, breathing techniques, and meditation or relaxation.

Overview

Yoga in its full form combines physical postures, breathing exercises, meditation, and a distinct philosophy. Yoga is intended to increase relaxation and balance the mind, body, and the spirit.

Early written descriptions of yoga are in Sanskrit, the classical language of India. The word "yoga" comes from the Sanskrit word yuj, which means "yoke or union." It is believed that this describes the union between the mind and the body. The first known text, *The Yoga Sutras,* was written more than 2,000 years ago, although yoga may have been practiced as early as 5,000 years ago. Yoga was originally developed as a method of discipline and attitudes to help people reach spiritual enlightenment. The Sutras outline eight limbs or foundations of yoga practice that serve as spiritual guidelines:

1. Yama (moral behavior)

2. Niyama (healthy habits)

3. Asana (physical postures)

4. Pranayama (breathing exercises)

5. Pratyahara (sense withdrawal)

6. Dharana (concentration)

7. Dhyana (contemplation)

8. Samadhi (higher consciousness)

The numerous schools of yoga incorporate these eight limbs in varying proportions. Hatha yoga, the most commonly practiced in the United States and Europe, emphasizes two of the eight limbs: Postures (asanas) and breathing exercises (pranayama). Some of the major styles of hatha yoga include Ananda, Anusara, Ashtanga, Bikram, Iyengar, Kripalu, Kundalini, and Viniyoga.

Use of Yoga for Health in the United States

According to the 2007 National Health Interview Survey (NHIS), which included a comprehensive survey of CAM use by Americans, yoga is one of the top 10 CAM modalities used. More than 13 million adults had used yoga in the previous year, and between the 2002 and 2007 NHIS, use of yoga among adults increased by 1 percent (or approximately 3 million people). The 2007 survey also found that more than 1.5 million children used yoga in the previous year.

People use yoga for a variety of health conditions including anxiety disorders or stress, asthma, high blood pressure, and depression. People also use yoga as part of a general health regimen—to achieve physical fitness and to relax.

The Status of Yoga Research

Research suggests that yoga might do the following:

* Improve mood and sense of well-being

* Counteract stress

* Reduce heart rate and blood pressure

* Increase lung capacity

* Improve muscle relaxation and body composition

* Help with conditions such as anxiety, depression, and insomnia

* Improve overall physical fitness, strength, and flexibility

* Positively affect levels of certain brain or blood chemicals

More well-designed studies are needed before definitive conclusions can be drawn about yoga's use for specific health conditions.

Side Effects and Risks

Yoga is generally considered to be safe in healthy people when practiced appropriately. Studies have found it to be well tolerated, with few side effects.

People with certain medical conditions should not use some yoga practices. For example, people with disk disease of the spine, extremely high or low blood pressure, glaucoma, retinal detachment, fragile or atherosclerotic arteries, a risk of blood clots, ear problems, severe osteoporosis, or cervical spondylitis should avoid some inverted poses.

Although yoga during pregnancy is safe if practiced under expert guidance, pregnant women should avoid certain poses that may be problematic.

Training, Licensing, and Certification

There are many training programs for yoga teachers throughout the country. These programs range from a few days to more than 2 years. Standards for teacher training and certification differ depending on the style of yoga.

There are organizations that register yoga teachers and training programs that have complied with minimum educational standards. For example, one nonprofit group requires at least 200 hours of training, with a specified number of hours in areas including techniques, teaching methodology, anatomy, physiology, and philosophy. However, there are currently no official or well-accepted licensing requirements for yoga teachers in the United States.

If You Are Thinking about Yoga

- Do not use yoga as a replacement for conventional care or to postpone seeing a doctor about a medical problem.

- If you have a medical condition, consult with your health care provider before starting yoga.

- Ask about the physical demands of the type of yoga in which you are interested, as well as the training and experience of the yoga teacher you are considering.

- Look for published research studies on yoga for the health condition you are interested in.

Tell your health care providers about any complementary and alternative practices you use. Give them a full picture of what you do to manage your health. This will help ensure coordinated and safe care.

Long-Term Yoga Practice May Decrease Women's Stress

Recent research has shown that women who practice hatha yoga (a common type of yoga involving body postures, breath control, and meditation) regularly recover from stress faster than women who are considered yoga "novices." The research, supported in part by NCCAM and published in the February 2010 issue of the journal *Psychosomatic Medicine*, also showed that yoga may boost the mood of both yoga experts and novices.

Researchers at Ohio State University enrolled 25 women identified as yoga "experts" (practiced yoga regularly once or twice weekly for at least 2 years and at least twice weekly during the past year) and 25 novices (participated in yoga classes or home practice with yoga videos for 6 to 12 sessions). The researchers assessed participants' cardiovascular, inflammatory, and endocrine responses before and after they took part in three activities: yoga practice, slow walking on a treadmill, and passively watching a video. They also measured participants' physiologic responses before and after certain stress events.

Although differences in inflammatory or endocrine responses were not unique to the yoga sessions, the researchers found that the novices' blood had 41 percent higher levels of the cytokine interleukin-6 (IL-6) than those of the experts. IL-6 is a stress-related compound that is thought to play a role in certain conditions such as cardiovascular disease and type 2 diabetes. In addition, the novices' levels of C-reactive protein, which serves as a general marker for inflammation, were nearly five times that of the yoga experts. Experts had lower heart rates in response to stress events than novices. Yoga also boosted mood in both groups, while the other two interventions (walking, video) did not.

The researchers suggested that this study offers insight into how yoga and its related practices may affect health. Regularly performing yoga could have health benefits, which may only become evident after years of practice.

Source: Kiecolt-Glaser JK, Christian L, Preston H, et al. Stress, inflammation, and yoga practice. *Psychosomatic Medicine*. Feb 2010;72(2):113–121.

Chapter 42

Treating Depression

There is help for someone who has depression. Even in severe cases, depression is highly treatable. The first step is to visit a doctor. Your family doctor or a health clinic is a good place to start. A doctor can make sure that the symptoms of depression are not being caused by another medical condition. A doctor may refer you to a mental health professional.

The most common treatments of depression are psychotherapy and medication.

Psychotherapy: Several types of psychotherapy—or talk therapy—can help people with depression. There are two main types of psychotherapy commonly used to treat depression: Cognitive-behavioral therapy (CBT) and interpersonal therapy (IPT). CBT teaches people to change negative styles of thinking and behaving that may contribute to their depression. IPT helps people understand and work through troubled personal relationships that may cause their depression or make it worse.

For mild to moderate depression, psychotherapy may be the best treatment option. However, for major depression or for certain people, psychotherapy may not be enough. For teens, a combination of medication and psychotherapy may work the best to treat major depression and help keep the depression from happening again. Also, a study about treating depression in older adults found that those who got better

Excerpted from "Depression," by the National Institute of Mental Health (NIMH, www.nimh.nih.gov), part of the National Institutes of Health, 2007.

with medication and IPT were less likely to have depression again if they continued their combination treatment for at least two years.

Medications: Medications help balance chemicals in the brain called neurotransmitters. Although scientists are not sure exactly how these chemicals work, they do know they affect a person's mood. Types of antidepressant medications that help keep the neurotransmitters at the correct levels include the following:

- SSRIs (selective serotonin reuptake inhibitors)
- SNRIs (serotonin and norepinephrine reuptake inhibitors)
- MAOIs (monoamine oxidase inhibitors)
- Tricyclics

These different types of medications affect different chemicals in the brain.

Medications affect everyone differently. Sometimes several different types have to be tried before finding the one that works. If you start taking medication, tell your doctor about any side effects right away. Depending on which type of medication, possible side effects include the following:

- Headache
- Nausea
- Insomnia and nervousness
- Agitation or feeling jittery
- Sexual problems
- Dry mouth
- Constipation
- Bladder problems
- Blurred vision
- Drowsiness during the day

Are there other therapies?

St. John's wort: The extract from St. John's wort (*Hypericum perforatum*), a bushy, wild-growing plant with yellow flowers, has been used for centuries in many folk and herbal remedies. The National Institutes of Health conducted a clinical trial to determine the effectiveness of the herb in treating adults who have major depression. Involving 340 patients diagnosed with major depression, the trial found that St. John's wort was no more effective than a sugar pill (placebo) in treating major depression. Another study is looking at whether St. John's wort is effective for treating mild or minor depression.

Other research has shown that St. John's wort may interfere with other medications, including those used to control HIV infection. On February 10, 2000, the U.S. Food and Drug Administration (FDA) issued a Public Health Advisory letter stating that the herb may interfere with certain medications used to treat heart disease, depression, seizures, certain cancers, and organ transplant rejection. The herb also may interfere with the effectiveness of oral contraceptives. Because of these potential interactions, patients should always consult with their doctors before taking any herbal supplement.

Electroconvulsive therapy: For cases in which medication and/or psychotherapy does not help treat depression, electroconvulsive therapy (ECT) may be useful. ECT, once known as shock therapy, formerly had a bad reputation. But in recent years, it has greatly improved and can provide relief for people with severe depression who have not been able to feel better with other treatments.

ECT may cause short-term side effects, including confusion, disorientation, and memory loss. But these side effects typically clear soon after treatment. Research has indicated that after 1 year of ECT treatments, patients show no adverse cognitive effects.

What does the FDA say about antidepressants?

Despite the fact that SSRIs and other antidepressants are generally safe and reliable, some studies have shown that they may have unintentional effects on some people, especially young people. In 2004, the FDA reviewed data from studies of antidepressants that involved nearly 4,400 children and teenagers being treated for depression. The review showed that 4% of those who took antidepressants thought about or attempted suicide (although no suicides occurred), compared to 2% of those who took sugar pills (placebo).

This information prompted the FDA, in 2005, to adopt a "black box" warning label on all antidepressant medications to alert the public about the potential increased risk of suicidal thinking or attempts in children and teenagers taking antidepressants. In 2007, the FDA proposed that makers of all antidepressant medications extend the black box warning on their labels to include young patients up through age 24 who are taking these medications for depression treatment. A "black box" warning is the most serious type of warning on prescription drug labeling.

The warning also emphasizes that children, teenagers, and young adults taking antidepressants should be closely monitored, especially during the initial weeks of treatment, for any worsening depression, suicidal thinking, or behavior. These include any unusual changes in behavior such as sleeplessness, agitation, or withdrawal from normal social situations. Results of a review of pediatric trials between 1988 and 2006 suggested that the benefits of antidepressant medications likely outweigh their risks to children and adolescents with major depression and anxiety disorders. The study was funded in part by the National Institute of Mental Health.

How can I find treatment and who pays?

Most insurance plans cover treatment for depression. Check with your own insurance company to find out what type of treatment is covered. If you don't have insurance, local city or county governments may offer treatment at a clinic or health center, where the cost is based on income. Medicaid plans also may pay for depression treatment.

If you are unsure where to go for help, ask your family doctor. Others who can help include the following:

- Psychiatrists, psychologists, licensed social workers, or licensed mental health counselors

- Health maintenance organizations

- Community mental health centers

- Hospital psychiatry departments and outpatient clinics

- Mental health programs at universities or medical schools

- State hospital outpatient clinics

- Family services, social agencies, or clergy

- Peer support groups

- Private clinics and facilities

- Employee assistance programs

- Local medical and/or psychiatric societies

You can also check the phone book under "mental health," "health," "social services," "hotlines," or "physicians" for phone numbers and addresses. An emergency room doctor also can provide temporary help and can tell you where and how to get further help.

Chapter 43

Treating Anxiety Disorders

In general, anxiety disorders are treated with medication, specific types of psychotherapy, or both. Treatment choices depend on the problem and the person's preference. Before treatment begins, a doctor must conduct a careful diagnostic evaluation to determine whether a person's symptoms are caused by an anxiety disorder or a physical problem. If an anxiety disorder is diagnosed, the type of disorder or the combination of disorders that are present must be identified, as well as any coexisting conditions, such as depression or substance abuse. Sometimes alcoholism, depression, or other coexisting conditions have such a strong effect on the individual that treating the anxiety disorder must wait until the coexisting conditions are brought under control.

People with anxiety disorders who have already received treatment should tell their current doctor about that treatment in detail. If they received medication, they should tell their doctor what medication was used, what the dosage was at the beginning of treatment, whether the dosage was increased or decreased while they were under treatment, what side effects occurred, and whether the treatment helped them become less anxious. If they received psychotherapy, they should describe the type of therapy, how often they attended sessions, and whether the therapy was useful.

Excerpted from "Anxiety Disorders," by the National Institute of Mental Health (NIMH, www.nimh.nih.gov), part of the National Institutes of Health, 2009.

Often people believe that they have "failed" at treatment or that the treatment didn't work for them when, in fact, it was not given for an adequate length of time or was administered incorrectly. Sometimes people must try several different treatments or combinations of treatment before they find the one that works for them.

Medication

Medication will not cure anxiety disorders, but it can keep them under control while the person receives psychotherapy. Medication must be prescribed by physicians, usually psychiatrists, who can either offer psychotherapy themselves or work as a team with psychologists, social workers, or counselors who provide psychotherapy. The principal medications used for anxiety disorders are antidepressants, anti-anxiety drugs, and beta-blockers to control some of the physical symptoms. With proper treatment, many people with anxiety disorders can lead normal, fulfilling lives.

Antidepressants

Antidepressants were developed to treat depression but are also effective for anxiety disorders. Although these medications begin to alter brain chemistry after the very first dose, their full effect requires a series of changes to occur; it is usually about 4 to 6 weeks before symptoms start to fade. It is important to continue taking these medications long enough to let them work.

SSRIs: Some of the newest antidepressants are called selective serotonin reuptake inhibitors, or SSRIs. SSRIs alter the levels of the neurotransmitter serotonin in the brain, which, like other neurotransmitters, helps brain cells communicate with one another.

Fluoxetine (Prozac®), sertraline (Zoloft®), escitalopram (Lexapro®), paroxetine (Paxil®), and citalopram (Celexa®) are some of the SSRIs commonly prescribed for panic disorder, OCD, PTSD, and social phobia. SSRIs are also used to treat panic disorder when it occurs in combination with OCD, social phobia, or depression. Venlafaxine (Effexor®), a drug closely related to the SSRIs, is used to treat GAD. These medications are started at low doses and gradually increased until they have a beneficial effect.

SSRIs have fewer side effects than older antidepressants, but they sometimes produce slight nausea or jitters when people first start to take them. These symptoms fade with time. Some people also experience sexual dysfunction with SSRIs, which may be helped by adjusting the dosage or switching to another SSRI.

Tricyclics: Tricyclics are older than SSRIs and work as well as SSRIs for anxiety disorders other than OCD. They are also started at low doses that are gradually increased. They sometimes cause dizziness, drowsiness, dry mouth, and weight gain, which can usually be corrected by changing the dosage or switching to another tricyclic medication.

Tricyclics include imipramine (Tofranil®), which is prescribed for panic disorder and GAD, and clomipramine (Anafranil®), which is the only tricyclic antidepressant useful for treating OCD.

MAOIs: Monoamine oxidase inhibitors (MAOIs) are the oldest class of antidepressant medications. The MAOIs most commonly prescribed for anxiety disorders are phenelzine (Nardil®), followed by tranylcypromine (Parnate®), and isocarboxazid (Marplan®), which are useful in treating panic disorder and social phobia. People who take MAOIs cannot eat a variety of foods and beverages (including cheese and red wine) that contain tyramine or take certain medications, including some types of birth control pills, pain relievers (such as Advil®, Motrin®, or Tylenol®), cold and allergy medications, and herbal supplements; these substances can interact with MAOIs to cause dangerous increases in blood pressure. The development of a new MAOI skin patch may help lessen these risks. MAOIs can also react with SSRIs to produce a serious condition called "serotonin syndrome," which can cause confusion, hallucinations, increased sweating, muscle stiffness, seizures, changes in blood pressure or heart rhythm, and other potentially life-threatening conditions.

Anti-anxiety drugs: High-potency benzodiazepines combat anxiety and have few side effects other than drowsiness. Because people can get used to them and may need higher and higher doses to get the same effect, benzodiazepines are generally prescribed for short periods of time, especially for people who have abused drugs or alcohol and who become dependent on medication easily. One exception to this rule is people with panic disorder, who can take benzodiazepines for up to a year without harm.

Clonazepam (Klonopin®) is used for social phobia and GAD, lorazepam (Ativan®) is helpful for panic disorder, and alprazolam (Xanax®) is useful for both panic disorder and GAD.

Some people experience withdrawal symptoms if they stop taking benzodiazepines abruptly instead of tapering off, and anxiety can return once the medication is stopped. These potential problems have led some physicians to shy away from using these drugs or to use them in inadequate doses. Buspirone (BuSpar®), an azapirone, is a newer anti-anxiety medication used to treat GAD. Possible side effects include dizziness, headaches, and nausea. Unlike benzodiazepines, buspirone must be taken consistently for at least 2 weeks to achieve an anti-anxiety effect.

Beta-blockers: Beta-blockers, such as propranolol (Inderal®), which is used to treat heart conditions, can prevent the physical symptoms that accompany certain anxiety disorders, particularly social phobia. When a feared situation can be predicted (such as giving a speech), a doctor may prescribe a beta-blocker to keep physical symptoms of anxiety under control.

Psychotherapy

Psychotherapy involves talking with a trained mental health professional, such as a psychiatrist, psychologist, social worker, or counselor, to discover what caused an anxiety disorder and how to deal with its symptoms.

Cognitive-behavioral therapy (CBT) is very useful in treating anxiety disorders. The cognitive part helps people change the thinking patterns that support their fears, and the behavioral part helps people change the way they react to anxiety-provoking situations.

For example, CBT can help people with panic disorder learn that their panic attacks are not really heart attacks and help people with social phobia learn how to overcome the belief that others are always watching and judging them. When people are ready to confront their fears, they are shown how to use exposure techniques to desensitize themselves to situations that trigger their anxieties.

People with OCD who fear dirt and germs are encouraged to get their hands dirty and wait increasing amounts of time before washing them. The therapist helps the person cope with the anxiety that waiting produces; after the exercise has been repeated a number of times, the anxiety diminishes. People with social phobia may be encouraged to spend time in feared social situations without giving in to the temptation to flee and to make small social blunders and observe how people respond to them. Since the response is usually far less harsh than the person fears, these anxieties are lessened. People with PTSD may be supported through recalling their traumatic event in a safe situation, which helps reduce the fear it produces. CBT therapists also teach deep breathing and other types of exercises to relieve anxiety and encourage relaxation.

Exposure-based behavioral therapy has been used for many years to treat specific phobias. The person gradually encounters the object or situation that is feared, perhaps at first only through pictures or tapes, then later face to face. Often the therapist will accompany the person to a feared situation to provide support and guidance.

CBT is undertaken when people decide they are ready for it and with their permission and cooperation. To be effective, the therapy must be directed at the person's specific anxieties and must be tailored to his or her needs. There are no side effects other than the discomfort of temporarily increased anxiety.

CBT or behavioral therapy often lasts about 12 weeks. It may be conducted individually or with a group of people who have similar problems. Group therapy is particularly effective for social phobia. Often "homework" is assigned for participants to complete between sessions. There is some evidence that the benefits of CBT last longer than those of medication for people with panic disorder, and the same may be true for OCD, PTSD, and social phobia. If a disorder recurs at a later date, the same therapy can be used to treat it successfully a second time.

Medication can be combined with psychotherapy for specific anxiety disorders, and this is the best treatment approach for many people.

How to Get Help for Anxiety Disorders

If you think you have an anxiety disorder, the first person you should see is your family doctor. A physician can determine whether the symptoms that alarm you are due to an anxiety disorder, another medical condition, or both.

If an anxiety disorder is diagnosed, the next step is usually seeing a mental health professional. The practitioners who are most helpful with anxiety disorders are those who have training in cognitive-behavioral therapy and/or behavioral therapy, and who are open to using medication if it is needed.

You should feel comfortable talking with the mental health professional you choose. If you do not, you should seek help elsewhere. Once you find a mental health professional with whom you are comfortable, the two of you should work as a team and make a plan to treat your anxiety disorder together.

Remember that once you start on medication, it is important not to stop taking it abruptly. Certain drugs must be tapered off under the supervision of a doctor or bad reactions can occur. Make sure you talk to the doctor who prescribed your medication before you stop taking it. If you are having trouble with side effects, it's possible that they can be eliminated by adjusting how much medication you take and when you take it.

Most insurance plans, including health maintenance organizations (HMOs), will cover treatment for anxiety disorders. Check with your insurance company and find out. If you don't have insurance, the Health and Human Services division of your county government may offer mental health care at a public mental health center that charges people according to how much they are able to pay. If you are on public assistance, you may be able to get care through your state Medicaid plan.

Ways to Make Treatment More Effective

Many people with anxiety disorders benefit from joining a self-help or support group and sharing their problems and achievements with others. Internet chat rooms can also be useful in this regard, but any advice received over the internet should be used with caution, as internet acquaintances have usually never seen each other and false identities are common. Talking with a trusted friend or member of the clergy can also provide support, but it is not a substitute for care from a mental health professional.

Stress management techniques and meditation can help people with anxiety disorders calm themselves and may enhance the effects of therapy. There is preliminary evidence that aerobic exercise may have a calming effect. Since caffeine, certain illicit drugs, and even some over-the-counter cold medications can aggravate the symptoms of anxiety disorders, they should be avoided. Check with your physician or pharmacist before taking any additional medications.

The family is very important in the recovery of a person with an anxiety disorder. Ideally, the family should be supportive but not help perpetuate their loved one's symptoms. Family members should not trivialize the disorder or demand improvement without treatment. If your family is doing either of these things, you may want to show them this text so they can become educated allies and help you succeed in therapy.

Chapter 44

Treating Bipolar Disorder

To date, there is no cure for bipolar disorder. But proper treatment helps most people with bipolar disorder gain better control of their mood swings and related symptoms. This is also true for people with the most severe forms of the illness.

Because bipolar disorder is a lifelong and recurrent illness, people with the disorder need long-term treatment to maintain control of bipolar symptoms. An effective maintenance treatment plan includes medication and psychotherapy for preventing relapse and reducing symptom severity.

Medications

Bipolar disorder can be diagnosed and medications prescribed by people with an MD (doctor of medicine). Usually, bipolar medications are prescribed by a psychiatrist. In some states, clinical psychologists, psychiatric nurse practitioners, and advanced psychiatric nurse specialists can also prescribe medications. Check with your state's licensing agency to find out more.

Not everyone responds to medications in the same way. Several different medications may need to be tried before the best course of treatment is found.

Excerpted from "Bipolar Disorder," by the National Institute of Mental Health (NIMH, www.nimh.nih.gov), part of the National Institutes of Health, 2009.

Keeping a chart of daily mood symptoms, treatments, sleep patterns, and life events can help the doctor track and treat the illness most effectively. Sometimes this is called a daily life chart. If a person's symptoms change or if side effects become serious, the doctor may switch or add medications.

Mood stabilizing medications are usually the first choice to treat bipolar disorder. In general, people with bipolar disorder continue treatment with mood stabilizers for years. Except for lithium, many of these medications are anticonvulsants. Anticonvulsant medications are usually used to treat seizures, but they also help control moods.

Lithium (sometimes known as Eskalith or Lithobid) was the first mood-stabilizing medication approved by the U.S. Food and Drug Administration (FDA) in the 1970s for treatment of mania. It is often very effective in controlling symptoms of mania and preventing the recurrence of manic and depressive episodes.

Valproic acid or divalproex sodium (Depakote), approved by the FDA in 1995 for treating mania, is a popular alternative to lithium for bipolar disorder. It is generally as effective as lithium for treating bipolar disorder.

More recently, the anticonvulsant lamotrigine (Lamictal) received FDA approval for maintenance treatment of bipolar disorder.

Other anticonvulsant medications, including gabapentin (Neurontin), topiramate (Topamax), and oxcarbazepine (Trileptal) are sometimes prescribed. No large studies have shown that these medications are more effective than mood stabilizers.

Valproic acid, lamotrigine, and other anticonvulsant medications have an FDA warning. The warning states that their use may increase the risk of suicidal thoughts and behaviors. People taking anticonvulsant medications for bipolar or other illnesses should be closely monitored for new or worsening symptoms of depression, suicidal thoughts or behavior, or any unusual changes in mood or behavior. People taking these medications should not make any changes without talking to their health care professional.

People with bipolar disorder often have thyroid gland problems. Lithium treatment may also cause low thyroid levels in some people. Low thyroid function, called hypothyroidism, has been associated with rapid cycling in some people with bipolar disorder, especially women.

Because too much or too little thyroid hormone can lead to mood and energy changes, it is important to have a doctor check thyroid levels carefully. A person with bipolar disorder may need to take thyroid medication, in addition to medications for bipolar disorder, to keep thyroid levels balanced.

Valproic acid may increase levels of testosterone (a male hormone) in teenage girls and lead to polycystic ovary syndrome (PCOS) in women who begin taking the medication before age 20. PCOS causes a woman's eggs to develop into cysts, or fluid filled sacs that collect in the ovaries instead of being released by monthly periods. This condition can cause obesity, excess body hair, disruptions in the menstrual cycle, and other serious symptoms. Most of these symptoms will improve after stopping treatment with valproic acid. Young girls and women taking valproic acid should be monitored carefully by a doctor.

Atypical antipsychotic medications are sometimes used to treat symptoms of bipolar disorder. Often, these medications are taken with other medications. Atypical antipsychotic medications are called "atypical" to set them apart from earlier medications, which are called "conventional" or "first-generation" antipsychotics.

Olanzapine (Zyprexa), when given with an antidepressant medication, may help relieve symptoms of severe mania or psychosis. Olanzapine is also available in an injectable form, which quickly treats agitation associated with a manic or mixed episode. Olanzapine can be used for maintenance treatment of bipolar disorder as well, even when a person does not have psychotic symptoms. However, some studies show that people taking olanzapine may gain weight and have other side effects that can increase their risk for diabetes and heart disease. These side effects are more likely in people taking olanzapine when compared with people prescribed other atypical antipsychotics.

Aripiprazole (Abilify), like olanzapine, is approved for treatment of a manic or mixed episode. Aripiprazole is also used for maintenance treatment after a severe or sudden episode. As with olanzapine, aripiprazole also can be injected for urgent treatment of symptoms of manic or mixed episodes of bipolar disorder.

Quetiapine (Seroquel) relieves the symptoms of severe and sudden manic episodes. In that way, quetiapine is like almost all antipsychotics. In 2006, it became the first atypical antipsychotic to also receive FDA approval for the treatment of bipolar depressive episodes.

Risperidone (Risperdal) and ziprasidone (Geodon) are other atypical antipsychotics that may also be prescribed for controlling manic or mixed episodes.

Antidepressant medications are sometimes used to treat symptoms of depression in bipolar disorder. People with bipolar disorder who take antidepressants often take a mood stabilizer, too. Doctors usually require this because taking only an antidepressant can increase a person's risk of switching to mania or hypomania, or of developing

451

rapid cycling symptoms. To prevent this switch, doctors who prescribe antidepressants for treating bipolar disorder also usually require the person to take a mood-stabilizing medication at the same time.

Recently, a large-scale, NIMH-funded study showed that for many people, adding an antidepressant to a mood stabilizer is no more effective in treating the depression than using only a mood stabilizer.

Fluoxetine (Prozac), paroxetine (Paxil), sertraline (Zoloft), and bupropion (Wellbutrin) are examples of antidepressants that may be prescribed to treat symptoms of bipolar depression.

Some medications are better at treating one type of bipolar symptoms than another. For example, lamotrigine (Lamictal) seems to be helpful in controlling depressive symptoms of bipolar disorder.

Side Effects of These Medications

Before starting a new medication, people with bipolar disorder should talk to their doctor about the possible risks and benefits.

The psychiatrist prescribing the medication or pharmacist can also answer questions about side effects. Over the last decade, treatments have improved, and some medications now have fewer or more tolerable side effects than earlier treatments. However, everyone responds differently to medications. In some cases, side effects may not appear until a person has taken a medication for some time.

If the person with bipolar disorder develops any severe side effects from a medication, he or she should talk to the doctor who prescribed it as soon as possible. The doctor may change the dose or prescribe a different medication. People being treated for bipolar disorder should not stop taking a medication without talking to a doctor first. Suddenly stopping a medication may lead to "rebound," or worsening of bipolar disorder symptoms. Other uncomfortable or potentially dangerous withdrawal effects are also possible.

Psychotherapy

In addition to medication, psychotherapy, or "talk" therapy, can be an effective treatment for bipolar disorder. It can provide support, education, and guidance to people with bipolar disorder and their families. Some psychotherapy treatments used to treat bipolar disorder include the following:

1. Cognitive behavioral therapy (CBT) helps people with bipolar disorder learn to change harmful or negative thought patterns and behaviors.

2. Family-focused therapy includes family members. It helps enhance family coping strategies, such as recognizing new episodes early and helping their loved one. This therapy also improves communication and problem-solving.

3. Interpersonal and social rhythm therapy helps people with bipolar disorder improve their relationships with others and manage their daily routines. Regular daily routines and sleep schedules may help protect against manic episodes.

4. Psychoeducation teaches people with bipolar disorder about the illness and its treatment. This treatment helps people recognize signs of relapse so they can seek treatment early, before a full-blown episode occurs. Usually done in a group, psychoeducation may also be helpful for family members and caregivers.

A licensed psychologist, social worker, or counselor typically provides these therapies. This mental health professional often works with the psychiatrist to track progress. The number, frequency, and type of sessions should be based on the treatment needs of each person. As with medication, following the doctor's instructions for any psychotherapy will provide the greatest benefit.

Other Treatments

Electroconvulsive therapy (ECT)—For cases in which medication and/or psychotherapy does not work, electroconvulsive therapy (ECT) may be useful. ECT, formerly known as "shock therapy," once had a bad reputation. But in recent years, it has greatly improved and can provide relief for people with severe bipolar disorder who have not been able to feel better with other treatments.

Before ECT is administered, a patient takes a muscle relaxant and is put under brief anesthesia. He or she does not consciously feel the electrical impulse administered in ECT. On average, ECT treatments last from 30–90 seconds.

People who have ECT usually recover after 5–15 minutes and are able to go home the same day.

Sometimes ECT is used for bipolar symptoms when other medical conditions, including pregnancy, make the use of medications too risky. ECT is a highly effective treatment for severely depressive, manic, or mixed episodes, but is generally not a first-line treatment.

ECT may cause some short-term side effects, including confusion, disorientation, and memory loss. But these side effects typically clear soon after treatment. People with bipolar disorder should discuss possible benefits and risks of ECT with an experienced doctor.

Sleep medications—People with bipolar disorder who have trouble sleeping usually sleep better after getting treatment for bipolar disorder. However, if sleeplessness does not improve, the doctor may suggest a change in medications. If the problems still continue, the doctor may prescribe sedatives or other sleep medications.

People with bipolar disorder should tell their doctor about all prescription drugs, over-the-counter medications, or supplements they are taking. Certain medications and supplements taken together may cause unwanted or dangerous effects.

Herbal supplements—In general, there is not much research about herbal or natural supplements. Little is known about their effects on bipolar disorder. An herb called St. John's wort (*Hypericum perforatum*), often marketed as a natural antidepressant, may cause a switch to mania in some people with bipolar disorder. St. John's wort can also make other medications less effective, including some antidepressant and anticonvulsant medications. Scientists are also researching omega-3 fatty acids (most commonly found in fish oil) to measure their usefulness for long-term treatment of bipolar disorder. Study results have been mixed. It is important to talk with a doctor before taking any herbal or natural supplements because of the serious risk of interactions with other medications.

Getting Help

If you are unsure where to go for help, ask your family doctor. Others who can help are listed below.

- Mental health specialists, such as psychiatrists, psychologists, social workers, or mental health counselors

- Health maintenance organizations

- Community mental health centers

- Hospital psychiatry departments and outpatient clinics

- Mental health programs at universities or medical schools

- State hospital outpatient clinics

- Family services, social agencies, or clergy

- Peer support groups

- Private clinics and facilities
- Employee assistance programs
- Local medical and/or psychiatric societies

You can also check the phone book under "mental health," "health," "social services," "hotlines," or "physicians" for phone numbers and addresses. An emergency room doctor can also provide temporary help and can tell you where and how to get further help.

Chapter 45

Coping with Traumatic Stress Reactions

Coping with Traumatic Stress Reactions

When trauma survivors take direct action to cope with their stress reactions, they put themselves in a position of power. Active coping with the trauma makes you begin to feel less helpless.

Active coping means accepting the impact of trauma on your life and taking direct action to improve things. Active coping occurs even when there is no crisis. Active coping is a way of responding to everyday life. It is a habit that must be made stronger.

Know That Recovery Is a Process

Following exposure to a trauma most people experience stress reactions. Understand that recovering from the trauma is a process and takes time. Knowing this will help you feel more in control. Remember the following:

- Having an ongoing response to the trauma is normal.

- Recovery is an ongoing, daily process. It happens little by little. It is not a matter of being cured all of a sudden.

This chapter contains text from "Coping with Traumatic Stress Reactions," by the National Center for Posttraumatic Stress Disorder (NCPTSD, www.ptsd .va.gov), part of the Veterans Administration, June 15, 2010, and excerpted from "Coping with Crime Victimization," by the Federal Bureau of Investigation (FBI, www.fbi.gov). The FBI document is undated; reviewed by David A. Cooke, MD, FACP, November 22, 2010.

- Healing doesn't mean forgetting traumatic events. It doesn't mean you will have no pain or bad feelings when thinking about them.

- Healing may mean fewer symptoms and symptoms that bother you less.

- Healing means more confidence that you will be able to cope with your memories and symptoms. You will be better able to manage your feelings.

Positive Coping Actions

Certain actions can help to reduce your distressing symptoms and make things better. Plus, these actions can result in changes that last into the future. The following text contains some positive coping methods.

Learn about trauma and PTSD: It is useful for trauma survivors to learn more about common reactions to trauma and about post-traumatic stress disorder (PTSD). Find out what is normal. Find out what the signs are that you may need assistance from others. When you learn that the symptoms of PTSD are common, you realize that you are not alone, weak, or crazy. It helps to know your problems are shared by hundreds of thousands of others. When you seek treatment and begin to understand your response to trauma, you will be better able to cope with the symptoms of PTSD.

Talk to others for support: When survivors talk about their problems with others, something helpful often results. It is important not to isolate yourself. Instead make efforts to be with others. Of course, you must choose your support people with care. You must also ask them clearly for what you need. With support from others, you may feel less alone and more understood. You may also get concrete help with a problem you have.

Practice relaxation methods: Try some different ways to relax, including the following:

- Muscle relaxation exercises
- Breathing exercises
- Meditation
- Swimming, stretching, and yoga
- Prayer

- Listening to quiet music
- Spending time in nature

While relaxation techniques can be helpful, in a few people they can sometimes increase distress at first. This can happen when you focus attention on disturbing physical sensations and you reduce contact with the outside world. Most often, continuing with relaxation in small amounts that you can handle will help reduce negative reactions. You may want to try mixing relaxation in with music, walking, or other activities.

Distract yourself with positive activities: Pleasant recreational or work activities help distract a person from his or her memories and reactions. For example, art has been a way for many trauma survivors to express their feelings in a positive, creative way. Pleasant activities can improve your mood, limit the harm caused by PTSD, and help you rebuild your life.

Talking to your doctor or a counselor about trauma and PTSD: Part of taking care of yourself means using the helping resources around you. If efforts at coping don't seem to work, you may become fearful or depressed. If your PTSD symptoms don't begin to go away or get worse over time, it is important to reach out and call a counselor who can help turn things around. Your family doctor can also refer you to a specialist who can treat PTSD. Talk to your doctor about your trauma and your PTSD symptoms. That way, he or she can take care of your health better.

Many with PTSD have found treatment with medicines to be helpful for some symptoms. By taking medicines, some survivors of trauma are able to improve their sleep, anxiety, irritability, and anger. It can also reduce urges to drink or use drugs.

Coping with the Symptoms of PTSD

Here are some direct ways to cope with these specific PTSD symptoms.

Unwanted distressing memories, images, or thoughts:

- Remind yourself that they are just that, memories.
- Remind yourself that it's natural to have some memories of the trauma(s).
- Talk about them to someone you trust.

- Remember that, although reminders of trauma can feel overwhelming, they often lessen with time.

Sudden feelings of anxiety or panic: Traumatic stress reactions often include feeling your heart pounding and feeling lightheaded or spacey. This is usually caused by rapid breathing. If this happens, remember the following:

- These reactions are not dangerous. If you had them while exercising, they most likely would not worry you.

- These feelings often come with scary thoughts that are not true. For example, you may think, "I'm going to die," "I'm having a heart attack," or "I will lose control." It is the scary thoughts that make these reactions so upsetting.

- Slowing down your breathing may help.

- The sensations will pass soon and then you can go on with what you were doing.

Each time you respond in these positive ways to your anxiety or panic, you will be working toward making it happen less often. Practice will make it easier to cope.

Feeling like the trauma is happening again (flashbacks):

- Keep your eyes open. Look around you and notice where you are.

- Talk to yourself. Remind yourself where you are, what year you're in, and that you are safe. The trauma happened in the past, and you are in the present.

- Get up and move around. Have a drink of water and wash your hands.

- Call someone you trust and tell them what is happening.

- Remind yourself that this is a common response after trauma.

- Tell your counselor or doctor about the flashback(s).

Dreams and nightmares related to the trauma:

- If you wake up from a nightmare in a panic, remind yourself that you are reacting to a dream. Having the dream is why you are in a panic, not because there is real danger now.

- You may want to get up out of bed, regroup, and orient yourself to the here and now.

- Engage in a pleasant, calming activity. For example, listen to some soothing music.
- Talk to someone if possible.
- Talk to your doctor about your nightmares. Certain medicines can be helpful.

Difficulty falling or staying asleep:

- Keep to a regular bedtime schedule.
- Avoid heavy exercise for the few hours just before going to bed.
- Avoid using your sleeping area for anything other than sleeping or sex.
- Avoid alcohol, tobacco, and caffeine. These harm your ability to sleep.
- Do not lie in bed thinking or worrying. Get up and enjoy something soothing or pleasant. Read a calming book, drink a glass of warm milk or herbal tea, or do a quiet hobby.

Irritability, anger, and rage:

- Take a time out to cool off or think things over. Walk away from the situation.
- Get in the habit of exercise daily. Exercise reduces body tension and relieves stress.
- Remember that staying angry doesn't work. It actually increases your stress and can cause health problems.
- Talk to your counselor or doctor about your anger. Take classes in how to manage anger.
- If you blow up at family members or friends, find time as soon as you can to talk to them about it. Let them know how you feel and what you are doing to cope with your reactions.

Difficulty concentrating or staying focused:

- Slow down. Give yourself time to focus on what it is you need to learn or do.
- Write things down. Making "to do" lists may be helpful.
- Break tasks down into small do-able chunks.
- Plan a realistic number of events or tasks for each day.

- You may be depressed. Many people who are depressed have trouble concentrating. Again, this is something you can discuss with your counselor, doctor, or someone close to you.

Trouble feeling or expressing positive emotions:

- Remember that this is a common reaction to trauma. You are not doing this on purpose. You should not feel guilty for something you do not want to happen and cannot control.

- Make sure to keep taking part in activities that you enjoy or used to enjoy. Even if you don't think you will enjoy something, once you get into it, you may well start having feelings of pleasure.

- Take steps to let your loved ones know that you care. You can express your caring in little ways: write a card, leave a small gift, or phone someone and say hello.

A Final Word

Try using all these ways of coping to find which ones are helpful to you. Then practice them. Like other skills, they work better with practice.

Coping with Crime Victimization

Anyone can become a victim of a crime. Being a victim of a crime can be a very difficult and stressful experience. While most people are naturally resilient and over time will find ways to cope and adjust, there can be a wide range of after effects to a trauma. One person may experience many of the effects, a few, or none at all. Not everyone has the same reaction. In some people the reaction may be delayed days, weeks, or even months. Some victims may think they are going crazy, when they are having a normal reaction to an abnormal event.

Getting back to normal can be a difficult process after a personal experience of this kind, especially for victims of violent crime and families of murder victims. Learning to understand and feel more at ease with the intense feelings can help victims better cope with what happened.

Victims may need to seek help from friends, family, a member of the clergy, a counselor, or a victim assistance professional.

Potential Effects of Trauma

Some people who have been victims of crime may experience some of these symptoms. Seek medical advice if the symptoms persist.

Physical symptoms include the following:

- Nausea
- Tremors
- Chills or sweating
- Lack of coordination
- Heart palpitations or chest pains
- High blood pressure
- Headaches
- Sleep disturbances
- Stomach upset
- Dizziness
- Loss of appetite
- Startled responses

Emotional symptoms include the following:

- Anxiety
- Fear
- Guilt
- Grief
- Depression
- Sadness
- Anger
- Irritability
- Numbness
- Feeling lost, abandoned, and isolated
- Wanting to withdraw or hide

Mental symptoms include the following:

- Slowed thinking
- Confusion
- Disorientation

- Memory problems

- Intrusive memories or flashbacks

- Nightmares

- Inability to concentrate

- Difficulty in making decisions

Tips for Coping

These are some ideas that may help you cope with the trauma or loss:

- Find someone to talk with about how you feel and what you are going through. Keep the phone number of a good friend nearby to call when you feel overwhelmed or feel panicked.

- Allow yourself to feel the pain. It will not last forever.

- Keep a journal.

- Spend time with others, but make time to spend time alone.

- Take care of your mind and body. Rest, sleep, and eat regular, healthy meals.

- Re-establish a normal routine as soon as possible, but don't over-do.

- Make daily decisions, which will help to bring back a feeling of control over your life.

- Exercise, though not excessively and alternate with periods of relaxation.

- Undertake daily tasks with care. Accidents are more likely to happen after severe stress.

- Recall the things that helped you cope during trying times and loss in the past and think about the things that give you hope. Turn to them on bad days.

These are things to avoid:

- Be careful about using alcohol or drugs to relieve emotional pain.

- Becoming addicted not only postpones healing, but also creates new problems.

- Make daily decisions, but avoid making life-changing decisions in the immediate aftermath, since judgment may be temporarily impaired.

- Don't blame yourself—it wasn't your fault.

- Your emotions need to be expressed. Try not to bottle them up.

For some victims and families of victims, life is forever changed. Life may feel empty and hollow. Life doesn't mean what it used to. Part of coping and adjusting is redefining the future. What seemed important before may not be important now. Many victims find new meaning in their lives as a result of their experience. It is important to remember that emotional pain is not endless and that it will eventually ease. It is impossible to undo what has happened but life can be good again in time.

For family and friends of a victim of crime:

- Listen carefully.

- Spend time with the victim.

- Offer your assistance, even if they haven't asked for help.

- Help with everyday tasks like cleaning, cooking, caring for the family, and minding the children.

- Give them private time.

- Don't take their anger or other feelings personally.

- Don't tell them they are "lucky it wasn't worse"—traumatized people are not consoled by such statements.

- Tell them that you are sorry such an event has occurred to them and you want to understand and help them.

Chapter 46

PTSD Treatment

Today, there are good treatments available for posttraumatic stress disorder (PTSD). When you have PTSD, dealing with the past can be hard. Instead of telling others how you feel, you may keep your feelings bottled up. Yet talking with a therapist can help you get better.

Cognitive-behavioral therapy (CBT) is one type of counseling. It appears to be the most effective type of counseling for PTSD. There are different types of cognitive behavioral therapies such as cognitive therapy and exposure therapy. Two forms of cognitive-behavioral therapy include cognitive processing therapy (CPT) and prolonged exposure therapy (PE).

There is also a similar kind of therapy called eye movement desensitization and reprocessing (EMDR) that is used for PTSD. Medications have also been shown to be effective. A type of drug known as a selective serotonin reuptake inhibitor (SSRI), which is also used for depression, is effective for PTSD.

Cognitive Behavioral Therapy

What is cognitive therapy?

In cognitive therapy, your therapist helps you understand and change how you think about your trauma and its aftermath. Your

---

From "Treatment of PTSD," by Jessica Hamblen, PhD, by the National Center for Posttraumatic Stress Disorder (NCPTSD, www.ptsd.va.gov), part of the Veterans Administration, January 2010.

goal is to understand how certain thoughts about your trauma cause you stress and make your symptoms worse.

You will learn to identify thoughts about the world and yourself that are making you feel afraid or upset. With the help of your therapist, you will learn to replace these thoughts with more accurate and less distressing thoughts. You also learn ways to cope with feelings such as anger, guilt, and fear.

After a traumatic event, you might blame yourself for things you couldn't have changed. For example, a soldier may feel guilty about decisions he or she had to make during war. Cognitive therapy, a type of CBT, helps you understand that the traumatic event you lived through was not your fault.

What is exposure therapy?

In exposure therapy your goal is to have less fear about your memories. It is based on the idea that people learn to fear thoughts, feelings, and situations that remind them of a past traumatic event.

By talking about your trauma repeatedly with a therapist, you'll learn to get control of your thoughts and feelings about the trauma. You'll learn that you do not have to be afraid of your memories. This may be hard at first. It might seem strange to think about stressful things on purpose. But you'll feel less overwhelmed over time.

With the help of your therapist, you can change how you react to the stressful memories. Talking in a place where you feel secure makes this easier.

You may focus on memories that are less upsetting before talking about worse ones. This is called "desensitization," and it allows you to deal with bad memories a little bit at a time. Your therapist also may ask you to remember a lot of bad memories at once. This is called "flooding," and it helps you learn not to feel overwhelmed.

You also may practice different ways to relax when you're having a stressful memory. Breathing exercises are sometimes used for this.

What is EMDR?

Eye movement desensitization and reprocessing (EMDR) is another type of therapy for PTSD. Like other kinds of counseling, it can help change how you react to memories of your trauma.

While thinking of or talking about your memories, you'll focus on other stimuli like eye movements, hand taps, and sounds. For example, your therapist will move his or her hand near your face, and you'll follow this movement with your eyes.

Experts are still learning how EMDR works. Studies have shown that it may help you have fewer PTSD symptoms. But research also suggests that the eye movements are not a necessary part of the treatment.

What about medication for PTSD?

Selective serotonin reuptake inhibitors (SSRIs) are a type of antidepressant medicine. These can help you feel less sad and worried. They appear to be helpful, and for some people they are very effective. SSRIs include citalopram (Celexa), fluoxetine (such as Prozac), paroxetine (Paxil), and sertraline (Zoloft).

Chemicals in your brain affect the way you feel. When you have anxiety or depression you may not have enough of a chemical called serotonin. SSRIs raise the level of serotonin in your brain.

There are other medications that have been used with some success. Talk to your doctor about which medications are right for you.

Other Types of Treatment

In addition to CBT and SSRIs, some other kinds of counseling may be helpful in your recovery from PTSD.

What is group therapy?

Many people want to talk about their trauma with others who have had similar experiences.

In group therapy, you talk with a group of people who also have been through a trauma and who have PTSD. Sharing your story with others may help you feel more comfortable talking about your trauma. This can help you cope with your symptoms, memories, and other parts of your life.

Group therapy helps you build relationships with others who understand what you've been through. You learn to deal with emotions such as shame, guilt, anger, rage, and fear. Sharing with the group also can help you build self-confidence and trust. You'll learn to focus on your present life, rather than feeling overwhelmed by the past.

What is brief psychodynamic psychotherapy?

In this type of therapy, you learn ways of dealing with emotional conflicts caused by your trauma. This therapy helps you understand how your past affects the way you feel now.

Your therapist can help you do the following:

- Identify what triggers your stressful memories and other symptoms
- Find ways to cope with intense feelings about the past
- Become more aware of your thoughts and feelings, so you can change your reactions to them
- Raise your self-esteem

What is family therapy?

PTSD can impact your whole family. Your kids or your partner may not understand why you get angry sometimes, or why you're under so much stress. They may feel scared, guilty, or even angry about your condition.

Family therapy is a type of counseling that involves your whole family. A therapist helps you and your family communicate, maintain good relationships, and cope with tough emotions. Your family can learn more about PTSD and how it is treated.

In family therapy, each person can express his or her fears and concerns. It's important to be honest about your feelings and to listen to others. You can talk about your PTSD symptoms and what triggers them. You also can discuss the important parts of your treatment and recovery. By doing this, your family will be better prepared to help you.

You may consider having individual therapy for your PTSD symptoms and family therapy to help you with your relationships.

Length of Treatment

Some people are in treatment for PTSD for 3 to 6 months. If you have other mental health problems as well as PTSD, treatment for PTSD may last for 1 to 2 years or longer.

PTSD and Other Disorders

It is very common to have PTSD at the same time as another mental health problem. Depression, alcohol or substance abuse problems, panic disorder, and other anxiety disorders often occur along with PTSD. In many cases, the PTSD treatments described in the preceding text will also help with the other disorders. The best treatment results occur when both PTSD and the other problems are treated together rather than one after the other.

Finding a Therapist

There are many ways to find a therapist. You can start by asking friends and family if they can recommend anyone. Be aware, though, that someone else's therapist might not have skills in treating trauma survivors.

Another way to locate a therapist is to make some phone calls. When you call, say that you are trying to find a provider who specializes in helping trauma survivors.

- Contact your local mental health agency or family doctor.

- Call your state psychological association.

- Call the psychology department at a local college.

- Call the National Center for Victims of Crime's toll-free information and referral service at 800-FYI-CALL (394-2255). This service uses agencies from across the country that support crime victims.

- If you work for a large company, call the human resources office to see if they make referrals.

- If you are a member of a Health Maintenance Organization (HMO), call to find out about mental health services. Some mental health services are listed in the phone book. In the blue Government pages, look in the "County Government Offices" section. In that section, look for "Health Services (Dept. of)" or "Department of Health Services." Then in that section, look under "Mental Health."

- In the yellow pages, therapists are listed under "counseling," "psychologists," "social workers," "psychotherapists," "social and human services," or "mental health."

- Information can also be found using the internet. You may find a list of therapists in your area. Some lists include the therapists' areas of practice. Listed below are some suggested websites:

  - Center for Mental Health Services Locator (http://mentalhealth .samhsa.gov/databases): This services locator is on the Substance Abuse and Mental Health Services Administration (SAMHSA) website.

  - Anxiety Disorders Association of America (www.adaa.org): This organization offers a referral network.

- ABCT Find a Therapist Service (www.abct.org): The Association for Advancement of Behavioral and Cognitive Therapies (ABCT, formerly AABT) maintains a database of therapists.

- Sidran (www.sidran.org): This site offers a referral list of therapists, as well as a fact sheet on how to choose a therapist for PTSD and dissociative disorders.

Your health insurance may pay for mental health services. Also, some services are available at low cost according to your ability to pay.

Choosing a Therapist

There are a many things to consider in choosing a therapist. Some practical issues are location, cost, and what insurance the therapist accepts. Other issues include the therapist's background, training, and the way he or she works with people.

Some people meet with a few therapists before deciding which one to work with. Most, however, try to see someone known in their area. Then they go with that person unless a problem occurs. Either way, here is a list of questions you may want to ask a possible therapist.

- What is your education? Are you licensed? How many years have you been practicing?

- What are your special areas of practice?

- Have you ever worked with people who have been through trauma? Do you have any special training in PTSD treatment?

- What kinds of PTSD treatments do you use? Have they been proven effective for dealing with my kind of problem or issue?

- What are your fees? (Fees are usually based on a 45-minute to 50-minute session.) Do you have any discounted fees? How much therapy would you recommend?

- What types of insurance do you accept? Do you file insurance claims? Do you contract with any managed care organizations? Do you accept Medicare or Medicaid insurance?

Goals for Therapy

When you begin therapy, you and your therapist should decide together what goals you hope to reach in therapy. Not every person with

PTSD will have the same treatment goals. For instance, not all people with PTSD are focused on reducing their symptoms.

Some people want to learn the best way to live with their symptoms and how to cope with other problems associated with PTSD. Perhaps you want to feel less guilt and sadness? Perhaps you would like to work on improving your relationships at work, or communication issues with your friends and family.

Your therapist should help you decide which of these goals seems most important to you, and he or she should discuss with you which goals might take a long time to achieve.

Your therapist should give you a good explanation for the therapy. You should understand why your therapist is choosing a specific treatment for you, how long they expect the therapy to last, and how they see if it is working. The two of you should agree at the beginning that this plan makes sense for you and what you will do if it does not seem to be working. If you have any questions about the treatment your therapist should be able to answer them.

You should feel comfortable with your therapist and feel you are working as a team to tackle your problems. It can be difficult to talk about painful situations in your life, or about traumatic experiences that you have had. Feelings that emerge during therapy can be scary and challenging. Talking with your therapist about the process of therapy, and about your hopes and fears in regard to therapy, will help make therapy successful.

If you do not like your therapist or feel that the therapist is not helping you, it might be helpful to talk with another professional. In most cases, you should tell your therapist that you are seeking a second opinion.

Chapter 47

Helping a Family Member with PTSD

When someone has posttraumatic stress disorder (PTSD), it can change family life. The person with PTSD may act differently and get angry easily. He or she may not want to do things you used to enjoy together.

You may feel scared and frustrated about the changes you see in your loved one. You also may feel angry about what's happening to your family, or wonder if things will ever go back to the way they were. These feelings and worries are common in people who have a family member with PTSD.

It is important to learn about PTSD so you can understand why it happened, how it is treated, and what you can do to help. But you also need to take care of yourself. Changes in family life are stressful, and taking care of yourself will make it easier to cope.

How can I help?

You may feel helpless, but there are many things you can do. Nobody expects you to have all the answers.

Here are ways you can help:

- Learn as much as you can about PTSD. Knowing how PTSD affects people may help you understand what your family member is going through. The more you know, the better you and your family can handle PTSD.

From "Helping a Family Member Who Has PTSD," by the National Center for Posttraumatic Stress Disorder (NCPTSD, www.ptsd.va.gov), part of the Veterans Administration, June 15, 2010.

- Offer to go to doctor visits with your family member. You can help keep track of medicine and therapy, and you can be there for support.

- Tell your loved one you want to listen and that you also understand if he or she doesn't feel like talking.

- Plan family activities together, like having dinner or going to a movie.

- Take a walk, go for a bike ride, or do some other physical activity together. Exercise is important for health and helps clear your mind.

- Encourage contact with family and close friends. A support system will help your family member get through difficult changes and stressful times.

Your family member may not want your help. If this happens, keep in mind that withdrawal can be a symptom of PTSD. A person who withdraws may not feel like talking, taking part in group activities, or being around other people. Give your loved one space, but tell him or her that you will always be ready to help.

How can I deal with anger or violent behavior?

Your family member may feel angry about many things. Anger is a normal reaction to trauma, but it can hurt relationships and make it hard to think clearly. Anger also can be frightening.

If anger leads to violent behavior or abuse, it's dangerous. Go to a safe place and call for help right away. Make sure children are in a safe place as well.

It's hard to talk to someone who is angry. One thing you can do is set up a time-out system. This helps you find a way to talk even while angry. Here's one way to do this.

- Agree that either of you can call a time-out at any time.

- Agree that when someone calls a time-out, the discussion must stop right then.

- Decide on a signal you will use to call a time-out. The signal can be a word that you say or a hand signal.

- Agree to tell each other where you will be and what you will be doing during the time-out. Tell each other what time you will come back.

While you are taking a time-out, don't focus on how angry you feel. Instead, think calmly about how you will talk things over and solve the problem.

After you come back, try these strategies:

- Take turns talking about solutions to the problem. Listen without interrupting.

- Use statements starting with "I," such as "I think" or "I feel." Using "you" statements can sound accusing.

- Be open to each other's ideas. Don't criticize each other.

- Focus on things you both think will work. It's likely you will both have good ideas.

- Together, agree which solutions you will use.

How can I communicate better?

You and your family may have trouble talking about feelings, worries, and everyday problems. Here are some ways to communicate better:

- Be clear and to the point.

- Be positive. Blame and negative talk won't help the situation.

- Be a good listener. Don't argue or interrupt. Repeat what you hear to make sure you understand, and ask questions if you need to know more.

- Put your feelings into words. Your loved one may not know you are sad or frustrated unless you are clear about your feelings.

- Help your family member put feelings into words. Ask, "Are you feeling angry? Sad? Worried?"

- Ask how you can help.

- Don't give advice unless you are asked.

If your family is having a lot of trouble talking things over, consider trying family therapy. Family therapy is a type of counseling that involves your whole family. A therapist helps you and your family communicate, maintain good relationships, and cope with tough emotions.

During therapy, each person can talk about how a problem is affecting the family. Family therapy can help family members understand and cope with PTSD.

Your health professional or a religious or social services organization can help you find a family therapist who specializes in PTSD.

How can I take care of myself?

Helping a person with PTSD can be hard on you. You may have your own feelings of fear and anger about the trauma. You may feel guilty because you wish your family member would just forget his or her problems and get on with life. You may feel confused or frustrated because your loved one has changed, and you may worry that your family life will never get back to normal.

All of this can drain you. It can affect your health and make it hard for you to help your loved one. If you're not careful, you may get sick yourself, become depressed, or burn out and stop helping your loved one.

To help yourself, you need to take care of yourself and have other people help you. Try the following:

- Don't feel guilty or feel that you have to know it all. Remind yourself that nobody has all the answers. It's normal to feel helpless at times.

- Don't feel bad if things change slowly. You cannot change anyone. People have to change themselves.

- Take care of your physical and mental health. If you feel yourself getting sick or often feel sad and hopeless, see your doctor.

- Don't give up your outside life. Make time for activities and hobbies you enjoy. Continue to see your friends.

- Take time to be by yourself. Find a quiet place to gather your thoughts and "recharge."

- Get regular exercise, even just a few minutes a day. Exercise is a healthy way to deal with stress.

- Eat healthy foods. When you are busy, it may seem easier to eat fast food than to prepare healthy meals. But healthy foods will give you more energy to carry you through the day.

- Remember the good things. It's easy to get weighed down by worry and stress. But don't forget to see and celebrate the good things that happen to you and your family.

How can I get help?

During difficult times, it is important to have people in your life who you can depend on. These people are your support network. They can help you with everyday jobs, like taking a child to school, or by giving you love and understanding.

You may get support from the following:

- Family members
- Friends, coworkers, and neighbors
- Members of your religious or spiritual group
- Support groups
- Doctors and other health professionals

Chapter 48

Preventing Suicide

Suicide is a major, preventable public health problem. In 2007, it was the 10th leading cause of death in the United States, accounting for 34,598 deaths. The overall rate was 11.3 suicide deaths per 100,000 people. An estimated 11 attempted suicides occur per every suicide death.

Suicidal behavior is complex. Some risk factors vary with age, gender, or ethnic group and may occur in combination or change over time.

What are the risk factors for suicide?

Research shows that risk factors for suicide include the following:

- Depression and other mental disorders or a substance abuse disorder, often in combination with other mental disorders (More than 90 percent of people who die by suicide have these risk factors.)

- Prior suicide attempt

- Family history of mental disorder or substance abuse

- Family history of suicide

- Family violence, including physical or sexual abuse

Excerpted from "Suicide in the U.S.: Statistics and Prevention," by the National Institute of Mental Health (NIMH, www.nimh.nih.gov), part of the National Institutes of Health, July 27, 2009.

- Firearms in the home, the method used in more than half of suicides

- Incarceration

- Exposure to the suicidal behavior of others, such as family members, peers, or media figures

However, suicide and suicidal behavior are not normal responses to stress; many people have these risk factors, but are not suicidal. Research also shows that the risk for suicide is associated with changes in brain chemicals called neurotransmitters, including serotonin. Decreased levels of serotonin have been found in people with depression, impulsive disorders, and a history of suicide attempts, and in the brains of suicide victims.

Are women or men at higher risk?

Suicide was the seventh leading cause of death for males and the 15th leading cause of death for females in 2007.

Almost four times as many males as females die by suicide.

Firearms, suffocation, and poison are by far the most common methods of suicide, overall. However, men and women differ in the method used, as shown in Table 48.1.

Table 48.1. Differences in Methods of Suicide Used by Men and Women

Suicide by:	Males (%)	Females (%)
Firearms	56	30
Suffocation	24	21
Poisoning	13	40

Is suicide common among children and young people?

In 2007, suicide was the third leading cause of death for young people ages 15 to 24. Of every 100,000 young people in each age group, the following number died by suicide:

- Children ages 10 to 14—0.9 per 100,000

- Adolescents ages 15 to 19—6.9 per 100,000

- Young adults ages 20 to 24—12.7 per 100,000

As in the general population, young people were much more likely to use firearms, suffocation, and poisoning than other methods of suicide, overall. However, while adolescents and young adults were more likely to use firearms than suffocation, children were dramatically more likely to use suffocation.

There were also gender differences in suicide among young people, as follows:

- Nearly five times as many males as females ages 15 to 19 died by suicide.

- Just under six times as many males as females ages 20 to 24 died by suicide.

Are older adults at risk?

Older Americans are disproportionately likely to die by suicide.

- Of every 100,000 people ages 65 and older, 14.3 died by suicide in 2007. This figure is higher than the national average of 11.3 suicides per 100,000 people in the general population.

- Non-Hispanic white men age 85 or older had an even higher rate, with 47 suicide deaths per 100,000.

Are some ethnic groups or races at higher risk?

Of every 100,000 people in each of the following ethnic/racial groups below, the following number died by suicide in 2007.

- Highest rates:
  - American Indian and Alaska Natives—14.3 per 100,000
  - Non-Hispanic Whites—13.5 per 100,000
- Lowest rates:
  - Hispanics—6.0 per 100,000
  - Non-Hispanic Blacks—5.1 per 100,000
  - Asian and Pacific Islanders—6.2 per 100,000

What are some risk factors for nonfatal suicide attempts?

- As noted, an estimated 11 nonfatal suicide attempts occur per every suicide death. Men and the elderly are more likely to have fatal attempts than are women and youth.

- Risk factors for nonfatal suicide attempts by adults include depression and other mental disorders, alcohol and other substance abuse, and separation or divorce.

- Risk factors for attempted suicide by youth include depression, alcohol or other drug use disorder, physical or sexual abuse, and disruptive behavior.

- Most suicide attempts are expressions of extreme distress, not harmless bids for attention. A person who appears suicidal should not be left alone and needs immediate mental health treatment.

What can be done to prevent suicide?

Research helps determine which factors can be modified to help prevent suicide and which interventions are appropriate for specific groups of people. Before being put into practice, prevention programs should be tested through research to determine their safety and effectiveness. For example, because research has shown that mental and substance abuse disorders are major risk factors for suicide, many programs also focus on treating these disorders as well as addressing suicide risk directly.

Studies showed that a type of psychotherapy called cognitive therapy reduced the rate of repeated suicide attempts by 50 percent during a year of follow-up. A previous suicide attempt is among the strongest predictors of subsequent suicide, and cognitive therapy helps suicide attempters consider alternative actions when thoughts of self-harm arise.

Specific kinds of psychotherapy may be helpful for specific groups of people. For example, a treatment called dialectical behavior therapy reduced suicide attempts by half, compared with other kinds of therapy, in people with borderline personality disorder (a serious disorder of emotion regulation).

The medication clozapine is approved by the Food and Drug Administration for suicide prevention in people with schizophrenia. Other promising medications and psychosocial treatments for suicidal people are being tested.

Since research shows that older adults and women who die by suicide are likely to have seen a primary care provider in the year before death, improving primary care providers' ability to recognize and treat risk factors may help prevent suicide among these groups. Improving outreach to men at risk is a major challenge in need of investigation.

What should I do if I think someone is suicidal?

If you think someone is suicidal, do not leave him or her alone. Try to get the person to seek immediate help from his or her doctor or the nearest hospital emergency room, or call 911. Eliminate access to firearms or other potential tools for suicide, including unsupervised access to medications.

If you are in a crisis and need help right away: Call this toll-free number, available 24 hours a day, every day: 800-273-TALK (8255). You will reach the National Suicide Prevention Lifeline, a service available to anyone. You may call for yourself or for someone you care about. All calls are confidential.

Part Five

Stress Management

Chapter 49

The Basics of Preventing and Managing Stress

Preventing and managing stress can help lower your risk of serious health problems like heart disease, high blood pressure, and depression. You can prevent or lessen stress by planning ahead and preparing for stressful events.

Some stress is hard to avoid. You can find ways to manage stress by doing the following:

- Noticing when you feel stressed
- Taking time to relax
- Getting active and eating healthy
- Talking to friends and family

What are the signs of stress?

When people are under stress, they may feel the following:

- Worried
- Irritable
- Depressed
- Unable to focus

Excerpted from "Manage Stress: The Basics," by the National Health Information Center (www.healthfinder.gov), May 13, 2010.

Stress also affects the body. Physical signs of stress include the following:

- Headaches
- Back pain
- Problems sleeping
- Upset stomach
- Weight gain or loss
- Tense muscles
- Frequent or more serious colds

Use this online tool to better understand your stress (http://www .mentalhealthamerica.net/llw/stressquiz.html).

What causes stress?

Stress is often caused by some type of change. Even positive changes, like marriage or a job promotion, can be stressful. Stress can be short-term or long-term.

Common causes of short-term stress include the following:

- Too much to do and not much time
- Lots of little problems in the same day (like a traffic jam or running late)
- Getting lost
- Having an argument

Common causes of longer-term stress include the following:

- Divorce or problems in a marriage
- Death of a loved one
- Illness
- Caring for someone who is sick
- Problems at work
- Money problems

What are the benefits of managing stress?

Managing stress can help you do the following:

- Sleep better
- Control your weight
- Get sick less often and heal faster
- Lessen neck and back pain
- Be in a better mood
- Get along better with family and friends

How can I feel less stressed?

Being prepared and in control of your situation will help you feel less stress.

Follow these tips for preventing and managing stress.

- **Plan your time.** Think ahead about how you are going to use your time. Write a to-do list and decide which tasks are the most important. Be realistic about how long each thing will take.

- **Prepare yourself.** Prepare ahead of time for stressful events like a job interview or a hard conversation with a loved one.

  - Picture the event in your mind.
  - Stay positive.
  - Imagine what the room will look like and what you will say.
  - Have a back-up plan.

- **Relax with deep breathing.**

- **Relax your muscles.** Stress causes tension in your muscles. Try stretching or taking a hot shower to help you relax.

- **Get active.** Physical activity can help prevent and manage stress. It can also help relax your muscles and improve your mood. Aim for 2 hours and 30 minutes a week of moderate aerobic activity, like walking fast or biking. Be sure to exercise for at least 10 minutes at a time. Do strengthening activities (like sit-ups or lifting weights) at least 2 days a week.

- **Eat healthy.** Give your body plenty of energy by eating fruits, vegetables, and protein.

- **Drink alcohol only in moderation.** Don't use alcohol and drugs to manage your stress. If you choose to drink, drink only in moderation. This means no more than one drink a day for women or two drinks a day for men.

491

- **Talk to friends and family.** Tell your friends and family if you are feeling stressed. They may be able to help.

- **Get help if you need it.** Stress is a normal part of life. But if your stress doesn't go away or keeps getting worse, you may need help. Over time, stress can lead to serious problems like depression, posttraumatic stress disorder (PTSD), or anxiety. If you are feeling down or hopeless, talk to a doctor about depression. If you are feeling anxious, find out how to get help for anxiety. A mental health professional (like a psychologist or social worker) can help treat these conditions with talk therapy (called psychotherapy) or medicines.

Lots of people need help dealing with stress—it's nothing to be ashamed of.

Chapter 50

Developing Resilience: The Most Important Defense against Stress

Resilience

Resilience is the ability to:

- bounce back;
- take on difficult challenges and still find meaning in life;
- respond positively to difficult situations;
- rise above adversity;
- cope when things look bleak;
- tap into hope;
- transform unfavorable situations into wisdom, insight, and compassion; and
- endure.

Resilience refers to the ability of an individual, family, organization, or community to cope with adversity and adapt to challenges or change. It is an ongoing process that requires time and effort and engages people in taking a number of steps to enhance their response

This chapter contains text excerpted from "Resilience," by the Substance Abuse and Mental Health Services Administration (SAMHSA, mentalhealth.samhsa.gov), part of the U.S. Department of Health and Human Services, 2009, and excerpted from "Resilience Factor Low in Depression, Protects Mice From Stress," by the National Institutes of Health (NIH, www.nih.gov), May 16, 2010.

to adverse circumstances. Resilience implies that after an event, a person or community may not only be able to cope and recover, but also change to reflect different priorities arising from the experience and prepare for the next stressful situation.

- Resilience is the most important defense people have against stress.

- It is important to build and foster resilience to be ready for future challenges.

- Resilience will enable the development of a reservoir of internal resources to draw upon during stressful situations.

Research has shown that resilience is ordinary, not extraordinary, and that people regularly demonstrate being resilient.

- Resilience is not a trait that people either have or do not have.

- Resilience involves behaviors, thoughts, and actions that can be learned and developed in anyone.

- Resilience is tremendously influenced by a person's environment.

Resilience changes over time. It fluctuates depending on how much a person nurtures internal resources or coping strategies. Some people are more resilient in work life, while others exhibit more resilience in their personal relationships. People can build resilience and promote the foundations of resilience in any aspect of life they choose.

What is individual or personal resilience?

Individual resilience is a person's ability to positively cope after failures, setbacks, and losses. Developing resilience is a personal journey. Individuals do not react the same way to traumatic or stressful life events. An approach to building resilience that works for one person might not work for another. People use varying strategies to build their resilience. Because resilience can be learned, it can be strengthened. Personal resilience is related to many factors including individual health and well-being, individual aspects, life history and experience, and social support.

Along with the factors listed above, there are several attributes that have been correlated with building and promoting resilience. The American Psychological Association reports the following attributes regarding resilience:

- The capacity to make and carry out realistic plans
- Communication and problem-solving skills
- A positive or optimistic view of life
- Confidence in personal strengths and abilities
- The capacity to manage strong feelings, emotions, and impulses

What is family resilience?

Family resilience is the coping process in the family as a functional unit. Crisis events and persistent stressors affect the whole family, posing risks not only for individual dysfunction, but also for relational conflict and family breakdown. Family processes mediate the impact of stress for all of its members and relationships, and the protective processes in place foster resilience by buffering stress and facilitating adaptation to current and future events. Following are the three key factors in family resilience:

- Family belief systems foster resilience by making meaning in adversity, creating a sense of coherence, and providing a positive outlook.

- Family organization promotes resilience by facilitating flexibility, capacity to adapt, connectedness and cohesion, emotional and structural bonding, and accessibility to resources.

- Family communication enhances resilience by engaging clear communication, open and emotional expressions, trust and collaborative problem solving, and conflict management.

How does culture influence resilience?

Cultural resilience refers to a culture's capacity to maintain and develop cultural identity and critical cultural knowledge and practices. Along with an entire culture fostering resilience, the interaction of culture and resilience for an individual also is important. An individual's culture will have an impact on how the person communicates feelings and copes with adversity. Cultural parameters are often embedded deep in an individual. A person's cultural background may influence one deeply in how one responds to different stressors. Assimilation could be a factor in cultural resilience, as it could be a positive way for a person to manage his/her environment. However, assimilation could create conflict between generations, so it could be seen as positive or negative depending on the individual and culture. Because of this, coping strategies are going to be different. With growing cultural diversity, the public has greater access to a number of different approaches to building resilience. It is something that can be built using approaches that make sense within each culture and tailored to each individual.

How is personal resilience built?

Developing resilience is a personal journey. People do not react the same way to traumatic events. Some ways to build resilience include the following actions:

- Making connections with others
- Looking for opportunities for self-discovery
- Nurturing a positive view of self
- Accepting that change is a part of living
- Taking decisive actions
- Learning from the past

The ability to be flexible is a great skill to obtain and facilitates resilience growth. Getting help when it is needed is crucial to building resilience. It is important to try to obtain information on resilience from books or other publications, self-help or support groups, and online resources.

What can be done to promote family resilience?

Developing family resilience, like individual resilience, is different for every family. The important idea to keep in mind is that an underlying stronghold of family resilience is cohesion, a sense of belonging, and communication. It is important for a family to feel that when their world is unstable they have each other. This sense of bonding and trust is what fuels a family's ability to be resilient. Families that learn how to cope with challenges and meet individual needs are more resilient to stress and crisis. Healthy families solve problems with cooperation, creative brainstorming, openness to others, and emphasis on the role of social support and connectedness (versus isolation) in family resiliency. Resilience is exercised when family members demonstrate behaviors such as confidence, hard work, cooperation, and forgiveness. These are factors that help families withstand stressors throughout the family life cycle.

Developing resilience is a personal journey. All people do not react the same to traumatic and stressful life events. An approach to building resilience that works for one person might not work for another. People use varying strategies.

Resilience involves maintaining flexibility and balance in life during stressful circumstances and traumatic events. Being resilient does not mean that a person does not experience difficulty or distress. Emotional pain and sadness are common in people who have suffered major adversity or trauma in their lives.

Stress can be dealt with proactively by building resilience to prepare for stressful circumstances, while learning how to recognize symptoms of stress. Fostering resilience or the ability to bounce back from a stressful situation is a proactive mechanism to managing stress.

Resilience Factor Low in Depression, Protects Mice From Stress

Scientists have discovered a mechanism that helps to explain resilience to stress, vulnerability to depression, and how antidepressants work. The new findings, in the reward circuit of mouse and human brains, have spurred a high tech dragnet for compounds that boost the action of a key gene regulator there, called deltaFosB.

A molecular main power switch—called a transcription factor—inside neurons, deltaFosB turns multiple genes on and off, triggering the production of proteins that perform a cell's activities.

"We found that triggering deltaFosB in the reward circuit's hub is both necessary and sufficient for resilience; it protects mice from developing a depression-like syndrome following chronic social stress," explained Eric Nestler, MD, of the Mount Sinai School of Medicine, who led the research team, which was funded by the National Institute of Health's National Institute of Mental Health (NIMH).

"Antidepressants can reverse this social withdrawal syndrome by boosting deltaFosB. Moreover, deltaFosB is conspicuously depleted in brains of people who suffered from depression. Thus, induction of this protein is a positive adaptation that helps us cope with stress, so we're hoping to find ways to tweak it pharmacologically," added Nestler, who also directs the ongoing compound screening project.

Nestler and colleagues reported the findings that inspired the hunt online May 16, 2010 in the journal *Nature Neuroscience*.

"This search for small molecules that augment the actions of deltaFosB holds promise for development of a new class of resilience-boosting treatments for depression," said NIMH director Thomas R. Insel. "The project, funded under the American Recovery and Reinvestment Act of 2009, is a stunning example of how leads from rodent experiments can be quickly followed up and translated into potential clinical applications."

DeltaFosB is more active in the reward hub, called the nucleus accumbens, than in any other part of the brain. Chronic use of drugs of abuse—or even natural rewards like excess food, sex, or exercise—can gradually induce increasing levels of this transcription factor in the reward hub. Nestler and colleagues have shown that this increase in deltaFosB can eventually lead to lasting changes in cells that increase rewarding responses to such stimuli, hijacking an individual's reward circuitry—addiction.

The new study in mice and human postmortem brains confirms that the same reward circuitry is similarly corrupted (though to a lesser degree than with drugs of abuse) in depression via effects of stress on deltaFosB.

Depressed patients often lack motivation and the ability to experience reward or pleasure—and depression and addiction often go together. Indeed, mice susceptible to the depression-like syndrome show enhanced responses to drugs of abuse, the researchers have found.

But the similarity ends there. For, while an uptick in deltaFosB promotes addiction, the researchers have determined that it also protects against depression-inducing stress. It turns out that stress triggers the transcription factor in a different mix of nucleus accumbens cell types—working through different receptor types—than do drugs and natural rewards, likely accounting for the opposite effects.

The researchers explored the workings of deltaFosB in a mouse model of depression.

Much as depressed patients characteristically withdraw from social contact, mice exposed to aggression by a different dominant mouse daily for 10 days often become socially defeated; they vigorously avoid other mice, even weeks later. Key findings in the brain's reward hub include the following:

- The amount of deltaFosB induced by the stress determined susceptibility or resilience to developing the depression-like behaviors. It counteracted the strong tendency to learn an association, or generalize, the aversive experience to all mice.

- Induction of deltaFosB was required for the antidepressant fluoxetine (Prozac) to reverse the stress-induced depression-like syndrome.

- Prolonged isolation from environmental stimuli reduced levels of deltaFosB, increasing vulnerability to depression-like behaviors.

- Among numerous target genes regulated by deltaFosB, a gene that makes a protein called the AMPA [alpha-amino-3-hydroxy-5-methyl-4-isoxazolepropionic acid] receptor is critical for resilience—or protecting mice from the depression-like syndrome. The AMPA receptor is a protein on neurons that boosts the cell's activity when it binds to the chemical messenger glutamate.

- Increased activity of neurons triggered by heightened sensitivity of AMPA receptors to glutamate increased susceptibility to stress-induced depression-like behavior.

- Induction of deltaFosB calmed the neurons and protected against depression by suppressing AMPA receptors' sensitivity to glutamate.

- Postmortem brain tissue of depressed patients contained only about half as much deltaFosB as that of controls, suggesting that poor response to antidepressant treatment may be traceable, in part, to weak induction of the transcription factor.

Reduced deltaFosB in the reward hub likely helps to account for the impaired motivation and reward behavior seen in depression, said Nestler. Boosting it appears to enable an individual to pursue goal-directed behavior despite stress.

The high-tech screening for molecules that boost DeltaFosB, supported by the Recovery Act grant, could lead to development of medications that would help people cope with chronic stress. The molecules could also potentially be used as telltale tracers in brain imaging to chart depressed patients' treatment progress by reflecting changes in deltaFosB, said Nestler.

Source: DeltaFosB in brain reward circuits mediates resilience to stress and antidepressant responses. Vialou V, Robison AJ, LaPlant QC, Covington III HE, Dietz DM, Ohnishi YN, Mouson E, Rush III AJ, Watts EL, Wallace DL, Iniguez SD, Ohnishi YH, Steiner MA, Warren B, Krishnan V, Neve RL, Ghose S, Beron O, Tamminga CA, Nestler EJ. *NatNeurosci.* Epub 2010 May 16.

Chapter 51

How to Say No:
Asserting Yourself Can
Reduce Stress

Saying No

Many people have great difficulty saying no to others. Even people who are quite assertive in other situations may find themselves saying yes to things that they really don't want to do. Now saying yes to something you don't really want to do can be appropriate in some situations. For example in a work situation if your boss asks you to do something and you don't really want to it wouldn't be appropriate to practice your assertiveness skills and say no. You may get the sack. What we are talking about here is if you find yourself saying yes in other situations. For example, if a friend asks you to do something which is a real inconvenience for you and you say yes, or if you find yourself volunteering for all sorts of jobs to the point that you are over-loaded.

The Effects of Not Being Able to Say No

If you say yes when you really mean no, resentment and anger can build up towards the person you have said yes to, even though they have done nothing wrong. You can also become increasingly frustrated and disappointed with yourself. And if you are taking on more that you can cope with, you can become over-worked and highly stressed. In the long term not being assertive in this way can decrease your self-esteem and lead to depression and anxiety.

At the other end of the spectrum some people are able to say no but do so in an aggressive manner without consideration or respect for the other person. This may result in people disliking you or being angry and resentful.

Neither of these situations is good assertive communication.

Unhelpful Beliefs: Why Is It Hard to Say No?

We are all born assertive. Anyone who has spent any time around a toddler knows that they have no trouble saying no. However as we grow older we learn from our environment and our experience that it is not always appropriate to say no. We can end up with a number of unhelpful beliefs about saying no that make it difficult for us to use this word. Some of these beliefs are listed in the following text. See if any apply to you:

Unhelpful Beliefs about Saying No

- Saying no is rude and aggressive.
- Saying no is unkind, uncaring, and selfish.
- Saying no will hurt and upset others and make them feel rejected.
- If I say no to somebody they won't like me anymore.
- Other's needs are more important than mine.
- I should always try and please others and be helpful.
- Saying no over little things is small minded and petty.

See if you can think of any others.

Changing Your Thinking: More Helpful Beliefs about Saying No

The unhelpful thoughts in the preceding text are not facts. They are just thoughts or opinions that we have learned. Each of them can be replaced by a more helpful thought or opinion about saying no. In the following text we have listed some of these:

- Other people have the right to ask and I have the right to refuse.
- When you say no you are refusing a request, not rejecting a person.

- When we say yes to one thing we are actually saying no to something else. We always have a choice and we are constantly making choices.

- People who have difficulty saying no usually overestimate the difficulty that the other person will have in accepting the refusal. We are not trusting that they can cope with hearing no. By expressing our feelings openly and honestly, it actually liberates the other person to express their feelings. By saying no to somebody it allows them to say no to your requests while still being able to ask for further requests.

See if you can think of any others; try and come up with alternatives for your own unhelpful beliefs about saying no.

Remember that sometimes to come up with a new thought you will need to do a Thought Diary or a Behavioral Experiment. These techniques can be applied to your beliefs about saying no as they can to any unassertive belief. You may not immediately believe these new beliefs or thoughts. This is normal. You have been thinking the old thoughts probably for a long time so it will take some time for these new thoughts to become as automatic as the old ones were. Keep practicing and you will get there.

Changing Your Behavior: How to Say No

So you have now worked through some of your unhelpful thoughts about saying no but you may still not be really sure how to go about it. There are some basic principles you can apply when you want to say no. These are:

1. Be straightforward and honest but not rude so that you can make the point effectively.

2. As a rule keep it brief.

3. Tell the person if you are finding it difficult.

4. Be polite—say something like "thank you for asking . . ."

5. Speak slowly with warmth otherwise no may sound abrupt.

6. Don't apologize and give elaborate reasons for saying no. It is your right to say no if you don't want to do things.

7. Remember that it is better in the long run to be truthful than breed resentment and bitterness within yourself.

8. When saying no take responsibility for it. Don't blame or make excuses. Change "I can't" to "I don't want to."

Ways of Saying No

There are also a number of ways you can say no. Some of these are more appropriate in particular situations. Trevor Powell describes six ways of saying no. These are described in the following text:

1. **The direct no.** When someone asks you to do something you don't want to do, just say no. The aim is to say no without apologizing. The other person has the problem but you do not have to allow him or her to pass it on to you. This technique can be quite forceful and can be effective with salespeople.

2. **The reflecting no.** This technique involves acknowledging the content and feeling of the request, then adding your assertive refusal at the end. For example "I know you want to talk to me about organizing the annual department review, but I can't do lunch today." Or "I know you're looking forward to a walk this afternoon but I can't come."

3. **The reasoned no.** In this technique you give a very brief and genuine reason for why you are saying no. For example "I can't have lunch with you because I have a report that needs to be finished by tomorrow."

4. **The rain check no.** This is not a definite no. It is a way of saying no to the request at the present moment but leaves room for saying yes in the future. Only use it if you genuinely want to meet the request. For example "I can't have lunch with you today, but I could make it sometime next week."

5. **The inquiring no.** As with the rain check no this is not a definite no. It is a way of opening up the request to see if there is another way it could be met. For example "Is there any other time you'd like to go?"

6. **The broken record no.** This can be used in a wide range of situations. You just repeat the simple statement of refusal over and over again. No explanation, just repeat it. It is particularly good for persistent requests. For example:

   Dave: No, I can't have lunch with you.

   Kate: Oh, please, it won't take long.

   Dave: No, I can't have lunch with you.

Kate: Oh, go on, I'll pay.

Dave: No, I can't have lunch with you.

Summary

- Saying no can be difficult for a lot of people.

- As toddlers we don't have any trouble saying no but as we learn from our environment and our experience we can start to have trouble with it.

- Saying yes when we really mean no can lead to stress, resentment, and anger.

- If we have trouble saying no it is often because we hold a number of unhelpful beliefs about saying no. These can be changed by realizing that they are just opinions and not facts. You can also use a Thought Diary or behavioral experiments to change your unhelpful beliefs.

- There are some guidelines to saying no. These include keeping it brief, being clear, and being honest.

- There are some different ways to say no. These include the direct no, the inquiring no, the rain check no, the reasoned no, and the broken record no.

About This Text

Contributors

Fiona Michel (MPsych[1] PhD[2])
Centre for Clinical Interventions

Dr. Anthea Fursland (PhD[2])
Centre for Clinical Interventions

Note: [1]Master of Psychology (Clinical Psychology), [2]Doctor of Philosophy (Clinical Psychology)

We would also like to thank Paula Nathan for her contribution to these modules.

Background

The concepts and strategies in the modules have been developed from evidence based psychological practice, primarily Cognitive-Behavior Therapy (CBT). CBT is a type of psychotherapy that is based on the theory that unhelpful negative emotions and behaviors are strongly influenced by problematic cognitions (thoughts). This can be found in the following:

Beck, A.T., Rush, A. J., Shaw, B.F., & Emery, G. (1979). *Cognitive Therapy of Depression.* New York: Guildford.

Clark, D. M. (1986). A cognitive approach to panic. *Behaviour Research and Therapy,* 24, 461–470.

Clark, D. M. & Wells, A. (1995). A cognitive model of social phobia. In R. Heimberg, M. Liebowitz, D.A.

References

These are some of the professional references used to create this module:

Alberti, R. & Emmons, M. (1974). *Your Perfect Right.* Impact, San Luis Obispo, California.

Back, R & Back, K. (1986). *Assertiveness at Work—A Practical Guide to Handling Awkward Situations.* McGraw Hill, London.

Davis, M., Eshelman, E.R. & McKay, M. (2000). *The Relaxation and Stress Reduction Workbook, Fourth Edition.* Oakland, CA: New Harbinger Publications.

Gambrill, E.D. & Richey, L.A. (1975). An assertion inventory for use in assessment and research. *Behavior Therapy,* 6, 550–561.

Holland, S. & Ward, C. (1980). *Assertiveness: A Practical Approach.* Winslow Press, Biccstcr.

Linehan, M. (1979). Structured cognitive-behavioural treatment of assertion problems. In Kendall & Hollon, *Cognitive Behavioural Interventions* (pp205–240). Academic Press.

McKay, M & Fanning, P. (1995). *Self esteem, third edition.* St. Martin's Paperbacks, California.

Powell, T. (2000). *The Mental Health Handbook (revised edition).* Speechmark Publishing, Wesleyan University Press.

Smith, M.J. (1975). *When I Say No I Feel Guilty.* Dial, New York.

Wolpe, J. (1973). *The Practice of Behavior Therapy.* Pergamon Press, New York.

This text forms part of:

Michel, F. (2008). *Assert Yourself.* Perth, Western Australia: Centre for Clinical Interventions. ISBN: 0-9757995-5-X. Created: November, 2008.

Chapter 52

Healthy Habits
to Combat Stress

Chapter Contents

Section 52.1

Your Guide to Healthy Sleep

Excerpted from "Your Guide to Healthy Sleep," by the National Heart, Lung, and Blood Institute (NHLBI, www.nhlbi.nih.gov), part of the National Institutes of Health, November 2005. Reviewed by David A. Cooke, MD, FACP, November 22, 2010.

Think of everything you do during your day. Try to guess which activity is so important you should devote one third of your time to doing it. Probably the first things that come to mind are working, spending time with your family, or pursuing leisure activities. But there's something else you should be doing about one third of your time—sleeping.

Many people view sleep as merely a "down time" when their brain shuts off and their body rests. In a rush to meet work, school, family, or household responsibilities, people cut back on their sleep, thinking it won't be a problem, because all of these other activities seem much more important. But research reveals that a number of vital tasks carried out during sleep help to maintain good health and enable people to function at their best.

While you sleep, your brain is hard at work forming the pathways necessary for learning and creating memories and new insights. Without enough sleep, you can't focus and pay attention or respond quickly. A lack of sleep may even cause mood problems. In addition, growing evidence shows that a chronic lack of sleep increases the risk for developing obesity, diabetes, cardiovascular disease, and infections.

Despite the mounting support for the notion that adequate sleep, like adequate nutrition and physical activity, is vital to our well-being, people are sleeping less. The nonstop "24/7" nature of the world today encourages longer or nighttime work hours and offers continual access to entertainment and other activities. To keep up, people cut back on sleep. A common myth is that people can learn to get by on little sleep (such as less than 6 hours a night) with no adverse consequences. Research suggests, however, that adults need at least 7–8 hours of sleep each night to be well rested. Indeed, in 1910, most people slept 9 hours a night. But recent surveys show the average adult now sleeps less than 7 hours a night, and more than one third of adults report daytime sleepiness so severe that it interferes with work and social functioning at least a few days each month. As many as 70 million Americans may be affected by chronic sleep loss or sleep disorders, at an annual cost of $16 billion in health care expenses and $50 billion in lost productivity.

What Is Sleep?

Sleep was long considered just a uniform block of time when you are not awake. Thanks to sleep studies done over the past several decades, it is now known that sleep has distinct stages that cycle throughout the night in predictable patterns. How well rested you are and how well you function depend not just on your total sleep time but on how much of the various stages of sleep you get each night.

Your brain stays active throughout sleep, and each stage of sleep is linked to a distinctive pattern of electrical activity known as brain waves.

Sleep is divided into two basic types: rapid eye movement (REM) sleep and non-REM sleep (with four different stages). Typically, sleep begins with non-REM sleep. In stage 1 non-REM sleep, you sleep lightly and can be awakened easily by noises or other disturbances. During this first stage of sleep, your eyes move slowly, and your muscle activity slows. You then enter stage 2 non-REM sleep, when your eye movements stop. Your brain shows a distinctive pattern of slower brain waves with occasional bursts of rapid waves.

When you progress into stage 3 non-REM sleep, your brain waves become even slower, although they are still punctuated by smaller, faster waves. By stage 4 non-REM sleep, the brain produces extremely slow waves almost exclusively. Stages 3 and 4 are considered deep sleep, during which it is very difficult to be awakened. Children who wet the bed or sleep walk tend to do so during stages 3 or 4 of non-REM sleep. Deep sleep is considered the "restorative" part of sleep that is necessary for feeling well rested and energetic during the day.

During REM sleep, your eyes move rapidly in various directions, even though your eyelids remain closed. Your breathing also becomes more rapid, irregular, and shallow, and your heart rate and blood pressure increase. Dreaming typically occurs during REM sleep. During this type of sleep, your arm and leg muscles are temporarily paralyzed so that you cannot "act out" any dreams that you may be having.

The first period of REM sleep you experience usually occurs about an hour to an hour and a half after falling asleep. After that, the sleep stages repeat themselves continuously while you sleep. As the night progresses, REM sleep time becomes longer, while time spent in non-REM sleep stages 3 and 4 becomes shorter. By morning, nearly all your sleep time is spent in stages 1 and 2 of non-REM sleep and in REM sleep. If REM sleep is disrupted during one night, REM sleep time is typically longer than normal in subsequent nights until you catch up. Overall, almost one half your total sleep time is spent in stages 1 and 2 non-REM sleep and about one fifth each in deep sleep (stages 3 and 4 of non-REM sleep) and REM sleep. In contrast, infants spend half or more of their total sleep time in REM sleep. Gradually, as they mature, the percentage of total sleep time they spend in REM progressively decreases to reach the one-fifth level typical of later childhood and adulthood.

Why people dream and why REM sleep is so important are not well understood. It is known that REM sleep stimulates the brain regions used in learning and the laying down of memories. Animal studies suggest that dreams may reflect the brain's sorting and selectively storing important new information acquired during wake time. While this information is processed, the brain might revisit scenes from the day while pulling up older memories. This process may explain why childhood memories can be interspersed with more recent events during dreams. Studies show, however, that other stages of sleep besides REM are also needed to form the pathways in the brain that enable us to learn and remember.

What Makes You Sleep?

Although you may put off going to sleep in order to squeeze more activities into your day, eventually your need for sleep becomes overwhelming and you are forced to get some sleep. This daily drive for sleep appears to be due, in part, to a compound known as adenosine. This natural chemical builds up in your blood as time awake increases. While you sleep, your body breaks down the adenosine. Thus, this molecule may be what your body uses to keep track of lost sleep and to trigger sleep when needed. An accumulation of adenosine and other factors might explain why, after several nights of less than optimal amounts of sleep, you build up a sleep debt that you must make up by sleeping longer than normal. Because of such built-in molecular feedback, you can't adapt to getting less sleep than your body needs. Eventually, a lack of sleep catches up with you.

The time of day when you feel sleepy and go to sleep is also governed by your internal "biological clock" and environmental cues—the most important being light and darkness. Your biological clock is actually a tiny bundle of cells in your brain that responds to light signals received through your eyes. When darkness falls, the biological clock triggers the production of the hormone melatonin. This hormone makes you feel drowsy as it continues to increase during the night. Because of your biological clock, you naturally feel the most sleepy between midnight and 7 a.m. You may also feel a second and milder daily "low" in the midafternoon between 1 p.m. and 4 p.m. At that time, another rise occurs in melatonin production and might make you feel sleepy.

Your biological clock makes you the most alert during daylight hours and the most drowsy in the early morning hours. Consequently, most people do their best work during the day. Our 24/7 society, however, demands that some people work at night. Nearly one quarter of all workers work shifts that are not during the daytime, and more than two thirds of these workers have problem sleepiness and/or difficulty sleeping. Because their work schedules are at odds with powerful sleep-regulating cues like sunlight, night shift workers often find themselves drowsy at work, and they have difficulty falling or staying asleep during the daylight hours when their work schedules require them to sleep.

The fatigue experienced by night shift workers can be dangerous. Major industrial accidents—such as the Three Mile Island and Chernobyl nuclear power plant accidents and the Exxon Valdez oil spill—have been caused, in part, by mistakes made by overly tired workers on the night shift or an extended shift.

Night shift workers also are at greater risk of being in car crashes when they drive home from work. One study found that one fifth of night shift workers had a car crash or a near miss in the preceding year because of sleepiness on the drive home from work. Night shift workers are also more likely to have physical problems, such as heart disease, digestive disturbances, and infertility, as well as emotional problems. All of these problems may be related, at least in part, to the workers' chronic sleepiness.

Other factors can also influence your need for sleep, including your immune system's production of cellular hormones called cytokines. These compounds are made in large quantities in response to certain infectious diseases or chronic inflammation and may prompt you to sleep more than usual. The extra sleep may help you conserve the resources needed to fight the infection. Recent studies confirm that being well rested improves the body's responses to infection.

People are creatures of habit, and one of the hardest habits to break is the natural wake and sleep cycle. A number of physiological factors conspire to help you sleep and wake up at the same times each day. Consequently, you may have a hard time adjusting when you travel across time zones. The light cues outside and the clocks in your new location may tell you it is 8 a.m. and you should be active, but your body is telling you it is more like 4 a.m. and you should sleep. The end result is jet lag—sleepiness during the day, difficulty falling or staying asleep at night, poor concentration, confusion, nausea, and general malaise and irritability.

What Does Sleep Do for You?

A number of tasks vital to health and quality of life are linked to sleep, and these tasks are impaired when you are sleep deprived.

Learning, Memory, and Mood

Students who have trouble grasping new information or learning new skills are often advised to "sleep on it," and that advice seems well founded. Recent studies reveal that people can learn a task better if they are well rested. They also can remember better what they learned if they get a good night's sleep after learning the task than if they are sleep deprived. Volunteers had to sleep at least 6 hours to show improvement in learning, and the amount of improvement was directly tied to how much time they slept. In other words, volunteers who slept 8 hours outperformed those who slept only 6 or 7 hours. Other studies suggest that all the benefits of training for mentally challenging tasks are maximized after a good night's sleep, rather than immediately following the training or after sleeping for a short period overnight.

Many well-known artists and scientists claim to have had creative insights while they slept. Mary Shelley, for example, said the idea for her novel *Frankenstein* came to her in a dream. Although it has not been shown that dreaming is the driving force behind innovation, one study suggests that sleep is needed for creative problem solving. In that study, volunteers were asked to perform a memory task and then were tested 8 hours later. Those who were allowed to sleep for 8 hours immediately after receiving the task and before being tested were much more likely to find a creative way of simplifying the task and improving their performance compared to those who were awake the entire 8 hours before being tested.

Exactly what happens during sleep to improve our learning, memory, and insight isn't known. Experts suspect, however, that while people

512

sleep, they form or reinforce the pathways of brain cells needed to perform these tasks. This process may explain why sleep is needed for proper brain development in infants.

Not only is a good night's sleep required to form new learning and memory pathways in the brain, but sleep is also necessary for those pathways to work up to speed. Several studies show that lack of sleep causes thinking processes to slow down. Lack of sleep also makes it harder to focus and pay attention. Lack of sleep can make you more easily confused. Studies also find a lack of sleep leads to faulty decision making and more risk taking. A lack of sleep slows down your reaction time, which is particularly significant to driving and other tasks that require quick response. When people who lack sleep are tested by using a driving simulator, they perform just as poorly as people who are drunk. The bottom line is: Not getting a good night's sleep can be dangerous!

Even if you don't have a mentally or physically challenging day ahead of you, you should still get enough sleep to put yourself in a good mood. Most people report being irritable, if not downright unhappy, when they lack sleep. People who chronically suffer from a lack of sleep, either because they do not spend enough time in bed or because they have an untreated sleep disorder, are at greater risk of developing depression. One group of people who usually don't get enough sleep is mothers of newborns. Some experts think depression after childbirth (postpartum blues) is caused, in part, by a lack of sleep.

Your Heart

Sleep gives your heart and vascular system a much-needed rest. During non-REM sleep, your heart rate and blood pressure progressively slow as you enter deeper sleep. During REM sleep, your heart rate and blood pressure have boosted spikes of activity. Overall, however, sleep reduces your heart rate and blood pressure by about 10 percent.

If you don't get enough sleep, this nightly dip in blood pressure, which appears to be important for good cardiovascular health, may not occur. According to several studies, if your blood pressure does not dip during sleep, you are more likely to experience strokes, chest pain known as angina, an irregular heartbeat, and heart attacks. You are also more likely to develop congestive heart failure, a condition in which fluid builds up in the body because the heart is not pumping sufficiently. Failure to experience the normal dip in blood pressure during sleep can be related to insufficient sleep time, an untreated sleep disorder, or other factors. African Americans, for example, tend not to have as much of a dip in blood pressure during sleep. This difference may help to explain why they are more likely than Caucasians to have serious cardiovascular disease.

A lack of sleep also puts your body under stress and may trigger the release of more adrenaline, cortisol, and other stress hormones during the day. These hormones contribute to your blood pressure not dipping during sleep, thereby increasing the risk for heart disease. Inadequate sleep may also negatively affect your heart and vascular system by the increased production of certain proteins thought to play a role in heart disease. For example, some studies find that people who chronically do not get enough sleep have higher blood levels of C-reactive protein. Higher levels of this protein may suggest a greater risk of developing hardening of the arteries (atherosclerosis).

Your Hormones

When you were young, your mother may have told you that you need to get enough sleep to grow strong and tall. She may have been right! Deep sleep triggers more release of growth hormone, which fuels growth in children and boosts muscle mass and the repair of cells and tissues in children and adults. Sleep's effect on the release of sex hormones also encourages puberty and fertility. Consequently, women who work at night and tend to lack sleep are, therefore, more likely to have trouble conceiving or to miscarry.

Your mother also probably was right if she told you that getting a good night's sleep on a regular basis would help keep you from getting sick and help you get better if you do get sick. During sleep, your body creates more cytokines—cellular hormones that help the immune system fight various infections. Lack of sleep can reduce the ability to fight off common infections. Research also reveals that a lack of sleep can reduce the body's response to the flu vaccine. For example, sleep-deprived volunteers given the flu vaccine produced less than half as many flu antibodies as those who were well rested and given the same vaccine.

Although lack of exercise and other factors are important contributors, the current epidemic of diabetes and obesity appears to be related, at least in part, to chronically getting inadequate sleep. Evidence is growing that sleep is a powerful regulator of appetite, energy use, and weight control. During sleep, the body's production of the appetite suppressor leptin increases, and the appetite stimulant ghrelin decreases. Studies find that the less people sleep, the more likely they are to be overweight or obese and prefer eating foods that are higher in calories and carbohydrates. People who report an average total sleep time of 5 hours a night, for example, are much more likely to become obese compared to people who sleep 7–8 hours a night.

A number of hormones released during sleep also control the body's use of energy. A distinct rise and fall of blood sugar levels during sleep appears to be linked to sleep stage. Not getting enough sleep overall or enough of each stage of sleep disrupts this pattern. One study found that, when healthy young men slept only 4 hours a night for 6 nights in a row, their insulin and blood sugar levels mimicked those seen in people who were developing diabetes. Another study found that women who slept less than 7 hours a night were more likely to develop diabetes over time than those who slept between 7 and 8 hours a night.

How Much Sleep Is Enough?

Animal studies suggest that sleep is as vital as food for survival. Rats, for example, normally live 2–3 years, but they live only 5 weeks if they are deprived of REM sleep and only 2–3 weeks if they are deprived of all sleep stages—a timeframe similar to death due to starvation. But how much sleep do humans need? To help answer that question, scientists look at how much people sleep when unrestricted, the average amount of sleep among various age groups, and the amount of sleep that studies reveal is necessary to function at your best.

When healthy adults are given unlimited opportunity to sleep, they sleep on average between 8 and 8.5 hours a night. But sleep needs vary from person to person. Some people appear to need only about 7 hours to avoid problem sleepiness whereas others need 9 or more hours of sleep. Sleep needs also change throughout the lifecycle. Newborns sleep between 16 and 18 hours a day, and children in preschool sleep between 10 and 12 hours a day. School-aged children and adolescents need at least 9 hours of sleep a night.

The hormonal influences of puberty tend to shift adolescents' biological clocks. As a result, teenagers are more likely to go to bed later than younger children and adults, and they tend to want to sleep later in the morning. This sleep–wake rhythm is contrary to the early-morning start times of many high schools and helps explain why most teenagers get an average of only 7–7.5 hours of sleep a night.

As people get older, the pattern of sleep also changes—especially the amount of time spent in the deep sleep stages. Children spend more time than adults in these sleep stages. This explains why children can sleep through loud noises and why they might not wake up when they are moved from the car to their beds. During adolescence, a big drop occurs in the amount of time spent in deep sleep, which is replaced by lighter, stage 2 sleep. Between young adulthood and midlife, the percentage of deep sleep falls again—from less than 20 percent to less than 5 percent, one study suggests—and is replaced with lighter sleep (stages 1 and 2). From midlife through late life, people's sleep has more interruptions by wakefulness during the night. This disruption causes older persons to lose more and more of stages 1 and 2 non-REM sleep as well as REM sleep.

Many older people complain of difficulty falling asleep, early morning awakenings, frequent and long awakenings during the night, daytime sleepiness, and a lack of refreshing sleep. Many sleep problems, however, are not a natural aspect of sleep in the elderly. Because older people are more likely to have many illnesses that can disrupt sleep, their sleep complaints often may be due, in part, to illnesses or the medications used to treat them. In fact, one study found that the prevalence of sleep problems is very low in healthy older adults. Other causes of some of older adults' sleep complaints are sleep apnea, restless legs syndrome, and other sleep disorders that become more common with age. Also, older people are more likely to have their sleep disrupted by the need to urinate during the night.

Some evidence shows that the biological clock shifts in older people, so they are more apt to go to sleep earlier at night and wake up earlier in the morning. No evidence indicates that older people can get by with less sleep than younger people. Poor sleep in older people is linked to excessive daytime sleepiness, attention and memory problems, depressed mood, and overuse of sleeping pills.

Despite variations in sleep quantity and quality, both related to age and between individuals, studies suggest that the optimal amount of sleep needed to perform adequately, avoid a sleep debt, and not have problem sleepiness during the day is about 7–8 hours for adults and 9 or more hours for school-aged children and adolescents. Similar amounts seem to be necessary to avoid further increasing the risk of developing obesity, diabetes, or cardiovascular disorders.

Quality of sleep is as important as quantity. People whose sleep is frequently interrupted or cut short may not get enough of both non-REM sleep and REM sleep. Both types of sleep appear to be crucial for learning and memory—and perhaps for all the other restorative benefits of healthy sleep, including the growth and repair of cells.

Many people try to make up for lost sleep during the week by sleeping more on the weekends. But if you have lost too much sleep, sleeping in on the weekend does not completely erase your sleep debt. Certainly, sleeping more at the end of the week does not make up for the hampered performance you most likely had at the beginning of or during that week. Just one night of inadequate sleep can adversely affect your functioning and mood during at least the next day.

Daytime naps are another strategy some people use to make up for lost sleep during the night. Some evidence shows that short naps (up to an hour) can make up, at least partially, for the sleep missed on the previous night and improve alertness, mood, and work performance. But naps don't substitute for a good night's sleep. One study found that a daytime nap after a lack of sleep at night did not fully restore levels of blood sugar to the pattern seen with adequate nighttime sleep. If a nap lasts longer than 1 hour, you may have a hard time waking up fully. In addition, late afternoon naps can make falling asleep at night more difficult.

What Disrupts Sleep?

Many factors can prevent a good night's sleep. These factors range from well-known stimulants, such as coffee, to certain pain relievers, decongestants, and other culprits. Many people depend on the caffeine in coffee, soft drinks (for example, colas), or tea to wake them up in the morning or to keep them awake. Caffeine is thought to block the cell receptors that adenosine uses to trigger its sleep inducing signals. In this way, caffeine fools the body into thinking it isn't tired. It can take as long as 6–8 hours for the effects of caffeine to wear off completely. Drinking a cup of coffee in the late afternoon consequently may prevent your falling asleep at night.

Nicotine is another stimulant that can keep you awake. Nicotine also leads to lighter than normal sleep. Heavy smokers also tend to wake up too early because of nicotine withdrawal. Although alcohol is a sedative that makes it easier to fall asleep, it prevents deep sleep and REM sleep, allowing only the lighter stages of sleep. People who drink alcohol also tend to wake up in the middle of the night when the effects of an alcoholic nightcap wear off.

Certain commonly used prescription and over-the-counter medicines contain ingredients that can keep you awake. These ingredients include decongestants and steroids. Many pain relievers taken by headache sufferers contain caffeine. Heart and blood pressure medications known as beta blockers can cause difficulty falling asleep and increase the number of awakenings during the night. People who have chronic asthma or bronchitis also have more problems falling asleep and staying asleep than healthy people, either because of their breathing difficulties or because of the medicines they take.

Other chronic painful or uncomfortable conditions—such as arthritis, congestive heart failure, and sickle cell anemia—can disrupt sleep, too. A number of psychological disorders—including schizophrenia, bipolar disorder, and anxiety disorders—are well known for disrupting sleep. Depression often leads to insomnia, and insomnia can cause depression. Some of these psychological disorders are more likely to disrupt REM sleep. Psychological stress also takes its toll on sleep, making it more difficult to fall asleep or stay asleep. People who feel stressed also tend to spend less time in deep sleep and REM sleep. Many people report having difficulties sleeping if, for example, they have recently lost a loved one, are undergoing a divorce, or are under stress at work.

Menstrual cycle hormones can affect how well women sleep. Progesterone is known to induce sleep and circulates in greater concentrations in the second half of the menstrual cycle. For this reason, women may sleep better during this phase of their menstrual cycle, but many women report trouble sleeping the night before their menstrual bleeding starts. This sleep disruption is probably related to the abrupt drop in progesterone levels in their bodies just before they begin to bleed. Women in their late forties and early fifties, however, report more difficulties sleeping (insomnia) than younger women. These difficulties may be because, as they near or enter menopause, they have lower concentrations of progesterone. Hot flashes in women of this age also may cause sleep disruption and difficulties.

Certain lifestyle factors may also deprive a person of needed sleep. Large meals or exercise just before bedtime can make it harder to fall asleep. Studies show that exercise in the evening delays the extra release of melatonin at night that helps the body fall asleep. Exercise in the daytime, on the other hand, is linked to improved nighttime sleep.

If you aren't getting enough sleep or aren't falling asleep early enough, you may be overscheduling activities that can prevent you from getting the quiet relaxation time you need to prepare for sleep. Most people report that it's easier to fall asleep if they have time to wind down into a less active state before sleeping. Relaxing in a hot bath before bedtime may help. In addition, your body temperature drops after a hot bath in a way that mimics, in part, what happens as you fall asleep. Probably for both these reasons, many people report that they fall asleep more easily after a hot bath.

Sleeping environment also can affect your sleep. Clear your bedroom of any potential sleep distractions, such as noises, bright lights, a television, or computer. Having a comfortable mattress and pillow can help promote a good night's sleep. You also sleep better if the temperature in your bedroom is kept on the cool side.

Tips for Getting a Good Night's Sleep

- Stick to a sleep schedule. Go to bed and wake up the same time each day. As creatures of habit, people have a hard time adjusting to altered sleep patterns. Sleeping later on weekends won't fully make up for the lack of sleep during the week and will make it harder to wake up early on Monday morning.

- Exercise is great but not too late in the day. Try to exercise at least 30 minutes on most days but not later than 5 or 6 hours before your bedtime.

- Avoid caffeine and nicotine. Coffee, colas, certain teas, and chocolate contain the stimulant caffeine, and its effects can take as long as 8 hours to wear off fully. Therefore, a cup of coffee in the late afternoon can make it hard for you to fall asleep at night. Nicotine is also a stimulant, often causing smokers to sleep only very lightly. In addition, smokers often wake up too early in the morning because of nicotine withdrawal.

- Avoid alcoholic drinks before bed. You may think having an alcoholic nightcap will help you sleep, but alcohol robs you of deep sleep and REM sleep, keeping you in the lighter stages of sleep. You also tend to wake up in the middle of the night when the effects of the alcohol have worn off.

- Avoid large meals and beverages late at night. A light snack is okay, but a large meal can cause indigestion that interferes with sleep. Drinking too many fluids at night can cause frequent awakenings to urinate.

- If possible, avoid medicines that delay or disrupt your sleep. Some commonly prescribed heart, blood pressure, or asthma medications, as well as some over-the-counter and herbal remedies for coughs, colds, or allergies, can disrupt sleep patterns. If you have trouble sleeping, talk to your doctor or pharmacist to see if any drugs you're taking might be contributing to your insomnia.

- Don't take naps after 3 p.m. Naps can help make up for lost sleep, but late afternoon naps can make it harder to fall asleep at night.

- Relax before bed. Don't overschedule your day so that no time is left for unwinding. A relaxing activity, such as reading or listening to music, should be part of your bedtime ritual.

- Take a hot bath before bed. The drop in body temperature after getting out of the bath may help you feel sleepy, and the bath can help you relax and slow down so you're more ready to sleep.

- Have a good sleeping environment. Get rid of anything that might distract you from sleep, such as noises, bright lights, an uncomfortable bed, or warm temperatures. You sleep better if the temperature in your bedroom is kept on the cool side. A TV or computer in the bedroom can be a distraction and deprive you of needed sleep.

- Having a comfortable mattress and pillow can help promote a good night's sleep.

- Have the right sunlight exposure. Daylight is key to regulating daily sleep patterns. Try to get outside in natural sunlight for at least 30 minutes each day. If possible, wake up with the sun or use very bright lights in the morning. Sleep experts recommend that, if you have problems falling asleep, you should get an hour of exposure to morning sunlight.

- Don't lie in bed awake. If you find yourself still awake after staying in bed for more than 20 minutes, get up and do some relaxing activity until you feel sleepy. The anxiety of not being able to sleep can make it harder to fall asleep.

- See a doctor if you continue to have trouble sleeping. If you consistently find yourself feeling tired or not well rested during the day despite spending enough time in bed at night, you may have a sleep disorder. Your family doctor or a sleep specialist should be able to help you.

Section 52.2

Exercise Can Help Control Stress

"Stress," © 2010 A.D.A.M., Inc. Reprinted with permission.

Exercise in combination with stress management techniques is extremely important for many reasons:

- Exercise is an effective distraction from stressful events.

- Exercise may directly blunt the harmful effects of stress on blood pressure and the heart (exercise protects the heart in any case).

Usually, a varied exercise regime is more interesting, and thus easier to stick to. Start slowly. Strenuous exercise in people who are not used to it can be very dangerous and any exercise program should be discussed with a physician. In addition, half of all people who begin a vigorous training regime drop out within a year. The key is to find activities that are exciting, challenging, and satisfying. The following are some suggestions:

- Sign up for aerobics classes at a gym.

- Brisk walking is an excellent aerobic exercise that is free and available to nearly anyone. Even short brisk walks can relieve bouts of stress.

- Swimming is an ideal exercise for many stressed people, including pregnant women, individuals with musculoskeletal problems, and those who suffer exercise-induced asthma.

- Yoga or Tai Chi can be very effective, combining many of the benefits of breathing, muscle relaxation, and meditation while toning and stretching the muscles. The benefits of yoga may be considerable. Numerous studies have found it beneficial for many conditions in which stress is an important factor, such as anxiety, headaches, high blood pressure, and asthma. It also elevates mood and improves concentration and the ability to focus.

521

As in other areas of stress management, making a plan and executing it successfully develops feelings of mastery and control, which are very beneficial in and of themselves. Start small. Just 10 minutes of exercise three times a week can build a good base for novices. Gradually build up the length of these every-other-day sessions to 30 minutes or more.

Section 52.3

Nutrition and Stress

"Nutrition and Stress," © 2010 Meals Matter. Reprinted with permission. Meals Matter is a public education website of the Dairy Council of California. For additional information, visit www.mealsmatter.org or www.dairycouncilofca.org.

Feeling wound-up, overworked, and exhausted? Do you feel a lack of focus or have trouble sleeping at night? Busy schedules can leave us stressed out, irritable, and run down.

When our lives get busy it is easy to overlook the importance of eating a balanced diet. Yet, good nutrition can make the difference between feeling great and energized, or cranky and tired.

Fight or Flight Response to Stress

When we feel threatened or under attack, brain chemicals and adrenal hormones that enable us to think quickly or to run away from a threat are released into the bloodstream.

This is our primitive "fight or flight response," which in the past helped us escape dangerous situations. These days, when we experience ongoing stress, these "fight or flight" chemicals are released continuously and can begin to interfere with the body's ability to stay in balance.

Brain Chemicals

Certain brain chemicals called neurotransmitters, such as serotonin, dopamine, and norepinephrine, dictate how we experience emotion and how we feel. Neurotransmitters generate feelings of happiness, mental alertness, and calmness. Deficiencies of the chemicals can lead to depression, irritability, anxiety, sleeplessness, and food cravings.

Neurotransmitters are derived in part from the foods we eat. So, a few simple dietary changes may help to increase their levels naturally and improve the body's response to stress, countering its effects on our health and moods.

Eating Behavior and Stress

Eating is a common response to stress. When we are under stress, we are more likely to skip meals or grab for our favorite high-calorie comfort foods. Eating favorite foods in moderation to help alleviate stress is probably fine. However, poor eating habits brought on by stress could lead to unwanted weight gain and poor health in the long term.

Dietary Stress-Fighters

Choosing balanced meals containing nutrient-rich foods, including complex carbohydrates, protein, and fat, that will slowly fuel our brain chemicals throughout the day is the ideal way to keep our bodies in balance during stressful periods.

Complex Carbohydrates

These increase the amount of serotonin in your brain, a powerful neurotransmitter that boosts your mood, calms you down, and helps you sleep. Food sources: fruits, vegetables, whole grains, and starchy foods.

Simple sugars (found in candy, syrups, table sugar, alcohol, and sweetened fruits), however, cause a brief spike in blood sugar which may make you feel better in the short term but can be followed by a quick drop in energy and leave you craving more.

Protein-Rich Foods

Eating them slows down the rate at which sugar is released into your bloodstream and keeps your blood sugar balanced. It also keeps you feeling full longer, making you less likely to grab for a high-calorie sweet snack. Food sources: dairy foods (cheese, milk, yogurt), eggs, fish, meats, legumes (beans and lentils), peanut butter, poultry, and tofu.

Essential Fats

These fats (a.k.a. omega-6 and omega-3 fatty acids) can only be obtained through our diet. They promote the flow of nutrients into cells and allow waste products to escape from the cells. Research shows that seafood such as salmon and other oily fish contain omega-3 fatty acids, which appear to help relieve mild depression.

Food sources: nuts (almonds, walnuts), oils (canola, flax, soybean), oily fish (salmon, sardines, tuna), and seeds (flax, pumpkin).

More dietary suggestions:

- Eat small meals and snacks that include protein-rich foods to maintain a stable blood sugar.

- Don't eliminate entire food groups—each food group provides its own unique nutrients.

- Avoid extremely low fat diets—some fat is needed for anti-depression.

- Have breakfast—skipping this important meal can lead to impulse snacking on sweets.

Exercise Improves Your Health

Physical activity has countless benefits, improving both physical and mental health. Try to get at least 30 minutes or more of moderate physical activity most days of the week.

If sleeplessness is a problem for you, it's best to exercise in the morning or during the day, rather than at night. Too much physical activity close to bedtime can rev up your metabolism and make it harder to fall asleep.

Section 52.4

Stress Levels Rise in Response to Caffeine

Penn State researchers have shown that a simple saliva test may offer a new way to probe the physical consequences of caffeine coupled with stress.

Laura Klein, associate professor of biobehavioral health, who led the study, explains that people's fight or flight response produces not only the familiar dry mouth, pounding heart, and sweaty palms that accompany a stressful experience but also body chemistry changes that could result in health consequences.

Using doses of caffeine equivalent to drinking 1 to 4 cups of coffee and an intense arithmetic test as stressors, Klein and her colleagues found a rise in the amount of alpha amylase, an enzyme secreted by the salivary glands, in the healthy young men who participated in the study.

The results verified, based on performance, that a moderate dose of caffeine—200 mg or about the amount in 2 cups of coffee—increased task performance and that doubling the amount of caffeine brings performance back down. The results also suggest that alpha amylase, which can be detected and measured via a new, non-invasive saliva test, provides a window on the biochemistry of the response not offered by cortisol alone which is commonly used to study the health consequences of stress.

The Penn State groups' results were detailed in a paper, "Effects of Caffeine and Stress on Salivary Alpha-Amylase in Young Men: A Salivary Biomarker of Sympathetic Activity," presented Thursday, March 2, [2006] at the annual meeting of American Psychosomatic Society in Denver. The authors are Klein; Courtney A. Whetzel and Jeanette M. Bennett, doctoral candidates in biobehavioral health; Frank E. Ritter, associate professor of information sciences and technology, psychology, and computer science and engineering; and Douglas A. Granger, associate professor of biobehavioral health and human development and family studies.

In the study, 45 healthy men, ages 18 to 30, who had not had any caffeine-containing food or medications for at least 4 hours, came to the laboratory and provided saliva samples. Fifteen minutes after providing the saliva sample, they were given one of three doses of caffeine: none; 200 mg (equivalent to 1 to 2 cups of coffee) or 400 mg (equivalent to 3 to 4 cups of coffee). Then all the participants completed a mental arithmetic test.

"The men had to count backwards from a four-digit number by sevens and 13s. When they made mistakes, I corrected them and told them to go faster. This went on for 20 minutes," Klein said.

Fifteen minutes after the test, the men provided another saliva sample. Their heart rate and blood pressure also were taken continuously throughout the testing period.

The researchers report that, as expected, blood pressure and heart rate increased in response to the arithmetic test and to caffeine. Alpha amylase levels in the participants' saliva also increased in response to caffeine and to stress, and these increases were positively associated with increased heart rate levels.

"Dependence and tolerance develop quickly to caffeine and other sympathomimetic substances, such as nicotine," Klein added. "These new results suggest that alpha amylase, along with other novel biomarkers, may enable us to understand withdrawal and tolerance to sympathomimetics as well as providing a window on their health consequences."

The study was supported by a grant from the Office of Naval Research on which Klein and Ritter are co-investigators and by the Penn State General Clinical Research Center. Co-author Granger developed the new salivary alpha amylase assay with a team of researchers at his company, Salimetrics LLC. Salimetrics assayed the alpha amylase samples used in the study.

Chapter 53

Stressful Situations: Tips for Coping

Chapter Contents

Section 53.1

Aggressive Driving

From "Are You an Aggressive Driver?" by the National Highway Traffic Safety Administration (NHTSA, www.nhtsa.gov), 1998. Reviewed by David A. Cooke, MD, FACP, November 8, 2010.

Is This You?

Do you do the following when driving?

- **Express frustration:** Taking out your frustrations on your fellow motorists can lead to violence or a crash.

- **Fail to pay attention when driving:** Reading, eating, drinking, or talking on the phone can be a major cause of roadway crashes.

- **Tailgate:** This is a major cause of crashes that can result in serious deaths or injuries.

- **Make frequent lane changes:** If you whip in and out of lanes to advance ahead, you can be a danger to other motorists.

- **Run red lights.** Do not enter an intersection on a yellow light. Remember flashing red lights should be treated as a stop sign.

- **Speed:** Going faster than the posted speed limit, being a "road racer," and going too fast for conditions are some examples of speeding.

Plan Ahead and Allow Yourself Extra Time

Use the following tips to avoid dangerous driving:

- **Concentrate.** Don't allow yourself to become distracted by talking on your cellular phone, eating, drinking, or putting on makeup.

- **Relax.** Tune the radio to your favorite relaxing music. Music can calm your nerves and help you to enjoy your time in the car.

- **Drive the posted speed limit.** Fewer crashes occur when vehicles are travelling at or about the same speed.

- **Identify alternate routes.** Try mapping out an alternate route. Even if it looks longer on paper, you may find it is less congested.

- **Use public transportation.** Public transportation can give you some much-needed relief from life behind the wheel.

- **Just be late.** If all else fails, just be late.

When Confronted with Aggressive Drivers

- **Get out of the way.** First and foremost make every attempt to get out of their way.

- **Put your pride aside.** Do not challenge them by speeding up or attempting to hold your own in your travel lane.

- **Avoid eye contact.** Eye contact can sometimes enrage an aggressive driver.

- **Ignore gestures.** Ignore gestures and refuse to return them.

- **Report serious aggressive driving.** You or a passenger may call the police. But, if you use a cell phone, pull over to a safe location.

Section 53.2

Caregiver Stress

From "Caregiver Stress," by the Office on Women's Health, part
of the U.S. Department of Health and Human Services, May 1, 2008.

What is a caregiver?

A caregiver is anyone who provides help to another person in need.
Usually, the person receiving care has a condition such as dementia,
cancer, or brain injury and needs help with basic daily tasks. Caregivers help with many things such as the following:

- Grocery shopping
- House cleaning
- Cooking
- Shopping
- Paying bills
- Giving medicine
- Bathing
- Using the toilet
- Dressing
- Eating

People who are not paid to provide care are known as informal
caregivers or family caregivers. The most common type of informal
caregiving relationship is an adult child caring for an elderly parent.
Other types of caregiving relationships include the following:

- Adults caring for other relatives, such as grandparents, siblings, aunts, and uncles
- Spouses caring for elderly husbands or wives
- Middle-aged parents caring for severely disabled adult children
- Adults caring for friends and neighbors

- Children caring for a disabled parent or elderly grandparent

Who are our nation's caregivers?

Most Americans will be informal caregivers at some point during their lives. During any given year, there are more than 44 million Americans (21% of the adult population) who provide unpaid care to an elderly or disabled person 18 years or older. Altogether, informal caregivers provide 80 percent of the long-term care in the United States.

- Sixty-one percent of caregivers are women.

- Most caregivers are middle-aged.

- Thirteen percent of caregivers are aged 65 years and older.

- Fifty-nine percent of informal caregivers have jobs in addition to caring for another person. Because of time spent caregiving, more than half of employed women caregivers have made changes at work, such as going in late, leaving early, or working fewer hours.

What is caregiver stress?

Caregiver stress is the emotional and physical strain of caregiving. It can take many forms. For instance, you may feel the following:

- Frustrated and angry taking care of someone with dementia who often wanders away or becomes easily upset

- Guilty because you think that you should be able to provide better care, despite all the other things that you have to do

- Lonely because all the time you spend caregiving has hurt your social life

- Exhausted when you go to bed at night

Caregiver stress appears to affect women more than men. About 75 percent of caregivers who report feeling very strained emotionally, physically, or financially are women.

Although caregiving can be challenging, it is important to note that it can also have its rewards. It can give you a feeling of giving back to a loved one. It can also make you feel needed and can lead to a stronger relationship with the person receiving care. About half of caregivers report that they appreciate life more as a result of their caregiving experience and caregiving has made them feel good about themselves.

Can caregiver stress affect my health?

Although most caregivers are in good health, it is not uncommon for caregivers to have serious health problems. Research shows that caregivers experience the following:

- Are more likely to have symptoms of depression or anxiety

- Are more likely to have a long-term medical problem, such as heart disease, cancer, diabetes, or arthritis

- Have higher levels of stress hormones

- Spend more days sick with an infectious disease

- Have a weaker immune response to the influenza, or flu, vaccine

- Have slower wound healing

- Have higher levels of obesity

- May be at higher risk for mental decline, including problems with memory and paying attention

One research study found that elderly people who felt stressed while taking care of their disabled spouses were 63 percent more likely to die within 4 years than caregivers who were not feeling stressed.

Part of the reason that caregivers often have health problems is that they are less likely to take good care of themselves. For instance, women caregivers, compared with women who are not caregivers, are less likely to get needed medical care, fill a prescription because of the cost, and get a mammogram.

Also, caregivers report that, compared with the time before they became caregivers, they are less likely to get enough sleep, cook healthy meals, and get enough physical activity.

How can I tell if caregiving is putting too much stress on me?

Caregiving may be putting too much stress on you if you have any of the following symptoms:

- Feeling overwhelmed

- Sleeping too much or too little

- Gaining or losing a lot of weight

- Feeling tired most of the time

- Loss of interest in activities you used to enjoy

- Becoming easily irritated or angered

- Feeling constantly worried

- Often feeling sad

- Frequent headaches, bodily pain, or other physical problems

- Abuse of alcohol or drugs, including prescription drugs

Talk to a counselor, psychologist, or other mental health professional right away if your stress leads you to physically or emotionally harm the person you are caring for.

What can I do to prevent or relieve stress?

To begin with, never dismiss your feelings as "just stress." Caregiver stress can lead to serious health problems and you should take steps to reduce it as much as you can.

Research shows that people who take an active, problem-solving approach to caregiving issues are less likely to feel stressed than those who react by worrying or feeling helpless. For instance, someone with dementia may ask the same question over and over again, such as, "Where is Mary?" A positive way of dealing with this would be to say, "Mary is not here right now," and then distract the person. You could say, "Let's start getting lunch ready," or involve the person in simple tasks, such as folding laundry.

Some hospitals offer classes that can teach you how to care for someone with the disease that your loved one is facing. To find these classes, ask your doctor, contact an organization that focuses on this disease, or call your local Area Agency on Aging. Other good sources of caregiving information include doctors and nurses, library books, and websites of disease-specific organizations.

Here are some more tips for reducing stress:

- Find out about caregiving resources in your community.

- Ask for and accept help. Be prepared with a mental list of ways that others can help you, and let the helper choose what she would like to do. For instance, one person might be happy to take the person you care for on a walk a couple times a week. Someone else might be glad to pick up some groceries for you.

- If you need financial help taking care of a relative, don't be afraid to ask family members to contribute their fair share.

- Say "no" to requests that are draining, such as hosting holiday meals.

- Don't feel guilty that you are not a "perfect" caregiver. Just as there is no "perfect parent," there is no such thing as a "perfect caregiver." You're doing the best you can.

- Identify what you can and cannot change. You may not be able to change someone else's behavior, but you can change the way that you react to it.

- Set realistic goals. Break large tasks into smaller steps that you can do one at a time.

- Prioritize, make lists, and establish a daily routine.

- Stay in touch with family and friends.

- Join a support group for caregivers in your situation, such as caring for someone with dementia. Besides being a great way to make new friends, you can also pick up some caregiving tips from others who are facing the same problems you are.

- Make time each week to do something that you want to do, such as go to a movie.

- Try to find time to be physically active on most days of the week, eat a healthy diet, and get enough sleep.

- See your doctor for a checkup. Tell her that you are a caregiver and tell her about any symptoms of depression or sickness you may be having.

- Try to keep your sense of humor.

If you work outside the home and are feeling overwhelmed, consider taking a break from your job. Employees covered under the federal Family and Medical Leave Act may be able to take up to 12 weeks of unpaid leave per year to care for relatives. Ask your human resources office about options for unpaid leave.

What caregiving services can I find in my community?

Caregiving services include the following:

- Transportation
- Meal delivery
- Home health care services (such as nursing or physical therapy)

- Non-medical home care services (such as housekeeping, cooking, or companionship)

- Home modification (changes to the home that make it easier for your loved one to perform basic daily tasks, such as bathing, using the toilet, and moving around)

- Legal and financial counseling

What can I do if I need a break?

Taking some time off from caregiving can reduce stress. Respite care provides substitute caregiving to give the regular caregiver a much-needed break. Various types of respite services are available:

- **In-home respite:** In this type of service, someone comes to your home to provide care. The type of care can range from simple companionship to nursing services.

- **Adult day-care centers:** Many adult day-care centers are located in churches or community centers. Some day-care centers provide care for both elderly adults and young children. During the day, the two groups meet for several hours to share in activities such as reading stories. This type of contact seems to benefit both young and old.

- **Short-term nursing homes:** If your loved one needs occasional nursing care and you must leave town for a couple weeks, some nursing homes will care for your loved one while you are gone.

- **Day hospitals:** Some hospitals provide medical care to patients during the day and then at night, the patient returns home.

What devices can I buy that will help me provide care?

There are devices that you can buy that can help you make sure that your loved one is safe. Here are some examples:

- Emergency response systems involve a button on a necklace, bracelet, or belt that your loved one wears. If she has an emergency and you are not home, she presses the button to alert a monitoring center. The center then alerts medical personnel and you. These systems are intended for people who can press the button and do not have dementia.

- An intercom system allows you to hear your loved one from another area of your home.

- A webcam is a video camera that allows you to see your loved one from another area of your home.

- Mobility monitors use a small transmitter to help keep track of people with dementia: When your loved one wearing a transmitter strapped to her ankle or wrist passes out of a set range, the transmitter alerts you that your loved one is wandering away.

Also, researchers are developing technologies to allow doctors and nurses to examine and treat patients from locations different than the patient's. This new field is called telemedicine. It uses a communication system, like the internet or two-way television, to collect medical information and provide instructions to the caregiver and patient. Telemedicine will be most useful in rural areas where few doctors are available. Some states already have limited telemedicine programs in operation.

How do I find out about caregiving services in my community?

Contact your local Area Agency on Aging (AAA) to learn about caregiving services where you live. AAAs are usually listed in the city or county government sections of the telephone directory under "Aging" or "Health and Human Services." The National Eldercare Locator, a service of the U.S. Administration on Aging, can also help you find your local AAA.

You might also want to consult with an eldercare specialist, a professional who specializes in aging-related issues. An eldercare specialist assists older adults and their family members by assessing their needs and identifying the best services and devices available to meet those needs. To find an eldercare specialist in your area, ask your doctor or local AAA.

How will I pay for home health care and other caregiving services?

Medicare, Medicaid, and private insurance companies will cover some of the costs of home health care. Other costs you will have to pay for yourself.

The costs of home care depends on what services you use. Non-medical workers like housekeepers are much less expensive than nurses or physical therapists. Also, some home care agencies are less expensive than others.

To find out if you are eligible for Medicare home health care services, read the free publication Medicare and Home Health Care (Publication No. CMS-10969), available at http://www.medicare.gov/Publications/Pubs/pdf/10969.pdf. You can also call your Regional Home Health Intermediary. To find the phone number, go to the Contacts Database of the Centers for Medicare & Medicaid Services at www.cms.hhs.gov/apps/contacts. You can also call 800-MEDICARE (800-633-4227).

To qualify for Medicaid, you must have a low income and few other assets. To find out if you qualify for Medicaid, call your State Medical Assistance Office. To find the phone number, go to the Contacts Database of the Centers for Medicare & Medicaid Services at: www.cms.hhs.gov/apps/contacts. You can also call 800-MEDICARE (800-633-4227).

Besides Medicare and Medicaid, there is another federal program, called the National Family Caregiver Support Program, that helps states provide services for family caregivers. To be eligible for the program, a caregiver must:

- care for an adult aged 60 years and older, or care for a person of any age with Alzheimer's disease or a related disorder,

- be a grandparent or relative 55 years of age or older who is the primary caregiver of a child under the age of 18; or

- be a grandparent or relative 55 years of age or older providing care to an adult, aged 18 to 59 years, with a disability.

Each state offers different amounts and types of services. These include the following:

- Information about available services

- Help accessing support services

- Individual counseling and organization of support groups

- Caregiver training

- Respite care

- Supplemental services, supplies, and equipment, such as home modifications, emergency response systems, nutritional supplements, incontinence supplies, etc.

To access services under the National Family Caregiver Support Program, contact your local Area Agency on Aging.

Section 53.3

Economic Hardship

From "Tips in a Time of Economic Crisis: Managing Your Stress," by the Substance Abuse and Mental Health Services Administration (SAMHSA, mentalhealth.samhsa.gov), part of the U.S. Department of Health and Human Services, 2009.

Many Americans rep ort experiencing heightened levels of stress during this time of financial crisis. Yet, few realize that this reaction to economic pressures closely resembles the psychological effects experienced after natural disasters, such as hurricanes, floods, wildfires, or even the terrorist attacks of 9/11.

Stress reduction and mental health promotion are as important now for people affected directly or indirectly by the financial crisis as for those who suffered from effects of natural or manmade disasters.

You Should Know

Nearly every day, each of us experiences stress of some kind. Feelings of stress come from reactions that our bodies have to challenges, pressures, and demands that are not a usual part of our daily lives. We may feel stress before taking a test or speaking in public, and elated after we're successful. Simple things such as missing the bus, being late for a meeting, or working under a deadline for a project may also cause us to feel stress. That short-term stress may make us feel worried or anxious, but is relatively harmless to our overall health status. We also may face long-term stress in the form of severe illness, divorce, unemployment, loss of a home, or trauma. These long-term stresses are real and increase our risk for some serious health problems.

Research suggests long-term stress can have serious effects. Stress triggers changes in our bodies and brains that may make us more likely to get sick. Problems we already have, such as high blood pressure, depression, anxiety, and diabetes can become worse. Over time, stress can become disabling, leading to stroke, heart attack, and even suicide.

Know the Signs of Stress

Stress may show itself in physical ways, including muscle tension and pain, headaches, stomach upset, or rapid heartbeat. Some of us may overeat; some may feel tired. Stress also can affect us emotionally. Anxiety, the jitters, and becoming short-tempered, forgetful, or unable to focus are all signs of stress.

While everyone reacts to stress differently, our bodies do send out signals to warn us when stress is becoming harmful. By paying attention to how our bodies and minds respond to stress—what our bodies are telling us—we can manage stress in better ways. And that can help reduce the risk to our long-term physical and emotional health.

Stress Reduction

Once we understand how we experience stress and how it affects the way we feel and act, we can take action. We can learn to manage our stress in healthy ways, before we feel overwhelmed.

Pay attention to body and mind:

- Recognize the early signs of stress.

- Work to stay positive; know that stress, depression, guilt, and anger are feelings that can be managed.

- Recall past solutions to similar problems and build on them.

Attend to your health:

- Get enough sleep.

- Eat healthy foods; drink water.

- Avoid alcohol.

- Don't use tobacco or illegal drugs.

- Get regular physical exercise.

Practice relaxation:

- Relax your body and mind. Use deep breathing, stretching, meditation, listening to music—whatever works.

- Pace yourself by alternating stressful tasks with pleasant activities.

- Take time to do nothing; just relax.

Set priorities:

- Make a list of things that need to be done.
- Identify how you will do each item on the list.
- Do the most important things first to help reduce stress.
- Do not be discouraged if goals can't be accomplished immediately.

Share your concerns:

- Talk with family and friends; share with them the situation, the challenges, and your feelings and worries.
- Share your concerns with individuals in similar situations; communicating ideas and solutions is a positive way to reduce stress.

Know When to Get Help

Even when we do everything we can to reduce our stress, sometimes things may become so overwhelming that we need to reach out to others for help. We shouldn't feel embarrassed to seek help if we haven't been able to overcome feelings of stress, depression, or anxiety on our own. And we shouldn't be afraid to help someone we care about do the same.

Talking helps. Reach out to partners, other family members, or close friends. Help can come from a faith community, your doctor, or a staff member at your workplace heath center. Referrals to mental health and substance abuse treatment professionals are readily available by contacting a local community mental health center or employee assistance program.

Most important, if thinking about suicide, get help immediately by calling 911 or 800-273-TALK (273-8255). If a friend or colleague threatens suicide, looks for ways to commit suicide, talks or writes about death or suicide, or feels rage, uncontrolled anger, or desires revenge, help them. Call 800-273-TALK immediately.

Section 53.4

Holiday Stress

Excerpted from "Successfully Managing Your Holiday Stress," by the
Employee Assistance Program, part of the U.S. Department of Justice's
Drug Enforcement Program (www.justice.gov/dea), 2008.

One humorous, but none-the-less true definition of insanity is "Doing the same thing over and over, but (unrealistically) expecting that there will be more satisfying results the next time we do it." Well, the holiday season is once again upon us, and despite the joy and excitement that they bring, many of us are beginning to re-experience that familiar, but uncomfortable feeling that we have a thousand things to do, but only enough time and money for 500 of them.

As December rolls around each year, many of us find that we experience increasing levels of stress and pressure as the demands and deadlines for shopping, sending cards, decorating, cooking, and planning gatherings draw ever nearer and we anticipate the arrival of relatives and friends. This seemingly paradoxical response to what is supposed to be a season of celebration has several names (and faces) including holiday stress, the holiday blues, and seasonal affective disorder and unfortunately is more common than most of us realize. What follows are some explanations of what causes this annual bout of seasonal discomfort and some suggestions on how to avoid becoming an annual casualty of this condition.

Cause #1: Social and Personal Expectations That You Should Be Merry

Just about everyone feels compelled to look and feel happy during the holidays. Often people feel just the opposite and ask themselves, "What's wrong with me?" The fact is that for many of us the holidays can be the most stressful or even saddest time of year.

Possible solutions: Give yourself permission to have honesty in your holiday emotions. Talk to a close friend, a pastor, or mentor, or other family members. Letting it out and understanding the roots of your feelings will help you to normalize this annual experience and the feelings that go with it.

541

Cause #2: Too Many Responsibilities

Crazy kids, too many presents, guests, cooking, obligatory gifts, decorations, cleaning, and financial pressures can lead to overload. This is a normal and not uncommon experience for many of us at this time of year.

Possible solutions: First, try making a list of everything you will attempt to get done in the weeks between Thanksgiving and New Year's Day. If just looking at the list makes you tired, it's time to cut back on the volume of things you are planning. Don't overcommit. Don't agree to do something just to be nice; particularly if it will make you feel not nice at all. If something doesn't sound like it will enhance your holiday or just can't be gotten to, drop it. No one else will ever know and you'll enjoy the holiday that much more.

Cause #3: Trying to Change or Control Other People

Yes, it's true—during the holidays your kids may be crazy with unrealistic expectations and greed, Dad may be grouchy about the family's cash flow, Mom may feel overloaded and dumped on, and the extended family may argue over who will host family celebrations. The holidays make us all act differently, and not necessarily for the better. Trying to point out and fix these undesirable changes in others often leads to World War III and a generally unpleasant holiday season.

Possible solutions: Within reason, grant yourself and others around you permission to react to the holidays any way you choose. Try not to sweat the small stuff because it's all small stuff. Realize that the only sane response to a crazy situation is to act crazy yourself. You have permission to be nuts. Also, remember the Serenity Prayer and what it says about knowing the difference between what you do and don't control. Do the best you can to change things, but often serenity is the best you'll get.

Cause #4: Unpleasant Memories (The Holiday Blues)

Many people have unpleasant recollections associated with the holidays, or find that the holidays cause them to grieve recent or even distant losses in their lives. This is a common experience and should not be taken as an indication that something is fundamentally wrong with them.

Possible solutions: While we can't (and shouldn't) forget the past, we can focus on memories without pain. Ease the healing process associated with grieving by sharing stories, family history, and pictures of those we have lost with the younger members of the family. Remember that positive memories have an even greater potential to bring joy than they do pain. If there have been unpleasant events in your past holidays, strive to establish new, enjoyable holiday experiences with family and friends to displace them.

Cause #5: Spontaneous Physical and Emotional Distress

Even when negative memories don't surface consciously, sometimes we are unknowingly exposed to trigger situations that unconsciously produce physical and/or emotional symptoms. These memories, and/or the vulnerability caused by doing too much may result in changes in sleep, mood, appetite, productivity, energy, as well as muscle tension, gastrointestinal discomfort, or other physical and/or emotional symptoms.

Possible solutions: Should you find yourself becoming symptomatic, remove yourself from your immediate surroundings and take some time to regroup and calm down. Try to understand what was triggering you. Often there is an unpleasant memory or association that was made in your mind by a trigger. Try also to reframe trigger situations in more objective, less emotional terms.

Cause #6: Insisting That Everything Must Go Perfectly and Blaming Yourself (or Others) When It Doesn't

During the holidays, there is a huge increase in our expectations for perfect outcomes and a parallel increase in the number of opportunities for things to go wrong. This combination virtually guarantees some disappointments for a majority of us, and for those of us who are perfectionistic is a recipe for disaster.

Possible solutions: Do an expectation inventory and reality check. Get rid of expectations that are unrealistically high or lack flexibility. Remember that during the holidays Murphy's Law is in overdrive: If something can go wrong, it will go wrong. By expecting and planning for problems, you will be far better able to cope.

Cause #7: Procrastination

Some people love the excitement of leaving many of their holiday tasks for the last minute. Others seem to go into denial that the calendar is actually moving, or that they have accomplished very few of

543

the dozens of things most of us need to accomplish at this time of year. Either one of these distortions could blindside us, leaving us buried in an avalanche of last-minute to-dos and maxing out our stress levels.

Possible solutions: Try approaching the holiday pressures of last-minute decorations, shopping, cooking, cleaning, and cards in the same way a great general anticipates a major battle—become a planner. List everything that has to get done and assign it a date or priority in that list. Accomplish a few tasks each day, every day, over an extended period. Demand help. Delegate tasks to other members of your family. Accept that some things may not get done and that some things may not get done your way. And again, remember that no one will notice what didn't get done unless you feel compelled to make it public.

Cause #8: Opening up Unresolved Family Conflicts

Sometimes bringing relatives together who rarely see each other can have an unpleasant consequence: Using the holidays to take up old, unresolved family business. Parents who treat their adult children as kids, siblings who resume unresolved disputes they last debated decades ago and relatives who keep a running tally on what gifts were given, their cost and whether someone was cheated are invariably a possibility in some high-energy families.

Possible solutions: If you think any of these might occur, have an action plan set up in advance. Have a strategy to resist getting drawn into old business. Stay positive, or better yet, use the holidays as a time of forgiveness and renewal. Make a concerted effort to make peace with family and friends with whom you have difficulties. Strive to keep everyone active (and distracted). Plan positive activities that minimize free time and redirect attention toward the mutually enjoyable sharing such as a concert, sporting event, play, movie, or church service. If you have house guests, plan for shorter stays (a 2–4 day maximum) or reserve motel rooms to ensure privacy and down time.

Cause #9: Going Broke for the Sake of Happiness

Many of us feel pressure during the holidays to spend beyond our means and without regard for our actual income. We also may lose track of expenses by counting the number of gifts we give or mentally compartmentalizing each purchase rather than watching the totals we are cumulatively spending. Building large credit card balances can cause holiday stress that will last for months (or years), and may derail other family financial goals such as saving for vacations, college, and retirement. Keeping up with the Jones and making the kids happy is tough (and expensive).

Possible solutions: Make sure that your holiday spending is determined by your budget and not by your guilt or need to impress others. Approach the holidays the way you would any big ticket purchase—with a budget. Identify how much you can afford to spend for the entire holiday and then divide it into categories such as travel, entertaining, food, and gifts. Make a list of each person you plan to give to and assign set a dollar amount against that name based on your budget. Stick to it. If you must use credit cards, spend no more than you can reasonable pay off in 3 months.

Section 53.5

Work Stress

Excerpted from "Exposure to Stress: Occupational Hazards in Hospitals," by the National Institute for Occupational Safety and Health (www.cdc.gov/niosh), part of the Centers for Disease Control and Prevention, July 2008.

Occupational stress has been a long-standing concern of the health care industry. Studies indicate that health care workers have higher rates of substance abuse and suicide than other professions and elevated rates of depression and anxiety linked to job stress. In addition to psychological distress, other outcomes of job stress include burnout, absenteeism, employee intent to leave, reduced patient satisfaction, and diagnosis and treatment errors.

What causes occupational stress?

The National Institute for Occupational Safety and Health (NIOSH) defines occupational stress as "the harmful physical and emotional responses that occur when the requirements of the job do not match the capabilities, resources, or needs of the worker."

The following workplace factors (job stressors) can result in stress:

- Job or task demands (work overload, lack of task control, role ambiguity)

- Organizational factors (poor interpersonal relations, unfair management practices)

- Financial and economic factors

- Conflict between work and family roles and responsibilities

- Training and career development issues (lack of opportunity for growth or promotion)

- Poor organizational climate (lack of management commitment to core values, conflicting communication styles, etc.)

Stressors common in health care settings include the following:

- Inadequate staffing levels

546

- Long work hours
- Shift work
- Role ambiguity
- Exposure to infectious and hazardous substances

Stressors vary among health care occupations and even within occupations, depending on the task being performed.

In general, studies of nurses have found the following factors to be linked with stress:

- Work overload
- Time pressure
- Lack of social support at work (especially from supervisors, head nurses, and higher management)
- Exposure to infectious diseases
- Needlestick injuries
- Exposure to work-related violence or threats
- Sleep deprivation
- Role ambiguity and conflict
- Understaffing
- Career development issues
- Dealing with difficult or seriously ill patients

Among physicians, the following factors are associated with stress:

- Long hours
- Excessive workload
- Dealing with death and dying
- Interpersonal conflicts with other staff
- Patient expectations
- Threat of malpractice litigation

The quality of patient care provided by a hospital may also affect health care worker stress. Beliefs about whether the institution provides high quality care may influence the perceived stress of job pressures and workload because higher quality care maybe reflected in greater support and availability of resources.

What are the potential adverse health effects of occupational stress?

Stress may be associated with the following types of reactions:

- Psychological (irritability, job dissatisfaction, depression)
- Behavioral (sleep problems, absenteeism)
- Physical (headache, upset stomach, changes in blood pressure)

An acute traumatic event could cause post-traumatic stress disorder (PTSD). Not every traumatized person develops full-blown or even minor PTSD.

Although individual factors (such as coping strategies) and social resources can modify the reaction to occupational stressors to some degree, working conditions can play a major role in placing workers at risk for developing health problems.

How can stress be controlled in the workplace?

As a general rule, actions to reduce job stress should give top priority to organizational changes that improve working conditions. But even the most conscientious efforts to improve working conditions are unlikely to eliminate stress completely for all workers. For this reason, a combination of organizational change and stress management is often the most successful approach for reducing stress at work.

The most effective way of reducing occupational stress is to eliminate the stressors by redesigning jobs or making organizational changes. Organizations should take the following measures:

- Ensure that the workload is in line with workers' capabilities and resources
- Clearly define workers' roles and responsibilities
- Give workers opportunities to participate in decisions and actions affecting their jobs
- Improve communication
- Reduce uncertainty about career development and future employment prospects
- Provide opportunities for social interaction among workers

The most commonly implemented organizational interventions in health care settings include the following:

- Team processes
- Multidisciplinary health care teams
- Multicomponent interventions

Team process or worker participatory methods give workers opportunities to participate in decisions and actions affecting their jobs. Workers receive clear information about their tasks and role in the department. Team-based approaches to redesign patient care delivery systems or to provide care (e.g., team nursing) have been successful in improving job satisfaction and reducing turnover, absenteeism, and job stress.

Multidisciplinary health care teams (e.g., composed of doctors, nurses, managers, pharmacists, psychologists, etc.) have become increasingly common in acute, long-term, and primary care settings. Teams can accomplish the following:

- Allow services to be delivered efficiently, without sacrificing quality
- Save time (a team can perform activities concurrently that one worker would need to provide sequentially)
- Promote innovation by exchanging ideas
- Integrate and link information in ways that individuals cannot

Multicomponent interventions are broad-based and may include the following:

- Risk assessment
- Intervention techniques
- Education

Successful organizational stress interventions have several things in common:

- Involving workers at all stages of the intervention
- Providing workers with the authority to develop, implement, and evaluate the intervention
- Significant commitment from top management and buy-in from middle management

- An organizational culture that supports stress interventions
- Periodic evaluations of the stress intervention

Without these components (in particular, management support) it is not likely that the intervention will succeed.

Occupational stress interventions can focus either on organizational change or the worker. Worker-focused interventions often consist of stress management techniques such as the following:

- Training in coping strategies
- Progressive relaxation
- Biofeedback
- Cognitive-behavioral techniques
- Time management
- Interpersonal skills

Another type of intervention that has shown promise for reducing stress among health care workers is innovative coping, or the development and application by workers of strategies like changes in work methods or skill development to reduce excessive demands.

The goal of these techniques is to help the worker deal more effectively with occupational stress. Worker-focused interventions have been the most common form of stress reduction in U.S. workplaces. Although worker interventions can help workers deal with stress more effectively, they do not remove the sources of workplace stress, and thus may lose effectiveness over time.

Mental health support intervention may be needed in the event of a significant event at a health care organization.

Conclusions

Health care occupations have long been known to be highly stressful and associated with higher rates of psychological distress than many other occupations. Health care workers are exposed to a number of stressors, ranging from work overload, time pressures, and lack of role clarity to dealing with infectious diseases and difficult and ill, helpless patients.

Such stressors can lead to physical and psychological symptoms, absenteeism, turnover, and medical errors. However, the literature points to both organizational and worker-focused interventions that can successfully reduce stress among health care workers. Although organizational interventions (because they address the sources of stress) are preferred, interventions that combine worker and organizational components may have the broadest appeal as they provide both long-term prevention and short-term treatment components.

Chapter 54

Other Stress Management Strategies

Chapter Contents

553

Section 54.1

Humor as Stress Relief

"Humor as Stress Relief," reprinted with permission from http://
hr.umich.edu/mhealthy. © 2007 Regents of the University of Michigan.

What are the health benefits of humor and laughter?

The sound of roaring laughter is far more contagious than any
cough, sniffle, or sneeze. Humor and laughter have many benefits—
and it's fun!

- People with a developed sense of humor typically have a stronger immune system.

- People who laugh heartily on a regular basis have lower standing blood pressure than the average person. When people have a good laugh, initially the blood pressure increases but then decreases to levels below normal. Breathing then becomes deeper which sends oxygen-enriched blood and nutrients throughout the body.

- Laughter can be a great workout for your diaphragm, abdominal, respiratory, facial, leg, and back muscles. It massages abdominal organs, tones intestinal functioning, and strengthens the muscles that hold the abdominal organs in place. It is estimated that hearty laughter can burn calories equivalent to several minutes on the rowing machine or the exercise bike.

- Laughter stimulates both sides of the brain to enhance learning. It eases muscle tension and psychological stress, which keeps the brain alert and allows people to retain more information. Laughing also elevates moods.

Striving to see humor in life and attempting to laugh at situations
rather than bemoan them will help improve your disposition and the
disposition of those around you. Your ability to laugh at yourself and
situations will help reduce your stress level and make life more enjoyable. Humor also helps you connect with others. People naturally
respond to the smiles and good cheer of those around them.

Tips for Adding More Humor and Laughter in Your Life

- Remind yourself to have fun.

- Spend time with those who help you see the bright side.

- Get regular doses of humor from various sources such as television sitcoms, movies, plays, or books.

Section 54.2

Pet Ownership Reduces Stress

"Healthy Reasons to Have a Pet," © 2009 Delta Society
(www.deltasociety.org). Reprinted with permission.

Compiled list of some research findings:

- Visits with a therapy dog helps heart and lung function by lowering pressures, diminishing release of harmful hormones, and decreases anxiety with hospitalized heart failure patients. (Cole, 2005)

- Displaying tanks of brightly colored fish may curtail disruptive behavior and improve eating habits of individuals with Alzheimer's disease. (Beck, 2002)

- Presence of a therapy dog can lower behavior distress in children during a physical examination at a doctor's office and may be useful in a variety of healthcare settings to decrease procedure-induced distress in children. (Nagengast, 1997, Hansen, 1999)

- Presence of a dog during dental procedures can reduce the stress of children who are distressed about coming to the dentist. (Havener, 2001)

- Animal-assisted therapy can effectively reduce the loneliness of residents in long-term care facilities. (Banks, 2002)

- People with borderline hypertension had lower blood pressure on days they took their dogs to work. (Allen, K. 2001)

- Seniors who own dogs go to the doctor less than those who do not. In a study of 100 Medicare patients, even the most highly stressed dog owners in the study had 21 percent fewer physician's contacts than non-dog owners. (Siegel, 1990)

- Activities of daily living (ADL) level of seniors who did not currently own pets deteriorated more on average than that of respondents who currently owned pets. (Raina, 1999)

- Seniors who own pets coped better with stressful life events without entering the healthcare system. (Raina, 1998)

- Pet owners have lower blood pressure. (Friedmann, 1983, Anderson 1992)

- Pet owners have lower triglyceride and cholesterol levels than non-owners. (Anderson, 1992)

- ACE [angiotensin-converting enzyme] inhibitors lower resting blood pressure but they do not diminish reactivity to mental stress. Pet ownership can lessen cardiovascular reactivity to psychological stress among hypertensive patients treated with a daily dose of Lisinopril. (Allen, 1999)

- Companionship of pets (particularly dogs) helps children in families adjust better to the serious illness and death of a parent. (Raveis, 1993)

- Pet owners feel less afraid of being a victim of crime when walking with a dog or sharing a residence with a dog. (Serpel, 1990)

- Pet owners have fewer minor health problems. (Friedmann, 1990, Serpel, 1990)

- Pet owners have better psychological well-being. (Serpel, 1990)

- Contact with pets develops nurturing behavior in children who may grow to be more nurturing adults. (Melson, 1990)

- Pet owners have a higher 1-year survival rates following coronary heart disease. (Friedman, 1980, 1995)

- Medication costs dropped from an average of $3.80 per patient per day to just $1.18 per patient per day in new nursing home facilities in New York, Missouri, and Texas that have animals and plants as an integral part of the environment. (Montague, 1995)

- Pets in nursing homes increase social and verbal interactions adjunct to other therapy. (Fick, 1992)

- Pet owners have better physical health due to exercise with their pets. (Serpel, 1990)

- Having a pet may decrease heart attack mortality by 3%. This translates into 30,000 lives saved annually. (Friedman, 1980)

- Dogs are preventive and therapeutic measures against everyday stress. (Allen, 1991)

- Pets decrease feeling of loneliness and isolation. (Kidd, 1994)

- Children exposed to humane education programs display enhanced empathy for humans compared with children not exposed to such programs. (Ascione, 1992)

- Positive self-esteem of children is enhanced by owning a pet. (Bergensen, 1989)

- Children's cognitive development can be enhanced by owning a pet. (Poresky, 1988)

- Seventy percent of families surveyed reported an increase in family happiness and fun subsequent to pet acquisition. (Cain, 1985)

- The presence of a dog during a child's physical examination decreases their stress. (Nadgengast, 1997, Baun, 1998)

- Children owning pets are more involved in activities such as sports, hobbies, clubs, or chores. (Melson, 1990)

- Children exposed to pets during the first year of life have a lower frequency of allergic rhinitis and asthma. (Hesselmar, 1999)

- Children with autism have more prosocial behaviors and less autistic behaviors such as self-absorption. (Redefer, 1989)

- Children who own pets score significantly higher on empathy and prosocial orientation scales than non-owners. (Vidovic, 1999)

- Pets fulfill many of the same support functions as humans for adults and children. (Melson, 1998)

- People who have AIDS [acquired immunodeficiency syndrome] who have pets have less depression and reduced stress. Pets are a major source of support and increase the perception of the ability to cope. (Siegel, 1999, Carmack, 1991)

Section 54.3

Social Support:
Who Can Give It and How to Get It

Excerpted and adapted from "Taking Time: Support for People with
Cancer," by the National Cancer Institute (NCI, www.cancer.gov),
part of the National Institutes of Health, November 9, 2009.

When you are stressed, it can be hard to ask for help to meet your
needs. To get the help you need, think about turning to family and
friends and people you meet in support groups.

No one needs to face stress alone. When people with stress seek and
receive help from others, they often find it easier to cope.

You may find it hard to ask for or accept help. After all, you are used
to taking care of yourself. Maybe you think that asking for help is a
sign of weakness. Or perhaps you do not want to let others know that
some things are hard for you to do. All these feelings are normal.

People feel good when they help others. However, your friends may
not know what to say or how to act when they're with you. Some people
may even avoid you. But they may feel more at ease when you ask
them something specific, like to cook a meal or pick up your children
after school. There are many ways that family, friends, and other people
who have stress-related disorders can help.

Family and Friends

Family and friends can support you in many ways. But, they may
wait for you to give them hints or ideas about what to do. Someone
who is not sure if you want company may call "just to see how things
are going." When someone says, "Let me know if there is anything I
can do," be honest. For example, tell this person if you need help with
an errand or a ride to the doctor's office.

Family members and friends can also do the following:

- Keep you company, give you a hug, or hold your hand

- Listen as you talk about your hopes and fears

- Help with rides, meals, errands, or household chores

- Go with you to doctor's visits or therapy sessions
- Tell other friends and family members ways they can help

Other People Who Have Stress-Related Disorders

Even though your family and friends help, you may also want to meet people who have stress-related disorders now or have had them in the past. Often, you can talk with them about things you can't discuss with others. People with stress understand how you feel and can do the following:

- Talk with you about what to expect
- Tell you how they cope with stress and live a normal life
- Help you learn ways to enjoy each day
- Give you hope for the future

Let your doctor or nurse know that you want to meet other people with stress-related disorders. You can also meet other people in the hospital, at your doctor's office, or through a support group.

Support groups are meetings for people with health disorders. They can be in person, by phone, or on the internet. These groups allow you and your loved ones to talk with others facing the same problems. Some support groups have a lecture as well as time to talk. Almost all groups have a leader who runs the meeting. The leader can be someone with a stress-related disorder or a counselor or social worker.

You may think that a support group is not right for you. Maybe you think that a group won't help or that you don't want to talk with others about your feelings. Or perhaps you're afraid that the meetings will make you sad or depressed.

Support groups may not be for everyone. Some people choose to find support in other ways. But many people find them very helpful. People in the groups often do the following:

- Talk about what it's like to have a stress-related disorder
- Help each other feel better, more hopeful, and not so alone
- Learn about what's new in treatment
- Share tips about ways to cope with stress

If you have a choice of support groups, visit a few and see what they are like. See which ones make sense for you. Although many groups are free, some charge a small fee. Find out if your health insurance pays for support groups.

Many hospitals, community groups, and schools offer support groups. Here are some ways to find groups near you:

- Call your local hospital and ask about its support programs.

- Ask your health care provider to suggest groups.

- Do an online search for groups.

- Look in the health section of your local newspaper for a listing of support groups.

Chapter 55

Stress Management for Children, Teens, and Families

Chapter Contents

Section 55.1

Stress Management Tips for Children and Teens

From "Stress Management for Children," by the Substance Abuse and Mental Health Services Administration (SAMHSA, www.samhsa.gov), part of the U.S. Department of Health and Human Services, July 16, 2008.

Children, teens, and their parents are under more stress than ever. Lists of "things to do" and "stars to reach for" grow longer. More to do means more stress to manage. This advice about stress management for children may seem ironic but holds true: When your child or teenager seems stressed by a busy schedule, schedule some time for free play.

Free play offers an excellent opportunity for parents to interact with their children and teenagers. Both children and their parents can realize benefits. Playtime is a great time for bonding, laughing, relaxing, and enjoying one another.

Playtime or unstructured downtime options are many and diverse—arts and crafts, hanging out with friends or instant messaging them via the computer, writing in a journal, cooking part of the family meal, or simply daydreaming. Children and adolescents benefit from unstructured but constructive, self-directed time to have fun. Obviously, organized sports with uniforms and the pressure to win do not count as free play. Watching television or video gaming doesn't count either.

Young people have less time for free play today because of busier lives and greater emphasis on academics and enrichment activities. Yet, according to the American Academy of Pediatrics (AAP), play is important in promoting healthy child development and maintaining strong parent bonds. Play "contributes to the cognitive, physical, social, and emotional well-being of children and youth," emphasizes the AAP.

What Is Stress?

Stress is a normal and necessary part of life. Stress can be positive or negative—depending on how someone handles the situation and the resources that are available. Also, what is stressful for one person may not be for another. For example, one person may view a stressful experience like changing schools as an exciting challenge. Someone else might feel nervous and insecure. How individuals handle stress differs, too. Most reactions fit into the categories of fight, flight, or freeze.

The consequences of stress are far reaching. Research shows a strong relationship between stress and substance abuse. Stress can alter a person's physiology and contribute to the development of such illnesses as high blood pressure, diabetes, and addiction. Children and adolescents who are stressed may show signs of emotional problems, aggressive behavior, shyness, anxiety, and fear in social situations.

Can Stress Be Managed?

Yes. Stress management for children and adolescents begins with recognizing the causes of stress. Some examples are a fight with a friend or a sibling, an upcoming test, a new school, a family conflict, and, of course, overscheduling. Choices about drinking, smoking, drugs, and sex, along with fears about violence, are common stressors for adolescents.

Symptoms of stress are not always obvious in children and youth. An adult might say, "I am stressed out." Instead, a young person may complain, "My stomach hurts."

Overscheduled children and adolescents are more likely to experience anxiety, especially about their performance. They may not want to go to school or participate in activities. They may experience sleep interruptions and changes in their eating patterns.

When stressors and symptoms occur, parents can use a variety of practical strategies such as changing their child's schedule or seeking mental health counseling. Parents can offer more unscheduled time for good, old-fashioned play. Play helps children and adolescents manage stress and reach their full potential.

Young people often are overscheduled with structured activities, according to Dr. T. Berry Brazelton, a well-known pediatrician and child development expert affiliated with Harvard Medical School. "They are missing the chance they have to dream, to fantasize, to make their own world work the way they want it. That to me is a very important part of childhood," he said in praising the AAP report.

What Are the Essential Components of Stress Management?

Parents and caregivers can help children manage stress by managing their schedules, promoting prosocial activities that benefit others as well as the individual, keeping the lines of communications open, and allowing unscheduled time for play and fun.

Establish a Daily Family Routine

Studies show that successful students have a family routine that includes eating meals together, a regular time for homework each afternoon or evening, and going to bed at a set time.

Just Say No

Set boundaries for your children. Children feel reassured and protected when guidelines are firm. Couching your "no" with care and concern is more likely to coax a cooperative response. Learn other ways to say "no," such as "Yes, after your homework is done." Help children learn to say no appropriately. This skill will be useful when difficult and stressful choices are presented during their teen years and throughout their lives.

Listen and Encourage

Listen to your child and encourage him to express his feelings, especially if you sense that he may be overwhelmed or experiencing stress. Respect her feelings and reassure her that everyone experiences nervousness, fear, and anxiety. It's okay to feel this way.

Offer Stress Safety Valves

Every child, teen, and adult needs a toolkit of stress safety valves— ways to relax or enjoy some downtime. Tried and true safety valves include taking a walk, listening to music, breathing slowly on a 1 to 10 count, even smiling at someone.

Help your children relieve some of the pressure they might be feeling by providing time and space for large-motor activities such as running and jumping. Having a special time and place for noisy activities is an excellent outlet for expressing aggression. Working with clay, hammering at a workbench, or engaging in other physically active play can help. Physical activity is a great way to relieve stress and an essential part of a healthy lifestyle.

Parents can model and teach their kids how to cope. Adolescents who feel stretched by the pressures of school, extracurricular activities, friends and family, and perhaps a part-time job can learn and practice stress management skills. For example, break a large task into smaller ones and take time out from stressful situations. Practicing healthy behaviors also helps in decreasing stress:

- Exercise and eat regularly.

- Avoid excess caffeine intake that can increase feelings of anxiety and agitation.

- Avoid alcohol, tobacco, and illegal drugs.

What Are Some Other Stress Management Tips?

Children who learn good stress management and good organizational skills can use them successfully today and forever. For example, by using a daily planner with a calendar and space for assignments, appointments, and other scheduled activities, your child can learn to plan ahead. And, make sure he marks in some moments for doing nothing at all, too.

Parents can serve as role models by managing their own stress and by setting priorities and limits, including bedtime. Scheduling time to talk and time to play helps both parents and their children handle stress.

Section 55.2

Helping Kids Cope in Times of Crisis

From "Helping Your Kids Cope in Times of Crisis," by the Substance Abuse and Mental Health Services Association (SAMHSA, www.samhsa.gov), part of the U.S. Department of Health and Human Services, September 13, 2008.

How can you help your kids deal with tough situations and make them feel safe in times of crisis? Children are exposed to traumatic events through TV, radio, newspapers, magazines, and even adult conversations that they overhear. The information can be scary to kids and they often need help managing what they've seen or heard. When you start talking with your children, you help them handle their feelings and you start a recovery of your own.

More than anything, children need to be assured that things will work out and be okay. They will seek comfort in knowing that parents, families, police, firefighters, faith organizations, doctors and nurses, and others care and are there to help and support the victims. When your child sees media coverage about a disaster, emphasize that many people are trained to help people and handle emergencies. Tell your child that these same people would be there if disaster struck your community.

How do you reassure your child? Here are some ideas on how to help kids cope in times of crisis:

- **Talk about the events.** Ask them what they know about the disaster, how it makes them feel, and what their concerns are.

- **Encourage them to say what is on their minds.** Answer their questions and help them understand what's going on.

- **Offer comfort.** Let your child know that it's OK after a disaster to feel scared about his own safety or sad about what has happened. Reassure him that sad feelings will get better as time goes by. You can tell him that even people who have lost a lot of important things will feel better someday. Offer comfort even if your child doesn't voice his fears out loud.

- **Respond in a positive way.** In speaking to your child, try to understand how she is feeling without making judgments. For instance, you might say, "Tell me what you're feeling," or "What you're saying is important to me. Let's talk about it." Try not to say things like, "Stop complaining," or "You should be over it by now."

- **Help children find ways to express themselves.** Writing a poem or drawing a picture can help your child express her feelings. Children can make cards to send to rescue workers to thank them for their hard work. Talk with your children about courage and let them know that police and community leaders are working to keep people safe.

- **Join with your neighbors in the relief effort.** Speak with your child's teachers, coaches, or other caregivers to learn about relief efforts in your community. See if there is anything you can do to help. They may be working to help support groups that are helping people affected by natural disasters and other crises. These groups include the following:

  - American Red Cross, 800-HELP-NOW, www.redcross.org

  - The Salvation Army, 800-SAL-ARMY, www.salvationarmyusa.org

  - United Way, 800-272-4630, national.unitedway.org

- **Volunteer together.** To provide goods and services to people in need, organizations need help from people. Money is not the only way to donate. Take some time out after school and work so that you and your children can help these groups with tasks such as putting together and sending out packages. Try local faith organizations or community groups.

- **Surround children with people they love.** Now is a good time to be with family and close friends. Creating a safe and caring environment can be the best thing for your kids in times of crisis, fear, and anxiety.

- **Turn off the TV and radio.** Try to reduce your children's media access, especially when media replay tragic events. Letting your kids see minute-to-minute coverage will only upset them and add to their anxiety and stress.

Some children may be affected by crisis more deeply than others. In fact, some children may need more help, including the aid of mental health professionals. Parents and caregivers, too, may benefit from help. These are normal feelings.

Section 55.3

Nature Helps Kids Deal with Stress

"A room with a view helps rural children deal with life's stresses, Cornell researchers report," April 24, 2003, by Susan S. Lang, *Cornell Chronicle.* Reprinted with permission. Reviewed by David A. Cooke, MD, FACP, November 8, 2010.

A room with a view—a green one, that is—can help protect children against stress, according to a study by two Cornell University environmental psychologists. Nature in or around the home, they say, appears to be a significant factor in protecting the psychological well-being of children in rural areas.

"Our study finds that life's stressful events appear not to cause as much psychological distress in children who live in high-nature conditions compared with children who live in low-nature conditions," says Nancy Wells, assistant professor of design and environmental analysis in the New York State College of Human Ecology at Cornell. "And the protective impact of nearby nature is strongest for the most vulnerable children—those experiencing the highest levels of stressful life events."

The study is published in the May 2003 issue of *Environment and Behavior* (Vol. 35:3, 311–330). Wells and Cornell colleague Gary Evans assessed the degree of nature in and around the homes of 337 rural children in grades 3 through 5 by calculating the number of live plants indoors, the amount of nature in the window views and the material of the outdoor yard (grass, dirt, or concrete). Their assessment was based on a "naturalness scale of residential environments" that they developed in 2000. In addition, they used standardized scales to measure stress in the children's lives, parents' reports of their children's stressed behavior, and the children's self-ratings of psychological well-being. The researchers then controlled for socioeconomic status and income.

"Our data also suggest little ceiling effect with respect to the benefits of exposure to the nature environment," the researchers note. "Even in a rural setting with a relative abundance of green landscape, more appears to be better when it comes to bolstering children's resilience against stress or adversity."

In 2000, Wells conducted a study that found that being close to nature also helps boost a child's attention span. "When children's cognitive functioning was compared before and after they moved from poor- to better-quality housing that had more green spaces around, profound differences emerged in their attention capacities even when the effects of the improved housing were taken into account," says Wells. Other studies, she notes, also support the theory that green spaces might help restore children's ability to focus their attention, thereby bolstering their cognitive resources by allowing neural inhibitory mechanisms to rest and recover from use. "By bolstering children's attentional resources, green spaces may enable children to think more clearly and cope more effectively with life stress," Wells says.

Another possible explanation for the protective effect of being close to nature, Wells says, is that green spaces foster social interaction and thereby promote social support. One study, for example, shows that children and parents who live in places that allow for outdoor access have twice as many friends as those who have restricted outdoor access due to traffic.

The study was supported, in part, by the John D. and Catherine T. MacArthur Research Network on Socioeconomic Status and Health, the W.T. Grant Foundation, the College of Human Ecology at Cornell, the National Institute for Child Health and Human Development, a U.S. Department of Agriculture Hatch Grant, and the National Institute of Mental Health.

Section 55.4

Combating Parental Stress

From "Combating Parental Stress," by the Substance Abuse and Mental
Health Services Administration (SAMHSA, www.samhsa.gov), part of
the U.S. Department of Health and Human Services, February 20, 2007.

Has your daily "to-do" list gotten so long that it no longer fits on
a single piece of paper? Or do you have so much to do that you don't
even have time to make a to-do list? You're not alone. Parents today
are working longer hours and commuting greater distances to and
from work. Their days don't slow down when they get home. Kids'
after-school schedules can be jam-packed, making life busy—and often
stressful—for parents.

Why is there so much parental stress?

There is no single answer to this complex question. Many things
contribute to stress among parents, including the following:

- Having good childcare and knowing that their kids are safe during the hours when parents are away from them

- Facing major life events such as a divorce, death, and midlife
  crisis

- Having financial worries—from paying monthly bills to saving
  for a child's college education to giving financial help to aging
  parents

- Being unemployed or fearful of being laid off from work

- Facing nagging health problems

- Feeling the strain of caring for an aging parent, chronically sick
  child, or family member with special needs

Parents, like kids, also may be trying to do more in a single day.
Technology items like computers and cell phones were supposed to
help us save time—and they do! But instead of savoring that extra
time, parents often pack in more tasks and chores.

How does stress affect parents and families?

According to one study, parents (especially of older children) suffer from higher levels of depression than adults who do not have children. Parents often focus on caring for their children and forget to take care of themselves. When parents don't pay attention to their physical and mental health, they put themselves at risk for stress-related problems like tension headaches, chronic fatigue, and depression.

Research also shows that the emotional well-being of children is strongly linked to their parents' mental health. To put in plainly: Parents who are stressed out often have kids who are stressed out. Your kids learn how to cope with life's ups and downs by watching how you manage stress. If you manage it well, you'll not only feel better, but you'll be a model for your kids and teach them how to manage stress in their lives.

How can parents manage stress?

Make friends and build strong social networks. Studies have shown that having one or two close friends or even a large group of friendly acquaintances is vital to emotional health. Many people live far away from their extended family members, so look to friends to fill this emotional need. Being friends with other parents also can lead to timesaving benefits like carpooling to and from activities.

Prioritize your to-do list in order of importance. What has to get done today? What can be deleted? What can wait until tomorrow? Tackle today's things first and then come up with a game plan for getting everything else done. You might have to say, "I won't have time to mop the floor until Saturday," but that's OK. Just having a plan for getting things done can help relieve stress.

Make sure your to-do list includes a little personal time for yourself. Have coffee with an old friend, take a bath, go for a walk, read a book, or take a nap. The goal is to do things that renew and energize you. Don't let yourself get run down! When you take time to revitalize yourself, you have more to give to others.

Sometimes there seems to be no time for parents to destress and parents may feel guilty about calling a timeout for themselves. What parent has time for a break when there is homework to help with, recitals to attend, practices to drive to, and work to be done? Moms and dads spend most of their time trying to raise happy, healthy kids, but your kids want happy, healthy parents! If you're overstressed, you're probably not at your best-and your kids know it. So, call a personal timeout and address the stress. You'll be helping yourself and your family.

Chapter 56

Managing Stress in Later Life

Rose isn't sleeping well. Retirement from her demanding job has been disappointing. "Relax," her kids say, "you deserve it." But Rose feels tense and worried about her future. Her husband Mel, retired for 2 years, doesn't seem interested in traveling and talks about finding a new job. Rose feels strange not working. Wasn't retirement supposed to be fun?

As you grow older, you may dream of freedom to travel, new interests, economic comfort, and more time with friends and family. Reality seldom seems to match expectations. Both the losses and gains of new roles can be stressors. Leaving a job may mean more freedom but it also may involve losses of challenging work, relationships, daily routine, or a sense of security. Family needs keep changing too, sometimes in unexpected ways.

What you've learned from past experiences can help you manage new stresses. You can't eliminate stress, but you can make choices about how you will use your resources in new situations.

Sources of Stress

- Changing parent and grandparent roles
- Changing couple relationship

- Choosing meaningful roles and activities
- Financial uncertainty
- Physical changes or illness
- Grief
- Loneliness
- Maintaining independence

Relationships: With Your Spouse

Your partner may not experience the same stressors that you do or react in the same way. Talking together about your needs and being willing to try out new ways of doing things are good ways to manage stress. Use the strength of your long relationship as a resource during times of change.

- Make time to talk. Be clear about your needs and feelings.
- Take time to listen to your spouse.
- Stay flexible and be willing to take some risks.
- Use the experience you have gained from other difficult times.
- Plan things you both enjoy.

Relationships: With Your Adult Children

After 45 years of marriage Marge and Jim have lots of retirement plans, including spending time as international volunteers. Now sadness and anxiety over their daughter's divorce threatens their dreams. How can they help their daughter and grandchildren? How should they relate to their son-in-law?

You don't ever stop being a parent. Worry, disappointment, or sadness about family members can seem overwhelming, but it is important to let go of the need to solve an adult child's problems. Focus on the things you can do to show your support.

- Recognize that you cannot protect your family from pain.
- Keep communication open with your children and grandchildren.
- Find someone to talk to about your own feelings.
- Set boundaries for what you can do and how much you can do.
- Take care of your own health and relationships.

Relationships: Grandparenting

Grandparents provide a vital link between generations. Grandparenting is not a role you choose, but you can decide how to carry it out. Disagreements with your children about your grandparenting role are stressful. Long distance separation, conflicting responsibilities, or serving as a substitute parent are other sources of stress.

- Talk with your children about expectations.
- Value the role of grandparent; it fills a vital need.
- Seek support if you are a grandparent who is parenting.

Managing Resources

After years filled with the demands of family and employment, most retirees are delighted to have enough time to pursue the activities they like the most. Some people, however, find that they have too much time. Their days are long; they miss the demands of the world of work. If you are in this group, the key to successful time management is developing your own structure for your time. What are the things you want to accomplish in the next month or year? How do those long-term goals translate into daily objectives? Plan your day around those short-term objectives. One of the most effective ways to become involved in your community is to volunteer. Such activities not only can add structure to your life; they can be immensely satisfying as well.

Although not rich, most retirees have enough money to live comfortably. Nevertheless, many elderly individuals are concerned about their finances. For some, the question is, "Will my money last my lifetime?" For others, the issue is one of cash flow; there is too much month at the end of the money. The best way to guarantee that your retirement funds last as long as you do is to continue to invest in low-risk investments. Also, make sure your insurance coverage is adequate.

If financial resources are short, are there other resources that could be used to generate more income? Could you consider a part-time job? Are there assets that could be sold, with the proceeds reinvested in income-producing assets?

Grief and Stress

Roger hangs up the phone and stares at the stack of documents on his desk. The lawyer recommended by the Alzheimer's Association was helpful. He can't change the impact of devastating expenses for Peggy's care, but it helps to get good advice. Roger misses Peggy constantly. Their home of 50 years seems empty.

Grief with its resulting changes and decisions is a source of severe stress. Grief is a normal response to the death of loved ones and friends, long-term illness of a spouse, physical separation, or loss of cherished dreams. When losses are chronic and outcomes are not clear, as in a progressive illness, it is very hard to manage the continuing stress. You will need help from others as you grieve. You also may need to help people understand your situation.

- Ask for help from friends, church, or professionals.

- Accept support from neighbors, friends, and family.

- Allow yourself as much time to grieve as you need.

- Take special care of your health.

Loneliness and Stress

Loneliness is natural when you miss loved ones, leave your old home, or lose your sense of purpose. The way you think about your loneliness can affect how stressful it is for you. Blaming others or waiting for someone to notice your sadness takes the control away from you. Taking some action, no matter how small, helps.

- Get to know the people who live near you.

- Learn a new skill through adult education.

- Offer your time. Call the Retired Senior Volunteers Program.

- Enrich your long-distance relationships through letters.

Eat Well, Be Well

Although no specific food can cure or alleviate stress, eating well can help you feel your best. Eating to maintain your health and strength isn't complex or time-consuming either.

Maintain an eating routine. Set aside certain times of day to eat meals and snacks. Going without food, even if you don't think you are hungry, leads to feeling weak, sick, and confused. You may feel more interested in eating if you get together with others, for example at a congregate meal site at noon, or with a neighbor in the evening one or two times a week.

Keep it simple. A healthful diet includes a variety of foods every day. Focus on fruits and vegetables, low-fat dairy products, whole-grain breads and cereals, and lean meats.

If you have a health condition that requires you to eat a certain way, be sure to do it. Take care of yourself by eating right. Simple, healthful eating can help you feel capable, positive, and alert. You can take charge by doing something good for yourself.

- Remember to eat regular meals and snacks.
- Share meal times with others.
- Focus on fruits and vegetables.
- Limit high-fat foods.
- Keep a supply of convenient, low-calorie foods on hand.
- Build physical activity, such as walking, into your daily life.
- Drink 6–8 glasses of water each day.

Health Changes and Stress

Joe and Ellen have been farming for 55 years. Lately their children have been urging them to get a nice place in town. Joe's health is poor. Still, this farm is home. They feel trapped between what they love and their physical limitations.

It's painful to give up familiar things. Change is especially stressful when you feel others are choosing for you. It's important to help your family understand your feelings but also to accept their concerns for you.

- Learn about resources for help. Call your Area Agency on Aging.
- Discuss options with your whole family.
- Listen to others' feelings but be honest about your own needs.
- Take your time. Staying in place may be an option.
- Consider the consequences of choices for you and your family.

Part Six

Additional Help and Information

Chapter 57

Glossary of Terms Related to Stress and Stress-Related Disorders

acute: Refers to a disease or condition that has a rapid onset, marked intensity, and short duration.[1]

acute stress disorder (ASD): A mental disorder that can occur in the first month following a trauma. ASD may involve feelings such as not knowing where you are, or feeling as if you are outside of your body.[2]

addiction: A chronic, relapsing disease characterized by compulsive drug seeking and use and by long-lasting changes in the brain.[3]

antidepressant: A medication used to treat depression.[1]

anxiety disorder: Any of a group of illnesses that fill people's lives with overwhelming anxieties and fears that are chronic and unremitting. Anxiety disorders include panic disorder, obsessive-compulsive disorder, posttraumatic stress disorder, phobias, and generalized anxiety disorder.[1]

anxiety: An abnormal sense of fear, nervousness, and apprehension about something that might happen in the future.[1]

Definitions in this chapter were compiled from documents published by several public domain sources. Terms marked 1 are from publications by the National Institutes of Health (www.nih.gov); terms marked 2 are from the Department of Veterans Affairs (www.va.gov), terms marked 3 are from the National Institute on Drug Abuse (www.nida.nih.gov); terms marked 4 are from the National Cancer Institute (www.cancer.gov); terms marked 5 are from the Office on Women's Health (www.womenshealth.gov); and terms marked 6 are from the National Institute on Mental Health (www.nimh.nih.gov).

arousal: A traumatic reaction that makes a person feel nervous and on edge. The trauma memory might be so intense that it is hard to sleep or focus the mind. Some people become more jumpy or quick to anger. Others feel like they have to be more on guard.[2]

avoidance: One of the symptoms of posttraumatic stress disorder (PTSD). Those with PTSD avoid situations and reminders of their trauma.[2]

biofeedback: A method of learning to voluntarily control certain body functions such as heartbeat, blood pressure, and muscle tension with the help of a special machine. This method can help control pain.[4]

bipolar disorder: A depressive disorder in which a person alternates between episodes of major depression and mania (periods of abnormally and persistently elevated mood). Also referred to as manic depression.[1]

body image: How a person feels about how she or he looks.[5]

chronic: Refers to a disease or condition that persists over a long period of time.[1]

cognition: Conscious mental activity that informs a person about his or her environment. Cognitive actions include perceiving, thinking, reasoning, judging, problem solving, and remembering.[1]

cognitive behavioral therapy (CBT): A blend of two therapies—cognitive therapy (CT) and behavioral therapy. CT focuses on a person's thoughts and beliefs, how they influence a person's mood and actions, and aims to change a person's thinking to be more adaptive and healthy. Behavioral therapy focuses on a person's actions and aims to change unhealthy behavior patterns.[6]

comorbidity: The occurrence of two disorders or illnesses in the same person, either at the same time (co-occurring comorbid conditions) or with a time difference between the initial occurrence of one and the initial occurrence of the other (sequentially comorbid conditions).[3]

cortisol: A hormone made by the adrenal cortex (the outer layer of the adrenal gland). It helps the body use glucose (a sugar), protein, and fats. Cortisol made in the laboratory is called hydrocortisone. It is used to treat many conditions, including inflammation, allergies, and some cancers. Cortisol is a type of glucocorticoid hormone.[4]

counselor: A person who usually has a master's degree in counseling and has completed a supervised internship.[5]

depression (depressive disorders): A group of diseases including major depressive disorder (commonly referred to as depression), dysthymia, and bipolar disorder.[1]

Diagnostic and Statistical Manual of Mental Disorders, Fourth Edition (DSM-IV): A book published by the American Psychiatric Association that gives general descriptions and characteristic symptoms of different mental illnesses. Physicians and other mental health professionals use the *DSM-IV* to confirm diagnoses for mental illnesses.[1]

dialectical behavior therapy: Dialectical behavior therapy (DBT) is a form of cognitive behavioral therapy used to treat people with suicidal thoughts and actions and borderline personality disorder (BPD). The term "dialectical" refers to a philosophic exercise in which two opposing views are discussed until a logical blending or balance of the two extremes—the middle way—is found.[6]

disorder: An abnormality in mental or physical health.[1]

dopamine: A brain chemical, classified as a neurotransmitter, found in regions of the brain that regulate movement, emotion, motivation, and pleasure.[3]

dual diagnosis: A term used to describe the comorbidity of a drug use disorder and another mental illness.[3]

dysthymia: A depressive disorder that is less severe than major depressive disorder but is more persistent.[1]

eating disorders: Eating disorders, such as anorexia nervosa, bulimia nervosa, and binge-eating disorder, involve serious problems with eating. This could include an extreme decrease of food or severe overeating, as well as feelings of distress and concern about body shape or weight.[5]

electroconvulsive therapy (ECT): A treatment for severe depression that is usually used only when people do not respond to medications and psychotherapy. ECT involves passing a low-voltage electric current through the brain. The person is under anesthesia at the time of treatment.[1]

epinephrine: A hormone and neurotransmitter. Also called adrenaline.[4]

family-focused therapy: Family-focused therapy (FFT) includes family members in therapy sessions to improve family relationships, which may support better treatment results.[6]

hormone: Substance produced by one tissue and conveyed by the bloodstream to another to effect a function of the body, such as growth or metabolism.[5]

hypertension: Also called high blood pressure, it is having blood pressure greater than 150 over 90 mmHg (millimeters of mercury). Long-term high blood pressure can damage blood vessels and organs, including the heart, kidneys, eyes, and brain.[5]

insomnia: Not being able to sleep.[5]

interpersonal therapy (IPT): Most often used on a one-on-one basis to treat depression or dysthymia (a more persistent but less severe form of depression).[6]

magnetic resonance imaging (MRI): An imaging technique that uses magnetic fields to take pictures of the structure of the brain.[1]

major depressive disorder: A depressive disorder commonly referred to as depression. Depression is more than simply being sad; to be diagnosed with depression, a person must have five or more characteristic symptoms nearly every day for a 2-week period.[1]

mania: Feelings of intense mental and physical hyperactivity, elevated mood, and agitation.[1]

mental illness: A health condition that changes a person's thinking, feelings, or behavior (or all three) and that causes the person distress and difficulty in functioning.[1]

migraine: A medical condition that usually involves a very painful headache, usually felt on one side of the head. Besides intense pain, migraine also can cause nausea and vomiting and sensitivity to light and sound. Some people also may see spots or flashing lights or have a temporary loss of vision.[5]

mindfulness relaxation: A type of meditation based on the concept of being mindful, or having increased awareness, of the present. It uses breathing methods, guided imagery, and other practices to relax the body and mind and help reduce stress.[4]

mood stabilizers: Medications used as part of treatment for bipolar disorder.[6]

neurotransmitters: A chemical produced by neurons to carry messages from one nerve cell to another.[3]

obsessive-compulsive disorder (OCD): An anxiety disorder in which a person suffers from obsessive thoughts and compulsive actions, such as cleaning, checking, counting, or hoarding. The person becomes trapped in a pattern of repetitive thoughts and behaviors that are senseless and distressing but very hard to stop.[5]

parasympathetic nervous system: The part of the nervous system that slows the heart, dilates blood vessels, decreases pupil size, increases digestive juices, and relaxes muscles in the gastrointestinal tract.[4]

panic disorder: An anxiety disorder in which a person suffers from sudden attacks of fear and panic. The attacks may occur without a known reason, but many times they are triggered by events or thoughts that produce fear in the person, such as taking an elevator or driving. Symptoms of the attacks include rapid heartbeat, chest sensations, shortness of breath, dizziness, tingling, and feeling anxious.[5]

phobia: An intense fear of something that poses little or no actual danger. Examples of phobias include fear of closed-in places, heights, escalators, tunnels, highway driving, water, flying, dogs, and injuries involving blood.[1]

posttraumatic stress disorder (PTSD): A disorder that develops after exposure to a highly stressful event (e.g., wartime combat, physical violence, or natural disaster). Symptoms include sleeping difficulties, hypervigilance, avoiding reminders of the event, and re-experiencing the trauma through flashbacks or recurrent nightmares.[3]

psychiatrist: A medical doctor (MD) who specializes in treating mental diseases. A psychiatrist evaluates a person's mental health along with his or her physical health and can prescribe medications.[1]

psychiatry: The branch of medicine that deals with identifying, studying, and treating mental, emotional, and behavioral disorders.[1]

psychologist: A mental health professional who has received specialized training in the study of the mind and emotions. A psychologist usually has an advanced degree such as a PhD.[1]

psychotherapy: A treatment method for mental illness in which a mental health professional (psychiatrist, psychologist, counselor) and a patient discuss problems and feelings to find solutions. Psychotherapy can help individuals change their thought or behavior patterns or understand how past experiences affect current behaviors.[1]

re-experiencing: A repeat of the feelings, bodily responses, and thoughts that occurred at the time of the traumatic event.[2]

schizophrenia: A chronic, severe, and disabling brain disease. People with schizophrenia often suffer terrifying symptoms such as hearing internal voices or believing that other people are reading their minds, controlling their thoughts, or plotting to harm them. These symptoms may leave them fearful and withdrawn. Their speech and behavior can be so disorganized that they may be incomprehensible or frightening to others.[1]

selective serotonin reuptake inhibitors (SSRIs): A group of medications used to treat depression. These medications cause an increase in the amount of the neurotransmitter serotonin in the brain.[1]

self-harm: Self-harm refers to a person's harming their own body on purpose. Other terms for self-harm are self-abuse or cutting. Overall, a person who self-harms does not mean to kill himself or herself.[2]

self-medication: The use of a substance to lessen the negative effects of stress, anxiety, or other mental disorders (or side effects of their pharmacotherapy). Self-medication may lead to addiction and other drug- or alcohol-related problems.[3]

serotonin: A neurotransmitter that regulates many functions, including mood, appetite, and sensory perception.[1]

stigma: A negative stereotype about a group of people.[1]

stress response: When a threat to life or safety triggers a primal physical response from the body, leaving a person breathless, heart pounding, and mind racing. From deep within the brain, a chemical signal speeds stress hormones through the bloodstream, priming the body to be alert and ready to escape danger. Concentration becomes more focused, reaction time faster, and strength and agility increase. When the stressful situation ends, hormonal signals switch off the stress response and the body returns to normal.[1]

sympathetic nervous system: The part of the body that increases heart rate, blood pressure, breathing rate, and pupil size. It also causes blood vessels to narrow and decreases digestive juices.[4]

syndrome: A group of symptoms or signs that are characteristic of a disease.[1]

trauma: A life-threatening event, such as military combat, natural disasters, terrorist incidents, serious accidents, or physical or sexual assault in adult or childhood.[2]

Chapter 58

Directory of Organizations for People with Stress-Related Disorders

Government Agencies That Provide Information about Stress-Related Disorders

Centers for Disease Control and Prevention (CDC)
1600 Clifton Road
Atlanta, GA 30333
Toll-Free: 800-CDC-INFO (232-4636)
TTY: 888-232-6348
Phone: 404-639-3311
Website: www.cdc.gov
E-mail: cdcinfo@cdc.gov

Federal Emergency Management Agency (FEMA)
U.S. Department of Homeland Security
500 C Street SW
Washington, DC 20472
Toll-Free: 800-621-FEMA (621-3362)
TTY: 800-462-7585
Phone: 202-646-2500
Website: www.fema.gov

Healthfinder®
National Health Information Center
P.O. Box 1133
Washington, DC 20013-1133
Toll-Free: 800-336-4797
Phone: 301-565-4167
Fax: 301-984-4256
Website:
www.healthfinder.gov
E-mail:
healthfinder@nhic.org

Resources in this chapter were compiled from several sources deemed reliable; all contact information was verified and updated in December 2010.

**National Cancer
Institute (NCI)**
NCI Office of Communications
and Education
Public Inquiries Office
6116 Executive Boulevard
Suite 300
Bethesda, MD 20892-8322
Toll-Free: 800-4-CANCER
(422-6237)
TTY: 800-332-8615
Website: www.cancer.gov
E-mail:
cancergovstaff@mail.nih.gov

**National Center for
Complementary and
Alternative Medicine
(NCCAM)**
National Institutes of Health
NCCAM Clearinghouse
P.O. 7923
Gaithersburg, MD 20898-7923
Toll-Free: 888-644-6226
TTY: 866-464-3615
Fax: 866-464-3616
Website: nccam.nih.gov
E-mail: info@nccam.nih.gov

**National Center for
Posttraumatic Stress
Disorder (NCPTSD)**
VA Medical Center (116D)
215 N. Main Street
White River Junction, VT 05009
Phone: 802-296-6300
Fax: 802-296-5135
Website: www.ptsd.va.gov
E-mail: ncptsd@va.gov

**National Digestive Diseases
Information Clearinghouse
(NDDIC)**
2 Information Way
Bethesda, MD 20892-3570
Toll-Free: 800-891-5389
TTY: 866-569-1162
Fax: 703-738-4929
Website: digestive.niddk.nih.gov
E-mail: nddic@info.niddk.nih.gov

**National Heart, Lung, and
Blood Institute (NHLBI)**
P.O. Box 30105
Bethesda, MD 20824-0105
Phone: 301-592-8573
TTY: 240-629-3255
Fax: 301-592-8563
Website: www.nhlbi.nih.gov
E-mail: nhlbiinfo@nhlbi.nih.gov

**National Institute of Allergy
and Infectious Diseases
(NIAID)**
6610 Rockledge Drive
MSC 6612
Bethesda, MD 20892-6612
Toll-Free: 866-284-4107
TDD: 800-877-8339
Fax: 301-402-3573
Website: www.niaid.nih.gov
E-mail:
ocpostoffice@niaid.nih.gov

National Institute of Arthritis and Musculoskeletal and Skin Diseases (NIAMS)
Information Clearinghouse
National Institutes of Health
1 AMS Circle
Bethesda, MD 20892-3675
Toll Free: 877-22-NIAMS
(226-4267)
Phone: 301-495-4484
TTY: 301–565–2966
Fax: 301-718-6366
Website: www.niams.nih.gov
E-mail: niamsinfo@mail.nih.gov

National Institute of Neurological Disorders and Stroke (NINDS)
NIH Neurological Institute
P.O. Box 5801
Bethesda, MD 20824
Toll-Free: 800-352-9424
Phone: 301-496-5751
TTY: 301-468-5981
Website: www.ninds.nih.gov
E-mail: braininfo@ninds.nih.gov

National Institute on Aging (NIA)
Building 31, Room 5C27
31 Center Drive, MSC 2292
Bethesda, MD 20892
Phone: 301-496-1752
TTY: 800-222-4225
Fax: 301-496-1072
Website: www.nia.nih.gov

National Institute on Alcohol Abuse and Alcoholism (NIAAA)
5635 Fishers Lane
MSC 9304
Bethesda, MD 20892-9304
Phone: 301-443-3860
Website: www.niaaa.nih.gov
E-mail: niaaaweb-r@exchange.nih.gov

National Institute on Drug Abuse (NIDA)
6001 Executive Boulevard
Room 5213
Bethesda, MD 20892-9561
Phone: 301-443-1124
Phone: 240-221-4007 (Spanish)
Website: www.drugabuse.gov
E-mail: information@nida.nih.gov

National Institute on Mental Health (NIMH)
Science Writing, Press, and
Dissemination Branch
6001 Executive Boulevard
Room 8184
MSC 9663
Bethesda, MD 20892-9663
Toll-Free: 866-615-6464
TTY: 866-415-8051
Phone: 301-443-4513
Fax: 301-443-4279
Website: www.nimh.nih.gov
E-mail: nimhinfo@nih.gov

National Institutes of Health (NIH)
9000 Rockville Pike
Bethesda, MD 20892
Phone: 301-496-4000
TTY: 301-402-9612
Website: www.nih.gov
E-mail: NIHinfo@od.nih.gov

National Women's Health Information Center (NWHIC)
Office on Women's Health
8270 Willow Oaks Corporate Drive
Fairfax, VA 22031
Washington, DC 20201
Toll-Free: 800-994-9662
Toll-Free TTY: 888-220-5446
Website: www.womenshealth.gov

Substance Abuse and Mental Health Services Administration (SAMHSA)
1 Choke Cherry Road
Rockville, MD 20857
Toll-Free: 877-SAMHSA-7
(726-4727)
TTY: 800-487-4889
Fax: 240-221-4292
Website: www.samhsa.gov
E-mail:
samhsainfo@samhsa.hhs.gov

U.S. Food and Drug Administration (FDA)
10903 New Hampshire Avenue
Silver Spring, MD 20993
Toll-Free: 888-INFO-FDA
(463-6332)
Website: www.fda.gov

U.S. National Library of Medicine (NLM)
8600 Rockville Pike
Bethesda, MD 20894
Toll-Free: 888-FIND-NLM
(346-3656)
TDD: 800-735-2258
Phone: 301-594-5983
Fax: 301-402-1384
Website: www.nlm.nih.gov
E-mail:
custserv@nlm.nih.gov

Private Agencies That Provide Information about Stress-Related Disorders

Academy for Guided Imagery
10780 Santa Monica Boulevard
Suite 290
Los Angeles, CA 90025
Toll-Free: 800-726-2070
Fax: 800-727-2070
Website: www
.academyforguidedimagery.com
E-mail: info@acadgi.com

American Academy of Child and Adolescent Psychiatry
3615 Wisconsin Avenue, NW
Washington, DC 20016-3007
Phone: 202-966-7300
Fax: 202-966-2891
Website: www.aacap.org

American Academy of Experts in Traumatic Stress
203 Deer Road
Ronkonkoma, NY 11749
Phone: 631-543-2217
Fax: 631-543-6977
Website: www.aaets.org
E-mail: info@aaets.org

American Academy of Family Physicians
P.O. Box 11210
Shawnee Mission, KS 66207-1210
Toll-Free: 800-274-2237
Phone: 913-906-6000
Fax: 913-906-6075
Website: www.aafp.org

American Association of Suicidology
5221 Wisconsin Avenue, NW
Washington, DC 20015
Phone: 202-237-2280
Fax: 202-237-2282
Website: www.suicidology.org

American Foundation for Suicide Prevention
120 Wall Street, 22nd Floor
New York, NY 10005
Toll-Free: 888-333-AFSP
(333-2377)
Phone: 212-363-3500
Fax: 212-363-6237
Website: www.afsp.org
E-mail: inquiry@afsp.org

American Heart Association
National Center
7272 Greenville Avenue
Dallas, TX 75231
Toll-Free: 800-AHA-USA-1
(242-8721)
Website: www.heart.org

American Institute for Cognitive Therapy
136 East 57th Street
Suite 1101
New York City, NY 10022
Phone: 212-308-2440
Website:
www.cognitivetherapynyc.com
E-mail: editor@
cognitivetherapynyc.com

American Institute of Stress
124 Park Avenue
Yonkers, NY 10703
Phone: 914-963-1200
Fax: 914-965-6267
Website: www.stress.org
E-mail: stress125@optonline.net

American Massage Therapy Association
500 Davis Street, Suite 900
Evanston, IL 60201-4695
Toll-Free: 877-905-0577
Phone: 847-864-0123
Fax: 847-864-5196
Website: www.amtamassage.org
E-mail: info@amtamassage.org

American Medical Association
515 North State Street
Chicago, IL 60654
Toll-Free: 800-621-8335
Website: www.ama-assn.org

American Music Therapy Association
8455 Colesville Road, Suite 1000
Silver Spring, MD 20910
Phone: 301-589-3300
Fax: 301-589-5175
Website: www.musictherapy.org
E-mail: info@musictherapy.org

American Psychiatric Association
1000 Wilson Boulevard, Suite 1825
Arlington, VA 22209
Toll-Free: 888-35-PSYCH
(357-7924)
Website: www.psych.org
E-mail: apa@psych.org

American Psychological Association
750 First Street NE
Washington, DC 20002-4242
Toll-Free: 800-374-2721
Phone: 202-336-5500
TDD/TTY: 202-336-6123
Website: www.apa.org

Anxiety Disorders Association of America
8730 Georgia Avenue
Silver Spring, MD 20910
Phone: 240-485-1001
Fax: 240-485-1035
Website: www.adaa.org

Anxiety Disorders Association of Canada
P.O. Box 117
Station Cote St-Luc
Montreal, Quebec H4V 2Y3
Phone: 514-484-0504
Toll-Free: 888-223-2252
Fax: 514-484-7892
Website: www.anxietycanada.ca
E-mail: contactus@
anxietycanada.ca

Association for Behavioral and Cognitive Therapies
305 7th Avenue, 16th Floor
New York, NY 10001
Phone: 212-647-1890
Fax: 212-647-1865
Website: www.abct.org
E-mail: mjeimer@abct.org

Association of Traumatic Stress Specialists
c/o MHANJ
88 Pompton Avenue
Verona, NJ 07044
Phone: 973-559-9200
Website: www.atss.info
E-mail: admin@atss.info

Biofeedback Certification International Alliance
10200 W 44th Avenue
Wheat Ridge, CO 80033-2840
Phone: 303-420-2902
Fax: 303-422-8894
Toll-Free: 866-908-8713
Website: www.bcia.org
E-mail: info@bcia.org

Cleveland Clinic
9500 Euclid Avenue
Cleveland, OH 44195
Toll-Free: 800-223-2273
TTY: 216-444-0261
Website: my.clevelandclinic.org

Depression and Bipolar Support Alliance
730 North Franklin Street
Suite 501
Chicago, IL 60654-7225
Toll-Free: 800-826-3632
Fax: 312-642-7243
Website: www.dbsalliance.org
E-mail: info@dbsalliance.org

Family Caregiver Alliance
180 Montgomery Street
Suite 900
San Francisco, CA 94104
Toll-Free: 800-445-8106
Phone: 415-434-3388
Website: www.caregiver.org
E-mail: info@caregiver.org

Freedom From Fear
308 Seaview Avenue
Staten Island, NY 10305
Phone: 718-351-1717
Fax: 718-980-5022
Website:
www.freedomfromfear.org
E-mail:
help@freedomfromfear.org

Imagery International
1574 Coburg Road, #555
Eugene, OR 97401-4802
Toll-Free: 866-494-9985
Website: www
.imageryinternational.org
E-mail: information@
imageryinternational.com

International OCD (Obsessive-Compulsive Disorder) Foundation
P.O. Box 961029
Boston, MA 02196
Phone: 617-973-5801
Fax: 617-973-5803
Website: www.ocfoundation.org
E-mail: info@ocfoundation.org

593

International Society for Traumatic Stress Studies
111 Deer Lake Road, Suite 100
Deerfield, IL 60015
Phone: 847-480-9028
Fax: 847-480-9282
Website: www.istss.org
E-mail: istss@istss.org

Iraq and Afghanistan Veterans of America
292 Madison Avenue, 10th Floor
New York, NY 10017
Phone: 212-982-9699
Fax: 212-982-8645
Website: www.iava.org

March of Dimes
National Office
1275 Mamaroneck Avenue
White Plains, NY 10605
Phone: 914-997-4488
Website: www.marchofdimes.com

Mental Health America
2000 North Beauregard Street
6th Floor
Alexandria, VA 22311
Toll-Free: 800-969-6642
Phone: 703-684-7722
Fax: 703-684-5968
Website: www.nmha.org
E-mail: infoctr@
mentalhealthamerica.net

National Alliance for Caregiving
4720 Montgomery Lane, 2nd Floor
Bethesda, MD 20814
Website: www.caregiving.org
E-mail: info@caregiving.com

National Alliance on Mental Illness
3803 North Fairfax Drive
Suite 100
Arlington, VA 22203
Toll-Free: 800-950-NAMI (6264)
Phone: 703-524-7600
Fax: 703-524-9094
Website: www.nami.org

National Center for Victims of Crime
2000 M Street NW, Suite 480
Washington, DC 20036
Phone: 202-467-8700
Fax: 202-467-8701
Website: www.ncvc.org

National Child Traumatic Stress Network
University of California at
Los Angeles
11150 West Olympic Boulevard
Suite 650
Los Angeles, CA 90064
Phone: 310-235-2633
Fax: 310-235-2612
Website: www.nctsn.org

National Eating Disorders Association
603 Stewart Street, Suite 803
Seattle, WA 98101
Toll-Free: 800-931-2237
Phone: 206-382-3587
Fax: 206-829-8501
Website:
www.nationaleatingdisorders.org
E-mail: info@
NationalEatingDisorders.org

National Family Caregivers Association

10400 Connecticut Avenue
Suite 500
Kensington, MD 20895-3944
Toll-Free: 800-896-3650
Phone: 301-942-6430
Fax: 301-942-2302
Website: www.nfcacares.org
E-mail:
info@thefamilycaregiver.org

National Headache Foundation

820 N. Orleans, Suite 217
Chicago, IL 60610
Toll-Free: 888-NHF-5552
(643-5552)
Phone: 312-274-2650
Website: www.headaches.org
E-mail: info@headaches.org

National Multiple Sclerosis Society

733 Third Avenue, 3rd Floor
New York, NY 10017
Toll-Free: 800-344-4867
Website:
www.nationalmssociety.org

National Organization for Victim Assistance

510 King Street, Suite 424
Alexandria, VA 22314
Toll-Free: 800-TRY-NOVA
(879-6682)
Website: www.trynova.org

National Psoriasis Foundation

6600 SW 92nd Avenue
Suite 300
Portland, OR 97223-7195
Toll-Free: 800-723-9166
Phone: 503-244-7404
Fax: 503-245-0626
Website: www.psoriasis.org
E-mail: getinfo@psoriasis.org

National Sleep Foundation

1522 K Street, NW
Suite 500
Washington, DC 20005
Phone: 202-347-3471
Fax: 202-347-3472
Website: www.sleepfoundation.org
E-mail: nsf@sleepfoundation.org

Nemours Foundation Center for Children's Health Media

1600 Rockland Road
Wilmington, DE 19803
Phone: 302-651-4000
Website: www.kidshealth.org
E-mail: info@kidshealth.org

PsychCentral

55 Pleasant Street
Suite 207
Newburyport, MA 01950
Phone: 978-992-0008
Website: www.psychcentral.com
E-mail:
talkback@psychcentral.com

Rape, Abuse, and Incest National Network
2000 L Street NW
Suite 406
Washington, DC 20036
Toll-Free: 800-656-HOPE
(656-4673)
Phone: 202-544-1034
Website: www.rainn.org
E-mail: info@rainn.org

Sidran Traumatic Stress Institute
P.O. Box 436
Brooklandville, MD 21022-0436
Phone: 410-825-8888
Fax: 410-560-0134
Website: www.sidran.org
E-mail: info@sidran.org

Social Phobia/Social Anxiety Association
2058 E. Topeka Drive
Phoenix, AZ 85024
Website: www.socialphobia.org

Suicide Awareness Voices of Education
8120 Penn Avenue South
Suite 470
Bloomington, MN 55431
Toll-Free: 800-273-8255
Phone: 952-946-7998
Website: www.save.org

Suicide Prevention Advocacy Network USA
1010 Vermont Avenue, NW
Suite 408
Washington, DC 20005
Phone: 202-449-3600
Fax: 202-449-3601
Website: www.spanusa.org
E-mail: info@spanusa.org

Transcendental Meditation Program
Website: www.tm.org

World Federation for Mental Health
12940 Harbor Drive
Suite 101
Woodbridge, VA 22192
Phone: 703-494-6515
Fax: 703-494-6518
Website: www.wfmh.org
E-mail: info@wfmh.com

Yoga Alliance
1701 Clarendon Boulevard
Suite 110
Arlington, VA 22209
Toll-Free: 888-921-YOGA
(921-9642)
Website: www.yogaalliance.org

Yoga Journal
Website: www.yogajournal.com

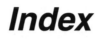

Index

Index

Page numbers followed by 'n' indicate a footnote. Page numbers in *italics* indicate a table or illustration.

599

Health Reference Series

Adolescent Health Sourcebook, 3rd Edition

Adult Health Concerns Sourcebook

AIDS Sourcebook, 5th Edition

Alcoholism Sourcebook, 3rd Edition

Allergies Sourcebook, 4th Edition

Alzheimer Disease Sourcebook, 5th Edition

Arthritis Sourcebook, 3rd Edition

Asthma Sourcebook, 3rd Edition

Attention Deficit Disorder Sourcebook

Autism & Pervasive Developmental Disorders Sourcebook, 2nd Edition

Back & Neck Sourcebook, 2nd Edition

Blood & Circulatory Disorders Sourcebook, 3rd Edition

Brain Disorders Sourcebook, 3rd Edition

Breast Cancer Sourcebook, 3rd Edition

Breastfeeding Sourcebook

Burns Sourcebook

Cancer Sourcebook for Women, 4th Edition

Cancer Sourcebook, 6th Edition

Cancer Survivorship Sourcebook

Cardiovascular Disorders Sourcebook, 4th Edition

Caregiving Sourcebook

Child Abuse Sourcebook, 2nd Edition

Childhood Diseases & Disorders Sourcebook, 2nd Edition

Colds, Flu & Other Common Ailments Sourcebook

Communication Disorders Sourcebook

Complementary & Alternative Medicine Sourcebook, 4th Edition

Congenital Disorders Sourcebook, 2nd Edition

Contagious Diseases Sourcebook, 2nd Edition

Cosmetic & Reconstructive Surgery Sourcebook, 2nd Edition

Death & Dying Sourcebook, 2nd Edition

Dental Care & Oral Health Sourcebook, 3rd Edition

Depression Sourcebook, 2nd Edition

Dermatological Disorders Sourcebook, 2nd Edition

Diabetes Sourcebook, 5th Edition

Diet & Nutrition Sourcebook, 4th Edition

Digestive Diseases & Disorder Sourcebook

Disabilities Sourcebook, 2nd Edition

Disease Management Sourcebook

Domestic Violence Sourcebook, 3rd Edition

Drug Abuse Sourcebook, 3rd Edition

Ear, Nose & Throat Disorders Sourcebook, 2nd Edition

Eating Disorders Sourcebook, 3rd Edition

Emergency Medical Services Sourcebook

Endocrine & Metabolic Disorders Sourcebook, 2nd Edition

Environmental Health Sourcebook, 3rd Edition

Ethnic Diseases Sourcebook

Eye Care Sourcebook, 4th Edition

Family Planning Sourcebook

Fitness & Exercise Sourcebook, 4th Edition

Food Safety Sourcebook

Forensic Medicine Sourcebook

Gastrointestinal Diseases & Disorders Sourcebook, 2nd Edition

Genetic Disorders Sourcebook, 4th Edition

Head Trauma Sourcebook

Headache Sourcebook

Health Insurance Sourcebook

Healthy Aging Sourcebook

Healthy Children Sourcebook

Healthy Heart Sourcebook for Women

Hepatitis Sourcebook

Household Safety Sourcebook

Hypertension Sourcebook

Immune System Disorders Sourcebook, 2nd Edition

Infant & Toddler Health Sourcebook

Infectious Diseases Sourcebook